Pocket Prescriber
Psychiatry

Pocket
Prescriber
Psychiatry

Edited by

Jonathan P Rogers MA MB BChir MRCP MRCPsych
NIHR Academic Clinical Fellow, Institute of Psychiatry, Psychology
and Neuroscience, King's College London, and South London
and Maudsley NHS Foundation Trust, London, UK

Cheryl CY Leung BSc (Hons) BMedSc BMBS
NIHR Academic Clinical Fellow, Institute of Psychiatry, Psychology
and Neuroscience, King's College London, and South London
and Maudsley NHS Foundation Trust, London, UK

Timothy RJ Nicholson MBBS BSc MSc PhD MRCP MRCPsych
Clinical Lecturer & NIHR Clinician Scientist, Institute of Psychiatry
Psychology & Neuroscience, King's College London, and Honorary Consultant
Neuropsychiatrist, South London & Maudsley NHS Foundation Trust

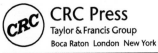

CRC Press
Taylor & Francis Group
Boca Raton London New York

CRC Press is an imprint of the
Taylor & Francis Group, an **informa** business

CRC Press
Taylor & Francis Group
6000 Broken Sound Parkway NW, Suite 300
Boca Raton, FL 33487-2742

© 2020 by Taylor & Francis Group, LLC
CRC Press is an imprint of Taylor & Francis Group, an Informa business

No claim to original U.S. Government works

Printed on acid-free paper
Printed by CPI Group (UK) Ltd, Croydon CR0 4YY

International Standard Book Number-13: 978-1-4441-7666-7 (Paperback)

Library of Congress Cataloging-in-Publication Data

Names: Rogers, Jonathan P., author. | Leung, Cheryl C. Y., editor. |
Nicholson, Timothy R. J., editor.
Title: Pocket prescriber psychiatry / edited by Jonathan P. Rogers, Cheryl C.Y. Leung,
Timothy R.J. Nicholson.
Description: Boca Raton : CRC Press, [2019] | Includes bibliographical references
and index.
Identifiers: LCCN 2019015207 (print) | LCCN 2019016846 (ebook) |
ISBN 9780429317330 (eBook) | ISBN 9781444176667 (pbk. : alk. paper)
Subjects: | MESH: Mental Disorders--drug therapy | Drug Prescriptions | Handbook
Classification: LCC RC454 (ebook) | LCC RC454 (print) | NLM WM 34 |
DDC 616.89--dc23
LC record available at https://lccn.loc.gov/2019015207

Visit the Taylor & Francis Web site at
http://www.taylorandfrancis.com

and the CRC Press Web site at
http://www.crcpress.com

CONTENTS

CONTRIBUTORS

Prof David S. Baldwin MA DM FRCPsych
Professor of Psychiatry
Faculty of Medicine
University of Southampton
Southampton, UK

Prof David Coghill BSc (Med Sci) MB
ChB, MD
Financial Markets Foundation Chair of
Developmental Mental Health
Departments of Paediatrics and Psychiatry
Faculty of Medicine
Dentistry and Health Sciences
University of Melbourne
Melbourne, Australia

Dr Fiona Cresswell MBChB BSc MRCP
DTM&H DipGUM PGCert Epi
Clinical PhD Fellow
Faculty of Infectious and Tropical Diseases
London School of Hygiene and Tropical
Medicine
London, UK

Dr Thomas Dewhurst MBBCh MRCPsych
Specialty Registrar in Psychiatry
South London and Maudsley NHS
Foundation Trust
London, UK

Dr Graham Fleming MBBS FRACGP
FCEM
Consultant in Emergency Medicine
King's College Hospital
London, UK

Prof Guy Goodwin FMedSci
Emeritus Professor of Psychiatry
Department of Psychiatry
University of Oxford
Oxford, UK

Prof Jeremy Hall MA MB BChir MPhil PhD
MRCPsych
Director
Neuroscience and Mental Health Research
Institute
Cardiff University
Cardiff, UK

Ms Jules Haste BSc DipClinPharm
MRPharmS, MCMHP
Principal Pharmacist
Sussex Partnership NHS Foundation Trust
Sussex, UK

Dr Frank Holloway FRCPsych
South London and Maudsley Hospital NHS
Foundation Trust
London, UK

Dr Jonathan Huntley PhD MBBS BA
Clinical Lecturer and Wellcome Trust
Clinical Fellow
Division of Psychiatry, University College London
and
Honorary Consultant Old Age Psychiatrist
Camden and Islington NHS Foundation Trust
London, UK

Dr Hind Khalifeh PhD BMBCh MRCPsych
NIHR Research Fellow and Hon Consultant
Psychiatrist
King's College London
and
South London and Maudsley NHS
Foundation Trust
London, UK

Dr Robin Kumar MBBS BSc (Hons) FRCA
Consultant Neuroanaesthetist
King's College Hospital
London, UK

Prof Anne Lingford-Hughes MA PhD BM
BCh FRCPsych
Professor of Addiction Biology
Imperial College London
and
Hon Consultant Psychiatrist
CNWL NHS Foundation Trust
London, UK

Dr James MacCabe BSc MB BS MSc
FRCPsych PhD
Reader in the Epidemiology of Psychosis
Institute of Psychiatry, Psychology and
Neuroscience
King's College London
London, UK

Prof R Hamish McAllister-Williams BSc MB ChB PhD MD FRCPsych
Professor of Affective Disorders
Institute of Neuroscience
Newcastle University
Newcastle upon Tyne, UK

Dr John DC Mellers MBBS (Melbourne) MRCPsych
Honorary Consultant Psychiatrist
Maudsley Hospital
Institute of Psychiatry, Psychology and Neuroscience
King's College London
London, UK

Dr Stirling Moorey BSc MBBS MA FRCPsych
Consultant Psychiatrist in CBT
South London and Maudsley NHS Foundation Trust
and
Visiting Senior Lecturer
Institute of Psychiatry, Psychology and Neuroscience
King's College London
London, UK

Prof John T O'Brien FMedSci
Foundation Professor of Old Age Psychiatry
Department of Psychiatry
University of Cambridge
Cambridge, UK

Mr Ian Osborne MPharm PgDip MRPharmS
Pharmacist
Pharmacy Department
Maudsley Hospital
and
Institute of Pharmaceutical Science
King's College London
London, UK

Dr Dene Robertson MB BS MRCGP MRCPsych
Consultant Psychiatrist, Clinical Director
Behavioural and Developmental Clinical Academic Group
South London and Maudsley NHS Foundation Trust
London, UK

Dr Tabish Saifee MRCP PhD
Consultant Neurologist and Senior Clinical Lecturer
The National Hospital for Neurology and Neurosurgery
London, UK

Dr Hugh Selsick BSc (Hon) MBBCh
Consultant in Psychiatry and Sleep Medicine
Insomnia Clinic
Royal London Hospital for Integrated Medicine and Sleep Disorder Centre
Guy's Hospital
London, UK

Prof Donald Singer BMedBiol MD FRCP FBPharmacolS
Professor of Clinical Pharmacology and Therapeutics
Fellowship of Postgraduate Medicine
London, UK

Prof John-Paul Taylor MBBS(Hons) PhD MRCPsych
Professor of Translational Dementia Research Institute of Neuroscience
and
Honorary Consultant in Old Age Psychiatry Northumberland, Tyne and Wear NHS Trust
Newcastle-Upon-Tyne, UK

Prof Peter Tyrer MD FRCPsych FMedSci
Emeritus Professor of Community Psychiatry
Imperial College London
London, UK

Dr Rachel Upthegrove MBBS FRCPsych PhD
Reader in Psychiatry and Youth Mental Health
Institute for Mental Health
University of Birmingham
Birmingham, UK

Dr Dan Wilson MB BChir MRCP
Consultant Physician
Department of Clinical Gerontology
King's College Hospital
London, UK

Prof Allan H. Young MB ChB MPhil PhD FRCPsych FRCPC FRSB
Director, Centre for Affective Disorders
Institute of Psychiatry, Psychology and Neuroscience
King's College London
London, UK

FOREWORD

Doctors are generally people who like books. Throughout our long training, we spend many hours with them (or perhaps now their electronic equivalents) attempting to turn the lead of the prose contained therein into the gold of clinical knowledge which should be in every clinician's brain as a bedrock of practice. However, our need to refresh and update this knowledge base never really ends for the active clinician, in training or not. To fill this need, many guidelines are available, but recently some of these have been bedevilled with controversy and have drifted somewhat from being the handy aid which the busy trainee and clinician requires. This fate has not befallen the *British Association for Psychopharmacology Guidelines* which remain as relevant and valued as ever for the guidance that they offer to the reader. The *BAP Guidelines* are based on expert opinion and high-quality evidence, are revised frequently and are free to download. The *BAP Guidelines* now also form the underpinning of evidence for this volume. The authors have worked hard to reconcile the mass of evidence with the need for brevity and have succeeded in this demanding task to produce a helpful text which all clinicians will find useful. This is to be greatly welcomed as such a practical compendium as the *Pocket Prescriber Psychiatry* will greatly aid the prescriber in psychiatry and find a welcome home in many pockets.

Professor Allan Young
MB ChB, MPhil, PhD, FRCPsych, FRCPC, FRSB
President, British Association for Psychopharmacology

ACKNOWLEDGEMENTS

This book is dedicated to Hannah for her kindness. We also wish to thank the inspiring teachers we have had who have influenced us over the years, particularly Mark Agius, Paul Wilkinson, Rupesh Adimulam, John Mellers, Robert Harland, Chris Kalafatis, Tom Pollak and Tony David.

Particular thanks go to the British Association for Psychopharmacology for their collaboration on this book and to Jeremy Hall, especially for coordinating this effort. Thanks also go to pharmacists who reviewed this manuscript: Loren Bailey, Stuart Benefield, Simone Brackenborough, Clare Brennan, Petrina Douglas-Hall, Paul Deslandes, Olubanke Dzahini, Ann McGinley, Emily Laing, Nickisha Patel, Sharanjeet Punny, Kalliopi Vallianatou and Seema Varma. We are particularly grateful to Ian Osborne, our lead pharmacist.

Thanks also go to David Taylor, Allan Young, Louise Howard, Clare Wilson, Bob Lepper, Gareth Owen, Ben Spencer and Allister Vale for their help and time. We are grateful to Jo Koster, Aoife McGrath, Kyle Meyer and Victoria Balque-Burns for their assistance with publishing.

STANDARD LAYOUT OF DRUGS

DRUG/TRADE NAME

Class/action: More information is given for generic forms, especially for the original and most commonly used drug(s) of each class.

Use: use^x (correlating to dose as follows).

CI: contraindications; **L** (liver failure), **R** (renal failure), **H** (heart failure), **P** (pregnancy), **B** (breastfeeding). *Allergy to active drug or any excipients (other substances in the preparation) assumed too obvious to mention.*

Caution: **L** (liver failure), **R** (renal failure), **H** (heart failure), **P** (pregnancy), **B** (breastfeeding), **E** (elderly patients). If a contraindication is given for a drug, it is assumed too obvious to mention that a caution is also inherently implied.

SE: side effects; listed in order of frequency encountered. Common/important side effects set in **bold**.

Warn: information to give to patients before starting drug.

Monitor: parameters that need to be monitored during treatment.

Interactions: included only if very common or potentially serious; ↑↓**P450** (induces/inhibits cytochrome P450 metabolism), **W+** (increases effect of warfarin), **W−** (decreases effect of warfarin).

Dose: dose^x (for use^x as previously mentioned). *NB: Doses are for adults only.*

Important points highlighted at end of drug entry.

Use/dose^{NICE}: National Institute for Health and Care Excellence (NICE) guidelines exist for the drug (basics often in the *British National Formulary* [BNF] – see https://www.nice.org.uk for full details).
Dose$^{BNF/SPC}$: Dose regimen complicated; please refer to BNF and/or SPC (Summary of Product Characteristics sheet; the manufacturer's information sheet enclosed with drug

packaging – can also be viewed at or downloaded from https://www.emc.medicines.org.uk). **Asterisks (*)** and **daggers (†)** denote links between information within local text.

Other sources:

BAP Guidance from the British Association for Psycho-pharmacology

MPG The Maudsley Prescribing Guidelines in Psychiatry, 13E

SIGN Scottish Intercollegiate Guidelines Network

UKTIS UK Teratology Information Service

UKDILAS UK Drugs in Lactation Advisory Service

NEPTUNE Novel Psychoactive Treatment: UK Network

Only relevant sections are included for each drug. **Trade names** (in **SOLID GREY** font) are given only if found regularly on drug charts or if non-proprietary (generic, non-trade-name) drug does not yet exist.

KEY

☠ Potential dangers highlighted with skull and crossbones

▼ New drug or new indication under intense surveillance by the Committee on Safety of Medicines (CSM): *important to report all suspected drug reactions via Yellow Card Scheme* (accurate as going to press: from May 2019 European Medicines Agency list)

☺ *Good for:* reasons to give a certain drug when choice exists

☹ *Bad for:* reasons to not give a certain drug when choice exists

⇒ Causes/goes to

∴ Therefore

Δ Change/disturbance

Ψ Psychiatric

↑ Increase/high

↓ Decrease/low

↑/↓ electrolytes refers to serum levels, unless stated otherwise.

DOSES

od	once daily	nocte	at night
bd	twice daily	mane	in the morning
tds	three times daily	prn	as required
qds	four times daily	stat	at once

ROUTES

im	intramuscular	po	oral
inh	inhaled	pr	rectal
iv	intravenous	sc	subcutaneous
ivi	intravenous infusion	top	topical
neb	via nebuliser	sl	sublingual

Routes are presumed po, unless stated otherwise.

LIST OF ABBREVIATIONS

5-ASA	5-aminosalicylic acid
5-HT	5-hydroxytryptamine (= serotonin)
A&E	accident and emergency
AAC	antibiotic-associated colitis
Ab	antibody
abdo	abdomen/abdominal
ABG	arterial blood gases
ABPM	ambulatory blood pressure monitoring
ACC	American College of Cardiology
ACCP	American College of Chest Physicians
ACE-i	angiotensin-converting enzyme (ACE) inhibitor
ACh	acetylcholine
ACS	acute coronary syndrome
ADP	adenosine diphosphate
AF	atrial fibrillation
Ag	antigen
AHA	American Heart Association
AKI	acute kidney injury
ALL	acute lymphoblastic leukaemia
ALP	alkaline phosphatase
ALS	adult life support (algorithms of the European Resuscitation Council)
ALT	alanine (-amino) transferase
AMI	acute myocardial infarction
AMTS	abbreviated mental test score (same as MTS)
ANA	anti-nuclear antigen
APTT	activated partial thromboplastin time
ARB	angiotensin receptor blocker
ARDS	adult respiratory distress syndrome
AS	aortic stenosis
ASAP	as soon as possible
assoc	associated
AST	aspartate transaminase
AV	arteriovenous

AVM	arteriovenous malformation
AVN	atrioventricular node
AZT	zidovudine
BAP	British Association for Psychopharmacology
BBB	bundle branch block
BCSH	British Committee for Standards in Haematology
BCT	broad complex tachycardia
BF	blood flow
BG	serum blood glucose in mmol/L; *see also* CBG (capillary blood glucose)
BHS	British Hypertension Society
BIH	benign intracranial hypertension
BIPAP	bilevel/biphasic positive airway pressure
BM	bone marrow (*NB:* BM is often used, confusingly, to signify finger-prick glucose; CBG [capillary blood glucose] is used for this purpose in this book)
BMI	body mass index = weight (kg)/height (m)^2
BNF	British National Formulary
BP	blood pressure
BPAD	bipolar affective disorder
BPH	benign prostatic hypertrophy
BTS	British Thoracic Society
Bx	biopsy
C	constipation
Ca	cancer (*NB:* calcium is abbreviated to Ca^{2+})
Ca^{2+}	calcium
CAH	congenital adrenal hyperplasia
CBF	cerebral blood flow
CBG	capillary blood glucose in mmol/L (finger-prick testing) (*NB:* BM is often used to denote this, but this is confusing and less accurate and thus not used in this book)
CCF	congestive cardiac failure
CCU	coronary care unit
cf	compared with
CI	contraindicated

CK	creatine kinase
CKD	chronic kidney disease
CLL	chronic lymphocytic leukaemia
CML	chronic myelogenous leukaemia
CMV	cytomegalovirus
CNS	central nervous system
CO	cardiac output
COCP	combined oral contraceptive pill
COPD	chronic obstructive pulmonary disease
COX	cyclo-oxygenase
CPR	cardiopulmonary resuscitation
CRF	chronic renal failure
CRP	C-reactive protein
CSF	cerebrospinal fluid
CSM	Committee on Safety of Medicines
CT	computerised tomography
CTO	Community Treatment Order
CVA	cerebrovascular accident
CVD	cardiovascular disease
CVP	central venous pressure
CXR	chest X-ray
D	diarrhoea
$D_{1/2/3 \dots}$	dopamine receptor subtype$_{1/2/3 \dots}$
D&V	diarrhoea and vomiting
DA	dopamine
DCT	distal convoluted tubule
dfx	defects
DI	diabetes insipidus
DIC	disseminated intravascular coagulation
DIGAMI	glucose, insulin and potassium intravenous infusion used in acute myocardial infarction
DKA	diabetic ketoacidosis
DM	diabetes mellitus
DMARD	disease-modifying anti-rheumatoid arthritis drug
DOAC	direct oral anticoagulant
dt	due to

DWI	diffusion-weighted (imaging); specialist magnetic resonance imaging (MRI) mostly used for stroke/transient ischaemic attack (TIA)
Dx	diagnosis
EØ	eosinophils
E'lyte	electrolyte
EBV	Epstein–Barr virus
ECG	electrocardiogram
ECT	electroconvulsive therapy
EF	ejection fraction
ENT	ear, nose and throat
EPSE	extrapyramidal side effects
ERC	European Resuscitation Council
ESC	European Society of Cardiology
esp	especially
ESR	erythrocyte sedimentation rate
exac	exacerbates
FBC	full blood count
Fe	iron
FFP	fresh frozen plasma
FGA	first generation antipsychotic
FHx	family history
FiO$_2$	inspired O$_2$ concentration
FMF	familial Mediterranean fever
FRIII	fixed rate intravenous insulin infusion
fx	effects
G6PD	glucose-6-phosphate dehydrogenase
GABA	γ-aminobutyric acid
GBS	Guillain–Barré syndrome
GCS	Glasgow Coma Scale
GFR	glomerular filtration rate
GI	gastrointestinal
GIK	glucose, insulin and K$^+$ infusion
GMC	General Medical Council (of United Kingdom)
GORD	gastro-oesophageal reflux disease
GTN	glyceryl trinitrate

GU	genitourinary
h	hour(s)
H(O)CM	hypertrophic (obstructive) cardiomyopathy
Hb	haemoglobin
HB	heart block
HBPM	home blood pressure monitoring
Hct	haematocrit
HDL	high-density lipoprotein
HF	heart failure
HHS	hyperosmolar hyperglycaemic state
HIV	human immunodeficiency virus
HLA	human leucocyte antigen
HMG-CoA	3-hydroxy-3-methyl-glutaryl coenzyme A
HONK	hyperosmolar non-ketotic state; *see also* HHS (hyperosmolar hyperglycaemic state)
HR	heart rate
hrly	hourly
HSV	herpes simplex virus
Ht	height
HTN	hypertension
HUS	haemolytic uraemic syndrome
Hx	history
IBD	inflammatory bowel disease
IBS	irritable bowel syndrome
IBW	ideal body weight
ICP	intracranial pressure
ICU	intensive care unit
IHD	ischaemic heart disease
IL-2	interleukin-2
im	intramuscular
inc	including
inh	inhaled
INR	international normalised ratio (prothrombin ratio)
IOP	intraocular pressure
ITP	immune/idiopathic thrombocytopenic purpura
ITU	intensive therapy unit

iv	intravenous
IVDU	intravenous drug user
ivi	intravenous infusion
Ix	investigation
JBDS	Joint British Diabetes Societies
JVP	jugular venous pressure
K+	potassium (serum levels unless stated otherwise)
LØ	lymphocytes
LA	long-acting
LBBB	left bundle branch block
LDL	low-density lipoprotein
LF	liver failure
LFTs	liver function tests
LMWH	low-molecular-weight heparin
LP	lumbar puncture
LVF	left ventricular failure
MØ	macrophages
mane	in morning
MAOI	monoamine oxidase inhibitor
MAP	mean arterial pressure
MCA	middle cerebral artery/Mental Capacity Act
MCV	mean corpuscular volume
metab	metabolised
MG	myasthenia gravis
MHA	Mental Health Act
MHRA	Medicines and Healthcare Products Regulatory Agency (UK)
MI	myocardial infarction
MMF	mycophenolate mofetil
MMSE	Mini-Mental State Examination (scored out of 30*)
MPG	The Maudsley Prescribing Guidelines in Psychiatry, 13th Edition
MR	modified release (drug preparation)†
MRI	magnetic resonance imaging
MRSA	methicillin-resistant *Staphylococcus aureus*
MS	multiple sclerosis

MTS	(abbreviated) Mental Test Score (scored out of 10*)
MUST	malnutrition universal screening tool
Mx	management
N	nausea
N&V	nausea and vomiting
NØ	neutrophils
NA	noradrenaline (norepinephrine)
Na$^+$	sodium (serum levels unless stated otherwise)
NBM	nil by mouth
NCT	narrow complex tachycardia
NDRI	noradrenaline and dopamine reuptake inhibitor
neb	via nebuliser
NEPTUNE	Novel Psychoactive Treatment: UK Network
NGT	nasogastric tube
NH	non-Hodgkin's (lymphoma)
NICE	National Institute for Health and Care Excellence
NIDDM	non-insulin-dependent diabetes mellitus
NIHSS	National (US) Institute of Health Stroke Scale
NIV	non-invasive ventilation
NMDA	N-methyl-D-aspartate
NMJ	neuromuscular junction
NMS	neuroleptic malignant syndrome
NO	nitric oxide
NPIS	National Poisons Information Service
NSAID	non-steroidal anti-inflammatory drug
NSTEMI	non-ST elevation myocardial infarction
NYHA	New York Heart Association
OCD	obsessive-compulsive disorder
OCP	oral contraceptive pill
OD	overdose (NB: od = once daily!)
OGD	oesophagogastroduodenoscopy
OTC	over-the-counter
p'way(s)	pathway(s)
PAN	polyarteritis nodosa
PBC	primary biliary cirrhosis

PCI	percutaneous coronary intervention (now preferred term for percutaneous transluminal coronary angioplasty [PTCA], which is a subtype of PCI)
PCOS	polycystic ovary syndrome
PCP	*Pneumocystis carinii* pneumonia
PCV	packed cell volume
PDA	patent ductus arteriosus
PE	pulmonary embolism
PEA	pulseless electrical activity
PEF	peak expiratory flow
PEG	percutaneous endoscopic gastrostomy
PG(x)	prostaglandin (receptor subtype x)
phaeo	phaeochromocytoma
PHx	past history (of)
PID	pelvic inflammatory disease
PML	progressive multifocal leukoencephalopathy
PMR	polymyalgia rheumatica
po	by mouth (oral)
PO_4	phosphate (serum levels, unless stated otherwise)
PPI	proton pump inhibitor
pr	rectal
prep(s)	preparation(s)
prn	as required
PSA	prostate-specific antigen
Pt	platelet(s)
PT	prothrombin time
PTH	parathyroid hormone
PTSD	post-traumatic stress disorder
PU	peptic ulcer
PUO	pyrexia of unknown origin
PVD	peripheral vascular disease
Px	prophylaxis
QT(c)	QT interval (corrected for rate)
RA	rheumatoid arthritis
RAS	renal artery stenosis

RBF	renal blood flow
r/f	refer
RF	renal failure
RID	relative infant dose
RLS	restless legs syndrome
ROSIER	recognition of stroke in emergency room scale for diagnosis of stroke/transient ischaemic attack (TIA)
RR	respiratory rate
RRT	renal replacement therapy
RSV	respiratory syncytial virus
RTI	respiratory tract infection
RV	right ventricle
RVF	right ventricular failure
Rx	treatment
SAH	subarachnoid haemorrhage
SAN	sinoatrial node
SBE	subacute bacterial endocarditis
sc	subcutaneous
SCLE	subacute cutaneous lupus erythematosus
SE(s)	side effect(s)
sec	second(s)
SGA	second generation antipsychotic
SIADH	syndrome of inappropriate antidiuretic hormone
SIGN	Scottish Intercollegiate Guidelines Network
SJS	Stevens-Johnson syndrome
sl	sublingual
SLE	systemic lupus erythematosus
SOA	swelling of ankles
SOB (OE)	shortness of breath (on exertion)
SPC	summary of product characteristic sheet (see page xi, refer box in 'Standard Layout of Drugs' in 'How to Use This Book')
spp	species
SR	slow/sustained release (drug preparation)
SSRI	selective serotonin reuptake inhibitor
SSS	sick sinus syndrome

STEMI	ST elevation myocardial infarction
supp	suppository
SVT	supraventricular tachycardia
Sx	symptoms
SZ	schizophrenia
$t_{\frac{1}{2}}$	half-life
T_3	triiodothyronine/liothyronine
T_4	thyroxine ($\uparrow/\downarrow$ T_4 = hyper-/hypothyroid)
TCA	tricyclic antidepressant
TE	thromboembolism
TEDS	thromboembolism deterrent stockings
TEN	toxic epidermal necrolysis
TFTs	thyroid function tests
TG	triglyceride
TIA	transient ischaemic attack
TIBC	total iron-binding capacity
TIMI score	risk score for unstable angina (UA)/non-ST elevation myocardial infarction (NSTEMI) named after thrombolysis in myocardial infarction (TIMI) trial
TNF	tumour necrosis factor
top	topical
TOXBASE	the primary clinical toxicology database of the National Poisons Information Service
TPMT	thiopurine methyltransferase
TPR	total peripheral resistance
TTA(s)	(drugs) to take away, i.e. prescriptions for inpatients on discharge/leave (aka TTO)
TTO(s)	*see also* TTA
TTP	thrombotic thrombocytopenic purpura
U&Es	urea and electrolytes
UA(P)	unstable angina (pectoris)
UC	ulcerative colitis
UDS	urine drug screen
UKTIS	UK Teratology Information Service
UKDILAS	UK Drugs in Lactation Advisory Service
URTI	upper respiratory tract infection

USS	Ultrasound scan
UTI	urinary tract infection
UV	ultraviolet
V	vomiting
VE(s)	ventricular ectopic(s)
VF	ventricular fibrillation
vit	vitamin
VLDL	very-low-density lipoprotein
VRIII	variable rate intravenous insulin infusion
VT	ventricular tachycardia
VTE	venous thromboembolism
VZV	varicella zoster virus (chickenpox/shingles)
w	with
w/in	within
w/o	without
WCC	white cell count
WE	Wernicke's encephalopathy
wk	week
wkly	weekly
WPW	Wolff–Parkinson–White syndrome
Wt	weight
xs	excess
ZE	Zollinger–Ellison syndrome

HOW TO PRESCRIBE SAFELY

Take time/care to ↓ risk to patients (and protect yourself).
Always check the following are correct for all prescriptions:
patient, indication and drug, **legible** format (generic name, clarity,
handwriting, **identifiable signature**, your contact number), dosage,
frequency, time(s) of day, date, duration of treatment, route of
administration.

DO

- Make a clear, accurate record in the notes of all medicines
  prescribed, and indication, written at the time of prescription.
- Complete allergy box and agreed relevant labels and e-alerts.
- Include on all drug charts and TTAs the patient's surname and
  given name, date of birth, date of admission and consultant
  (if possible use a printed label for patient details).
- **PRINT** (i.e. use uppercase) all drugs as approved (generic)
  names, e.g. 'IBUPROFEN' *not* **nurofen**'.
- State dose, route and frequency, giving strength of solutions/
  creams.
- Write microgram in full; avoid abbreviations such as mcg or µ.
- Abbreviate the word gram to 'g' (rather than 'gm' which is easily
  confused with mg).
- Write the word 'units' in full, preceded by a space; abbreviating
  to 'U' can be misread as zero (a 10-fold error).
- Document weight: guides dosing and GFR calculation.
- Write quantities <1 g in mg (e.g. 400 mg *not* 0.4 g).
- Write quantities <1 mg in micrograms (e.g. 200 micrograms *not*
  0.2 mg).
- Write quantities <1 microgram in nanograms (e.g. 500
  nanograms *not* 0.5 micrograms).
- Do not use trailing zeroes (10 mg *not* 10.0 mg).
- Precede decimal points with another figure (e.g. 0.8 mL *not*
  .8 mL), and only use decimals where unavoidable.
- Check and recheck calculations.

- Provide clear additional instructions, e.g. for monitoring, review of antibiotic route and duration, maximum daily/24 h dose for as required drugs.
- Specify solution to be used and duration of any iv infusions/injections.
- Avoid using abbreviated/non-standard drug names.
- Avoid writing 'T' (tablet sign) for non-tablet formulations, e.g. sprays.
- Amend a prescribed drug by drawing a line through it, date and initial this, then rewrite as new prescription.
- Review need for drugs when rewriting a drug chart.
- Check and count number of drugs when rewriting a drug chart.
- Check when prescribing unfamiliar drug(s)/doses or drugs you were familiar with but have not prescribed recently.

IMPORTANT FURTHER ADVICE

1 Make sure choice of drug and dose are right for the patient, their condition and significant comorbidity, with particular attention to age*, gender, ethnicity, renal or liver dysfunction, risk of drug-drug and drug-disease interactions and risks in pregnancy (and those of childbearing age who may become pregnant) and during breastfeeding. Anticipate possible effects of over-the-counter and herbal medicines and lifestyle (e.g. dietary salt and alcohol intake).

   *Although arbitrary, age older than 65 years denotes 'elderly', fx of age can occur earlier/later and are continuous across age spectrum.

2 Common settings where drug problems occur are often predictable if you understand relevant risks, pathology, routes of drug metabolism (liver, P450, renal, etc.) and drug mechanisms of action. Take particular care with
   - Renal or liver disease.
   - Pregnancy/breastfeeding: use safest options (in the United Kingdom consider consulting the UK Teratology Information Service [tel: 0344 8920909]).

- Prescribing or dispensing medicines that could be confused with others (e.g. sound or look similar). See MHRA for examples.
- NSAIDs/bisphosphonates and peptic ulcer disease.
- Asthma and β-blockers.
- Conditions worsened by antimuscarinic drugs (see p. 346, refer 'Cholinoceptors' in 'Side Effect Profiles' in 'Basic Psychopharmacology'): urinary retention/BPH, glaucoma, paralytic ileus.
- Rare conditions where drugs commonly pose risk, e.g. porphyria, myasthenia, G6PD deficiency, phaeo.

3 Always ensure informed consent; agreeing proposed prescriptions with the patient (or carer if patient has authorised their involvement in their care or has lost capacity); explaining proposed benefits, nature and duration of treatment; clarifying concerns; warning of possible, especially severe, adverse effects; highlighting recommended monitoring and review arrangements and stating what the patient should do in the event of a suspected adverse reaction. Only in extreme emergencies can it be justified to have not done this. For drugs with common potentially fatal/severe side effects, document that these risks have been explained to, and accepted by, the patient.

4 See legal advice on eligibility to prescribe and use unlicensed and off-label medicines, checking national guidance (in the UK, see MHRA and GMC guidance).

5 Make sure that you are being objective. Prescribing should be for the benefit of the patient not the prescriber.

6 Keep up to date about medicines you are prescribing and the related conditions you are treating.

7 Follow CSM guidance on reporting suspected adverse reactions to black triangle drugs and other medicines (see https://www.mhra.gov.uk for links to Yellow Card reporting scheme and downloads of details of reported adverse drug reactions for specific medicines).

8 Ensure continuity of care by keeping the patient's GP (or other preferred medical adviser) informed about prescribing, monitoring and follow-up arrangements and responsibilities.

9 Check that appropriate previous medicines are continued and over-the-counter and herbal medicine use is recorded.

10 Patient Group Directions: the GMC advises these should be limited to situations where there is a 'distinct advantage for patient care ... consistent with appropriate professional relationships and accountability'.

11 Deprescribing should be part of routine patient care. It concerns withdrawing or reducing the dose of medicines, supervised by a healthcare professional. Its aim is to improve outcomes, e.g. by minimising polypharmacy. Deprescribing needs counselling and shared decision-making with patients.

12 Keep up to date with GMC advice on prescribing (GMC guidelines: https://www.gmc-uk.org/ethical-guidance/ethical-guidance-for-doctors/prescribing-and-managing-medicines-and-devices).

13 All sedative medications may impair driving and the ability to operate machinery. Warn patients of this risk.

Common/useful drugs

ACAMPROSATE/CAMPRAL EC

Modifies GABA transmission ⇒ ↓pleasurable fx of alcohol ∴ ↓s craving and relapse rate.

Use: maintaining alcohol abstinence supported by counselling.

CI: **L** (if severe), **R/P/B**.

SE: GI upset, pruritus, rash, Δ libido.

Dose: 666 mg tds po if age 18–65 years (avoid outside this age range) and >60 kg (if <60 kg, give 666 mg mane then 333 mg noon and nocte). *Start ASAP after alcohol stopped. Usually give for 1 year.*

ACETYLCYSTEINE (*N*-ACETYLCYSTEINE, NAC)/PARVOLEX

Precursor of glutathione, which detoxifies metabolites of paracetamol.

Use: paracetamol OD.

Caution: asthma* and atopy.

SE: allergy: rash, bronchospasm*, anaphylactoid reactions (esp if ivi too quick**).

Dose: initially 150 mg/kg in 5% glucose 200 mL as ivi over 60 min, then 50 mg/kg in 500 mL over 4 h, then 100 mg/kg in 1 L over 16 h. *NB:* use max Wt of 110 kg for dose calculation, even if patient weighs more. Ensure not given too quickly**. See p. 383, refer 'Paracetamol Overdose' in 'Drug Toxicity Syndromes' in 'Emergencies' for Mx of paracetamol OD and treatment line graph.

ACICLOVIR (previously ACYCLOVIR)

Antiviral. Inhibits DNA polymerase *only in infected cells:* needs activation by viral thymidine kinase (produced by herpes species).

Use: *iv:* severe HSV or varicella zoster virus (VZV) infections, e.g. meningitis, encephalitis and in immunocompromised patients (esp HIV – also used for Px); *po/top:* mucous membrane, genital, eye infections.

Caution: dehydration*, **R/P/B**.

SE: at ↑doses: AKI, encephalopathy (esp if dehydrated*). Also hypersensitivity, seizures, GI upset, blood disorders, skin reactions (including photosensitivity), headache, fever, dyspnoea, many non-specific neurological symptoms, ↓Pt, ↓WBC. Rarely Ψ reactions and hepatotoxicity.

Interactions: ↑s fx/toxicity of theophylline/aminophylline.
Dose: 5 mg/kg tds ivi over 1 h (10 mg/kg tds ivi if HSV encephalitis or VZV in immunocompromised patients); po/top.^{SPC/BNF}

☠ ivi leaks ⇒ severe local inflammation/ulceration ☠.

ACIDEX
Alginate raft-forming oral suspension for acid reflux.
Dose: 10–20 mL after meals and at bedtime in patients over 12 years (*NB*: 3 mmol Na+/5 mL).

ACTIVATED CHARCOAL see Charcoal.

AGOMELATINE/VALDOXAN
Antidepressant: synthetic melatonin analogue; melatonin receptor (MT_1/MT_2) agonist (also $5\text{-}HT_{2C/B}$ antagonist); re-synchronises circadian rhythms and ↑s NA/DA in frontal cortex via $5\text{-}HT_{2C}$ antagonism.
Use: depression, esp if risk of inconsistent use (↓risk of withdrawal syndrome) or if prominent insomnia/sleep reversal.
CI: dementia, transaminases >3× upper limit of normal, and see interactions that follow, **L/B**.
Caution: Hx mania (bipolar), R/P/E.
SE: GI upset (N, D and C, abdo pain), **headache**, Δ LFTs (↑transaminases in 5%; usually transient), drowsiness, sweating, anxiety, suicidal behaviour.
Monitor: LFTs before and 3, 6, 12 and 24 wk after starting. Repeat if dose↑.
Interactions: levels ↑↑ by strong CYP1A2 inhibitors (e.g. fluvoxamine, ciprofloxacin – avoid), ↑ by moderate inhibitors (e.g. propranolol, enoxacin, oestrogens) and ↓ by smoking.
Dose: 25 mg nocte (can ↑ to 50 mg nocte after 2 wk).

ALENDRONATE (ALENDRONIC ACID)/FOSAMAX
Bisphosphonate: ↓s osteoclastic bone resorption.
Use: osteoporosis Rx and Px (esp if on corticosteroids).

CI: delayed GI emptying (esp achalasia and oesophageal stricture/other abnormalities), $\downarrow Ca^{2+}$, unable to sit/stand upright $\geq$30 min, **R** (if severe)/**P**/**B**.

Caution: upper GI disorders (inc gastritis/PU), **R**.

SE: oesophageal reactions*, GI upset/distension, $\downarrow Ca^{2+}$, $\downarrow PO_4$ (transient), PU, hypersensitivity (esp skin reactions), myalgia. Rarely osteonecrosis of jaw and femoral stress fractures (discontinue drug and should receive no further bisphosphonates).

Warn: take upright with full glass of water on an empty stomach; stay upright $\geq$30 min until breakfast* or other oral medicine. Stop tablets and seek medical attention if symptoms of oesophageal irritation. Dental review if dental hygiene poor.

Dose: 10 mg mane$^{SPC/BNF}$ (10 mg od dosing can be given as once-wkly 70 mg tablet *if for post-menopausal osteoporosis*. Once-wkly doses unlicensed in men but may $\uparrow$ compliance).

ALFACALCIDOL

1-α-hydroxycholecalciferol: partially activated vit D.
1-α-hydroxy group normally added by kidney, but still requires hepatic (25)-hydroxylation for full activation.

Use: severe vit D deficiency 2° to CRF.

CI/SE: $\uparrow Ca^{2+}$.

Caution: nephrolithiasis, breastfeeding, **E**/**P**/**B**.

Monitor: Ca^{2+} and PO_4: monitor levels wkly, watch for symptoms (esp N&V), rash, nephrocalcinosis.

Interactions: fx $\downarrow$d by barbiturates, anticonvulsants; $\uparrow$d by thiazides.

Dose: initially 1 microgram (= 1000 nanograms) od po; maintenance 250–1000 nanograms od po.
NB: $\downarrow$dose in elderly (initial dose 500 nanograms).

ALISKIREN

Direct renin inhibitor ($\downarrow$s angiotensinogen $\Rightarrow$ angiotensin I).

Use: essential HTN.

CI: angioedema, potent P-glycoprotein inhibitors (*ciclosporin, itraconazole, quinidine), **P**/**B**.

Caution: not recommended with ACE-i, ARBs, dehydration (risk of ↓BP), RAS, diuretics, ↓Na^+ diet, **↑K^+, moderate potent P-glycoprotein inhibitors (*ketoconazole, clari-/teli-/erythromycin, verapamil, amiodarone), DM***, R (if GFR <30 mL/min)/H/P/B/E.
SE: diarrhoea, dizziness, ↓BP, ↑K^+, ↓GFR. Rarely rash, angioedema, ↓Hb.
Monitor: U&Es esp **↑K^+ if taking ACE-i, ARBs, K^+ sparing diuretics, K^+ salts (inc dietary salt substitutes) or heparin. Check BG/HbA_{1C} regularly***.
Interactions: metab by/↓/↑P450 ∴ many; ↓s furosemide levels. Levels ↓ by irbesartan; levels ↑ by keto-/itraconazole. fx ↓ by NSAIDs. fx ↑ by P-glycoprotein inhibitors (see *CI/Caution).
Dose: initially 150 mg od, ↑ing to 300 mg od if required.

ALLOPURINOL

Xanthine oxidase inhibitor: ↓s uric acid synthesis.
Use: Px of gout, renal stones (urate or Ca^{2+} oxalate) and other ↑urate states (esp 2° to chemotherapy).
CI: acute gout: can worsen – do not start drug during attack (but do not stop drug if acute attack occurs during Rx).
Caution: R (↓dose), L (↓dose and monitor LFTs), P/B.
SE: GI upset, ☠ severe skin reactions ☠ (*stop if drug rash develops and allopurinol is implicated* – can reintroduce cautiously if mild reaction and no recurrence). Rarely neuropathy (and many non-specific neurological symptoms), blood disorders, RF, hepatotoxicity, gynaecomastia, vasculitis.
Warn: report rashes, maintain good hydration; ↑risk acute attacks just after initiating.
Interactions: ↑s fx/toxicity of azathioprine (and possibly other cytotoxics, esp ciclosporin), chlorpropamide and theophyllines. ↑levels of vidarabine and didanosine. Level ↓d by salicylates and probenecid. ↑rash with ampicillin and amoxicillin, W+.
Dose: initially 100 mg od po (↑ if required to max of 900 mg/day in divided doses of up to 300 mg) after food. Usual dose 300 mg/day.
NB: ↓dose if ↑s fx other drugs or LF or RF.
Initial Rx can ↑gout: give colchicine or NSAID (naproxen or ibuprofen – *not aspirin*) Px until ≥1 month after urate normalised.

ALPHAGAN see Brimonidine; α_2-agonist eye drops for glaucoma.

ALPRAZOLAM/XANAX

Short-acting benzodiazepine: GABA$_A$ receptor positive allosteric modulator.

Use: short-term use in anxiety.

CI: respiratory depression, marked neuromuscular respiratory weakness inc unstable myasthenia gravis, sleep apnoea, acute pulmonary insufficiency, chronic psychosis, depression (do not give alprazolam alone), **L** (if severe).

Caution: respiratory disease, muscle weakness (inc MG), Hx of drug/alcohol abuse, personality disorder, organic brain diseases, **R**/**P**/**B**/**E**.

SE: respiratory depression (rarely apnoea), drowsiness, dependence (problematic, as short half-life). Also ataxia, amnesia, headache, vertigo, GI upset, jaundice, ↓BP, ↓HR, visual/libido/urinary disturbances, blood disorders, paradoxical disinhibition in Ψ disorder.

Warn: sedation ↑ by alcohol. Do not stop suddenly, as can ⇒ withdrawal.

Interactions: levels ↑ by aprepitant, crizotinib, diltiazem, dronedarone, erythromycin, fluconazole, imatinib, isavuconazole, netupitant, nilotinib, posaconazole, verapamil.

Dose: 250–500 micrograms po tds, ↑ if necessary up to 3 mg po od (elderly: 250 micrograms bd/tds).

Not prescribable in NHS primary care.

ALUMINIUM HYDROXIDE

Antacid, PO_4-binding agent (↓s GI absorption).

Use: dyspepsia, ↑PO_4 (which can ↑risk of bone disease; esp good if secondary to RF, when ↑Ca^{2+} can occur dt ↑PTH, as other PO_4 binders often contain Ca^{2+}).

CI: ↓PO_4, porphyria.

SE: constipation*. Aluminium can accumulate in RF (esp on dialysis) ⇒ ↑risk of encephalopathy, dementia, osteomalacia.

L/R/H = Liver, Renal and Heart failure. E = elderly. P = pregnancy. B = breastfeeding.

Interactions: can ↓drug absorption, e.g. oral antibiotics (e.g. tetracyclines), digoxin and NSAIDs.
Dose: 1–2 (500 mg) tablets prn (qds often sufficient). ↑doses to individual requirements, esp if for ↑PO_4. Avoid within 2 h of drug of which absorption ↓d (see BNF). Also available as 475 mg capsules as **Alu-Caps** (contains ↓Na^+). Most effective taken with meals and at bedtime. Consider laxative Px*.

AMANTADINE

Weak DA agonist; ↑s release and ↓s reuptake of DA; NMDA antagonist. Also antiviral properties; ↓s release of viral nucleic acid.
Use: Parkinson's disease and dyskinesias[1]. Also used for fatigue in MS (unlicensed[NICE])[2].
CI: gastric ulcer (inc Hx of), epilepsy, **R** (if creatinine clearance <15 mL/min), **P/B**.
Caution: confused or hallucinatory states, **L/H/E**.
SE: confusion, hallucinations, pedal oedema NMS-like syndrome.
Warn: Can ↓skilled task performance (esp driving). Stop drug slowly*.
Interactions: memantine ↑risk of CNS toxicity, anticholinergics.
Dose: 100–400 mg daily[SPC/BNF,1]; 200 mg daily[2].[NICE] *NB:* ↓**dose in RF, E ≥ 65 years.**
NB: stop slowly*: risk of withdrawal syndrome.

AMFEBUTAMONE see Bupropion; aid to smoking cessation.

AMIODARONE

Class III antiarrhythmic: ↑s refractory period of conducting system; has ↓negative inotropic fx than other drugs and can give when others ineffective/CI.
Use: tachyarrhythmias: esp paroxysmal SVT, AF, atrial flutter, nodal tachycardias, VT and VF. Also in CPR/periarrest arrhythmias.
CI: ↓HR (sinus), sinoatrial HB, SAN disease or severe conduction disturbance w/o pacemaker, Hx of thyroid disease/iodine sensitivity, **P/B**.
Caution: porphyria, ↓K^+ (↑risk of torsades), **L/R/H/E**.
SE: *Acute:* N&V (dose-dependent), ↓**HR/BP**. *Chronic:* rarely but seriously ↑ or ↓T_4, interstitial lung disease (e.g. fibrosis, *but*

reversible if caught early), **hepatotoxicity, conduction disturbances** (esp ↓HR). *Common:* **malaise, fatigue,** photosensitive skin (rarely 'grey-slate'), corneal deposits ± 'night glare' (reversible), tremor, sleep disorders. *Less commonly:* optic neuritis (rare but can ↓vision), peripheral neuropathy, blood disorders, hypersensitivity.

Warn: avoid sunlight/use sunscreen (inc several months after stopping).

Monitor: TFTs and LFTs (baseline then 6 monthly). Also baseline K^+ and CXR (watch for ↑SOB/alveolitis).

Interactions: Drugs that ↑QT. ↑s fx of phenytoin and digoxin. Other class III and many class Ia antiarrhythmics, antipsychotics, TCAs, lithium, erythromycin, co-trimoxazole, antimalarials, nelfinavir, ritonavir ⇒ ↑risk of ventricular arrhythmias. Verapamil, diltiazem and β-blockers ⇒ ↑risk of ↓HR and HB; CYP3A4 inhibition with statins ↑myopathy, **W+**.

Dose: po: load with 200 mg tds in first wk, 200 mg bd in second wk, then (usually od) maintenance dose according to response (long $t_{1/2}$: months before steady plasma concentration). *NB: initiate in hospital or specialist outpatient service*; **iv:** (extreme emergencies only) 150–300 mg in 10–20 mL 5% glucose over ≥3 min (do not repeat for at least 15 min); **ivi:** 5 mg/kg over 20–120 min (max 1.2 g/day).

☠ iv doses: give via central line (if no time for insertion, give via largest Venflon possible) with ECG monitoring. Avoid giving if severe respiratory failure or ↓BP (unless caused by arrhythmia), as can worsen. Avoid iv boluses if CCF/cardiomyopathy ☠.

AMISULPRIDE/SOLIAN

Atypical antipsychotic with selective D_2 receptor binding; low dose preferentially blocks presynaptic autoreceptors, but high dose blocks post-synaptic receptors.

Use: acute psychotic episode in schizophrenia[1], schizophrenia with predominantly negative symptoms[2].

CI: CNS depression, phaeo, prolactin-dependent tumours **P/B**.

Caution: Parkinson's, drugs that ↑QTc, epilepsy, MG, phaeo, glaucoma (angle-closure), ↑prostate, severe respiratory disease, jaundice, blood disorders, DM.

A

Class SE: EPSE, ↑prolactin and assoc Sx, sedation, ↑Wt, ↑QTc, VTE, blood dyscrasias, ↓seizure threshold, NMS.

Monitor: ECG may be required, esp if (risk factors for) CVD or inpatient admission; prolactin concentration at start of therapy, 6 months and then yearly; physical health monitoring (cardiovascular disease risk) at least once/year.

Interactions: ↑risk of ↑QTc/torsade de pointes with β-blockers, calcium channel blockers, diuretics, stimulant laxatives, class 1A and III antiarrhythmics (e.g. quinidine, disopyramide, amiodarone, sotalol), ↑sedative fx of alcohol, ↓fx of levodopa, ropinirole.

Dose: 400–800 mg po od in two divided doses (maximum 1.2 g od)[1], 50–300 mg po od[2].

AMITRIPTYLINE

TCA: blocks reuptake of NA (and 5-HT).

Use: depression[1] (esp if insomnia, ↓appetite, psychomotor slowing or agitation prominent. *NB:* ↑danger in OD cf other antidepressants), neuropathic pain[2], migraine prophylaxis.

CI: recent MI (w/in 3 months), arrhythmias (esp HB), CCF, mania, porphyria **B**, **L** (if severe).

Caution: cardiac/thyroid disease, epilepsy*, glaucoma (angle-closure), ↑prostate, phaeo, porphyria, anaesthesia. Also Hx of mania, psychosis or urinary retention, **L/H/P/E**.

SE: antimuscarinic fx, cardiac fx (arrhythmias, HB, HR, postural ↓BP, dizziness, syncope: **dangerous in OD**), ↑Wt, **sedation** (often ⇒ 'hangover'), seizures. Rarely mania, fever, blood disorders, hypersensitivity, Δ LFTs, ↓Na⁺ (esp in elderly), agitation, confusion, serotonin syndrome, neuroleptic malignant syndrome.

Interactions: ☠ **MAOIs ⇒ HTN and CNS excitation. Never give with, or <2 wk after, MAOI** ☠. Levels ↑d by SSRIs, phenothiazines and cimetidine. ↑risk of arrhythmias with amiodarone, pimozide (is CI), thioridazine and some class I antiarrhythmics. ↑risk of paralytic ileus with antimuscarinics. ↑s sedative fx of alcohol.

Dose: initially 25 mg bd (daily dose of 10–25 mg in elderly), ↑if required to max 75 mg bd[1]; initially 10 mg nocte ↑ing if required to 75 mg nocte[2].

> 💀 Overdose is associated with high rate of fatality. TCA overdose ⇒ dilated pupils, arrhythmias, ↓BP, hypothermia, hyperreflexia, extensor plantar responses, seizures, respiratory depression and coma 💀.

AMLODIPINE/ISTIN

Ca^{2+} channel blocker (dihydropyridine): as nifedipine, but ⇒ no ↓contractility or ↑HF.

Use: HTN, angina (esp 'Prinzmetal's' = coronary vasospasm).

CI: ACS, cardiogenic shock, significant aortic stenosis, **P/B**.

Caution: BPH (poly-/nocturia), acute porphyria, **L**.

SE: as nifedipine but ↑ankle swelling and possibly ↓vasodilator fx (headache, flushing and dizziness).

Interactions: care with inducers of cytochrome 3A4; ↓simvastatin dose max 20 mg od; avoid grapefruit juice.

Dose: initially 5 mg od po (↑ if required to 10 mg). *NB:* consider ↓dose in **LF**.

AMOBARBITAL (= SODIUM AMYTAL)

Intermediate-acting barbiturate: binds to $GABA_A$ receptors at α/β subunits ⇒ ↑GABA fx.

Use: severe intractable insomnia in patients already taking barbiturates.

CI: respiratory impairment, sleep apnoea, CNS depression, porphyria, **L/R/B**.

Caution: risk of dependence, **E**.

SE: sedation, respiratory depression, headache, GI upset (C&V&N), ataxia, agitation, confusion, ↓HR, ↓BP.

Warn: Avoid with alcohol.

Interactions: ↑sedation and respiratory depression fx with alcohol; CNS depressant fx prolonged by MAOIs.

Dose: 100–200 mg po of the base or 60–200 mg of the sodium salt at bedtime.

☠ Increased hostility and aggression after barbiturates and alcohol usually indicates intoxication ☠.

AMOXICILLIN

Broad-spectrum penicillin; good GI absorption (can give po and iv).
Use: mild pneumonias[1] (esp community acquired), UTI, *Listeria* meningitis, Lyme disease (*Borrelia burgdorferi*) – erythema migrans[2] or involving cranial nerves[2] or Lyme arthritis[3], endocarditis Px and many ENT/dental/other infections. *Often used with clavulanic acid as co-amoxiclav.*
CI/Caution/SE/Interactions: see Ampicillin.
Dose: 500–1000 mg tds po/iv[1]; 1000 mg tds po for 21 days[2] or 28 days[3]; for other severe infections, see SPC/BNF (mild/moderate infections usually 250–500 mg tds po). *NB:* ↓**dose in RF.**

AMPICILLIN

Broad-spectrum penicillin for iv use: has ↓GI absorption cf amoxicillin, which is preferred po.
Use: meningitis (esp *Listeria*)[1], Px pre-operative or for endocarditis during invasive procedures if valve lesions/prostheses, respiratory tract/ENT infections (esp community-acquired pneumonia dt *Haemophilus influenzae* or *Streptococcus pneumoniae*), UTIs (not for blind Rx, as *Escherichia coli* often resistant).
CI: penicillin hypersensitivity (*NB:* cross-reactivity with cephalosporins).
Caution: EBV/CMV infections, ALL, CLL (all ↑risk of rash), R.
SE: rash (erythematous, maculopapular: often does not reflect true allergy) more common in RF or crystal nephropathy, **N&V&D** (rarely AAC), hypersensitivity, CNS/blood disorders.
Interactions: levels ↑ by probenecid. ↑risk of rash with allopurinol. Can ↓fx of OCP (warn patient); ↑levels of methotrexate, **W+.**
Dose: most indications 250 mg–1 g qds po, 500 mg qds im/iv[SPC/BNF] (meningitis 2 g 4-hrly ivi[1]). *NB:* ↓**dose in RF.**

ANTABUSE see Disulfiram; adjunct to alcohol withdrawal.

ANTACIDS see Alginates (e.g. **Acidex**, **Gastrocote**, **Gaviscon**, **Peptac** or **Co-magaldrox**.

APIXABAN/ELIQUIS

Oral anticoagulant; direct inhibitor of activated factor X (factor Xa)

Use: Px of venous thromboembolism following knee[1] or hip[2] replacement surgery, Rx of deep-vein thrombosis (DVT)[3], Rx of pulmonary embolism[3], Px of recurrent DVT[4] or PE[4], Px of stroke and systemic embolism in non-valvular AF and at ≥ 1 risk factor[5] (e.g. previous stroke or transient ischaemic attack [TIA], symptomatic HF, diabetes mellitus, hypertension, or ≥ 75 years of age).

CI: active, clinically significant bleeding, risk factors for major bleeding[BNF], **L** (if severe)/**R** (if severe)/ **P/B**.

Caution/Interactions: ☠ anaesthesia with post-operative indwelling epidural catheter (risk of paralysis), see BNF ☠; prosthetic heart valve (efficacy not established); **L**.

SE: anaemia, haemorrhage; nausea, skin reactions; administration site reactions; CNS haemorrhage, $\downarrow$BP; post-procedural haematoma, $\downarrow$Pt; wound complications.

Warn: carry alert card at all times.

Dose: start 12–24 hours after surgery – 2.5 mg bd po[1,2] for 10–14 days[1]; for 32–38 days[2]. Initially 10 mg bd for 7 days po, then maintenance 5 mg bd po[3]. 2.5 mg bd po, after completion of 6 months anticoagulant Rx[4]. 5 mg twice daily, reduce dose to 2.5 mg twice daily in patients with ≥ 2 of the following: ≥ 80 years of age, Wt <61 kg, or serum creatinine ≥ 133 micromol/L[5]. See SPC for how to change from, or to, other anticoagulants.

AQUEOUS CREAM Emulsifying ointment (phenoxyethanol in purified water). Topical cream used as emollient in dry skin conditions and as a soap substitute.

ARIPIPRAZOLE/ABILIFY

Atypical (third generation) antipsychotic; *partial* D_2 (and 5-HT_{1A}) agonist $\Rightarrow$ ↓dopaminergic neuronal activity. Also potent 5-HT_{2A} antagonist.

Use: schizophrenia, mania (Px and acute Rx).

CI: coma, CNS depression, phaeo, **B**.

Caution: cerebrovascular disease, Hx or ↑risk of seizures, family Hx of ↑QT, **L/P/E**.

SE: EPSE (esp akathisia/restlessness, although generally $\Rightarrow$ ↓EPSE than other antipsychotics), dizziness, sedation (or insomnia), blurred vision, fatigue, headache, GI upset, anxiety and ↑salivation. Rarely ↑HR, depression, orthostatic ↓BP. Very rarely skin/blood disorders, ↑QTc, DM, NMS, tardive dyskinesia, seizures and CVA.

Interactions: metab by P450 $\therefore$ many: most importantly levels ↑ by itraconazole, HIV protease inhibitors, fluoxetine, paroxetine and levels ↓ by carbamazepine, rifampicin, rifabutin, phenytoin, primidone, efavirenz, nevirapine and St John's wort.

Dose: 10–15 mg po od (max 30 mg/od); 5.25–15 (usually 9.75) mg im as single dose repeated after ≥2 h if required (max three injections/day or combined im/po dose of 30 mg/day). *NB:* ↓**dose in elderly.**

ASPIRIN

NSAID. Inhibits COX-1 and COX-2 $\Rightarrow$ ↓PG synthesis ($\therefore$ anti-inflammatory and antipyrexial) and ↓thromboxane A_2 ($\therefore$ anti-Pt aggregation).

Use: mild-to-moderate pain/pyrexia[1], IHD and thromboembolic CVA Px[2] and acute Rx[3].

CI: <16 years old, unless specifically indicated (can $\Rightarrow$ Reye's syndrome), PU (active or at analgesic dose PHx of), hypersensitivity to any NSAID, haemophilia, **R** (GFR <10 mL/min)/**L** (if severe)/**B**.

Caution: asthma, gout, any allergic disease*, dehydration, uncontrolled HTN, gout, G6PD deficiency, **L/R** (avoid if either severe)/**P/E**.

SE: GI irritation, bleeding (esp GI: ↑↑risk if also anticoagulated)**. Rarely hypersensitivity* (anaphylaxis, bronchospasm, skin reactions), AKI, hepatotoxicity, ototoxic in OD.

Interactions: ↑GI bleeding with anticoagulants**, other NSAIDs (avoid), SSRIs and SNRIs. **W+**. Can ⇒ ↑levels of methotrexate, ↑fx of anticonvulsants and ↓fx of spironolactone.

Dose: 300–900 mg 4–6 hrly (max 4 g/day)[1], 75 mg od[2], 300 mg stat[3].

Stop 7 days before surgery if significant bleeding is expected. If cardiac surgery or patient has ACS, consider continuing.

ATENOLOL

β-blocker: (mildly) cardioselective* ($\beta_1 > \beta_2$), ↑H_2O solubility ∴ ↓central fx** and ↑renal excretion***.

Use: HTN[1], angina[2], MI (within 12 h as early intervention)[3], arrhythmias[4].

CI/Caution/SE/Interactions: see Propranolol ⇒ ↓bronchospasm* (but avoid in all asthma/only use in COPD if no other choice) and ↓sleep disturbance/nightmares**.

Dose: 25–50 mg od po[1]; 100 mg od po[2]; 5 mg iv over 5 min, 50 mg po 15 min later, 50 mg po after 12 h, then 100 mg od po[3]; 50–100 mg od po[4] (for iv doses, see SPC/BNF). *NB:* consider ↓dose in RF***.

ATOMOXETINE

Noradrenaline reuptake inhibitor: exact mechanism unknown.

Use: ADHD.

CI: phaeo, severe cerebro-/cardiovascular disease, **H**.

Caution: ↑QTc, aggressive behaviour, cerebro-/cardiovascular disease, emotional lability, epilepsy, hostility, HTN, mania, psychosis, susceptibility to angle-closure glaucoma.

SE: Headache, GI upset, ↓appetite, ↓growth rate, cardiac fx (↑HR, ↑BP, postural ↓BP, syncope), somnolence, Δmood, dizziness, rash. *Uncommonly* suicidal behaviour, ↑QTc.

Monitor: Depression, anxiety, tics, pulse, BP, Wt, Ht and appetite at start, after each dose Δ and every 6 months.

Interactions: levels ↑ by bupropion, cinacalcet, fluoxetine, panobinostat, paroxetine, terbinafine; ↑risk of SE with dexamfetamine, lisdexamfetamine, MAOIs.

Dose: adult (70 kg+): initially 500 microgram/kg po od for 7 days, maintenance 1.2 mg/kg od (maximum 1.8 mg/kg od/120 mg od); adult (70 kg+): initially 40 mg po od for 7 days, maintenance 80–100 mg od (maximum 120 mg od), may be given as single dose om or in two divided doses with last dose no later than early evening.

ATORVASTATIN/LIPITOR

HMG-CoA reductase inhibitor.

Use/CI/Caution/SE: see Simvastatin.

Interactions: ↑risk of myopathy includes with ☠ fibrates ☠, daptomycin, ciclosporin, nicotinic acid, itra-/posaconazole. Levels ↑ by clari-/telithromycin.

Dose: initially 10 mg nocte (↑ if necessary, at intervals 1 ≥4 wks, to max 80 mg). In CVD and post ACS aim for 80 mg daily[NICE].

AZITHROMYCIN

Macrolide antibiotic: see Erythromycin.

Use: see Erythromycin (but with ↑activity against Gram −ve and ↓activity against Gram +ve organisms). Also genital chlamydia, Lyme disease (*Borrelia burgdorferi*) – erythema migrans ± non-focal symptoms and non-severe typhoid.

CI: as erythromycin, plus **L** (if severe).

Caution/SE/Interactions: as erythromycin (*NB:* ↑**P450** ∴ many interactions) but ⇒ ↓GI SEs.

Dose: 500 mg od po *for 3 days only* (continue for 7 days for typhoid); 500 mg od po for 17 days for Lyme disease; for GU infections 1 g od po *as single dose*.

AZOPT see Brinzolamide; eye drops for glaucoma.

AZT see Zidovudine; antiretroviral for HIV.

BACLOFEN

Skeletal muscle relaxant: ↓s spinal reflexes, general CNS inhibition at ↑doses.

Use: spasticity, if chronic/severe (esp 2° to MS or cord pathology).

CI: PU, porphyria, hereditary galactose intolerance.

Caution: Ψ disorders, epilepsy, Hx of PU, Parkinson's, porphyria, DM, hypertonic bladder sphincter, respiratory/cerebrovascular disease, L/R/P/E.

SE: sedation, ↓muscle tone, nausea, urinary dysfunction, GI upset, ↓BP. Others rare: ↑spasticity (*stop drug!*), multiple neurological/Ψ symptoms, cardiac/hepatic/respiratory dysfunction.

Warn: may ↓skilled tasks (esp driving), ↑s fx of alcohol.

Interactions: fx ↑ by TCAs. May ↑fx of antihypertensives.

Dose: 5 mg tds po (after food) ↑ing, if required, to max of 100 mg/day. *NB:* ↓dose in RF. In severe cases, can give by intrathecal pump (see SPC/BNF).

Stop gradually over ≥1–2 wk to avoid withdrawal symptoms: confusion, ↑spasticity, Ψ reactions, fits, ↑HR.

BACTROBAN see Mupirocin; topical antibiotic (esp for nasal MRSA). See local policy for infection control.

BECLOMETASONE

Inh corticosteroid: ↓s airway oedema and mucous secretions.

Use: chronic asthma not controlled by short-acting β₂ agonists alone.

Caution: TB (inc quiescent).

SE: oral candidiasis (2° to immunosuppression: ↓d by rinsing mouth with H_2O after use), **hoarse voice.** Rarely glaucoma, hypersensitivity. ↑doses may ⇒ adrenal suppression, Cushing's, ↓bone density, lower RTI, ↓growth (controversial).

Dose: 200–2000 micrograms daily inh (normally start at 200 micrograms bd). Use high-dose inhaler if daily requirements are >800 micrograms.[SPC/BNF] Specify named product for CFC metered disc inhalers, as dose ranges from 50 to 400 micrograms/delivery. CFC-free pressurized metered dose inhalers are not interchangeable.

Rarely ⇒ paradoxical bronchospasm: can be prevented by switching from aerosol to dry powder forms or by using inh β_2 agonists.

BECOTIDE see Beclometasone.

BENDROFLUMETHIAZIDE
Thiazide diuretic: ↓s Na^+ (and Cl) reabsorption from DCT ⇒ Na^+ and H_2O loss and stimulates K^+ excretion.
Use: oedema[1] (2° to HF or low-protein states), HTN[2] (in short term by ↓ing fluid volume and CO; in long term by ↓ing TPR); Px against renal stones in hypercalciuria[3].
CI: ↓K^+(refractory to Rx), ↓Na^+, ↑Ca^{2+}, Addison's disease, ↑urate (if symptoms), L/R (if either severe, otherwise caution).
Caution: porphyria, and can worsen gout, DM or SLE, P/B/E.
SE: dehydration (esp in elderly), ↓BP (esp postural), ↓K^+, GI upset, impotence, ↓Na^+, alkalosis (with ↓Cl), ↓Mg^{2+}, ↑Ca^{2+}, ↑urate/gout, ↑glucose, lipid metabolism (esp ↑cholesterol), rash, photosensitivity, blood disorders (inc ↓Pt, ↓NØ), pancreatitis, intrahepatic cholestasis, hypersensitivity reactions (inc severe respiratory and skin reactions), arrhythmias.
Interactions: ↑s lithium levels. fx ↓ by **NSAIDs** and oestrogens. If ↓K^+ can ↑toxic fx of many drugs (esp digoxin, NSAIDs, corticosteroids and many antiarrhythmics). ↑risk of ↓Na^+ with carbamazepine; ↑risk of ↓K^+ with amphotericin. ↑risk of allopurinol hypersensitivity.
Dose: initially 5–10 mg mane po[1], then ↓dose *frequency* (i.e. omit days) if possible; 2.5 mg od po[2,3] (little benefit from ↑doses).

BENPERIDOL
Potent butyrophenone typical antipsychotic: dopamine antagonist, selective for D_2 receptor; some weaker binding to 5-HT receptors.

Use: antisocial sexual behaviour.

CI: ↓GCS, phaeo.

Caution: Parkinson's, drugs that ↑QTc, epilepsy, MG, glaucoma (angle-closure), ↑prostate, severe respiratory disease, jaundice, blood disorders, DM, stroke risk factors, P.

Class SE: EPSE, ↑prolactin and assoc Sx, sedation, ↑Wt, QT prolongation, VTE, blood dyscrasias, ↓seizure threshold, NMS.

Warn: Photosensitivity at high doses. Extrapyramidal effects and withdrawal syndrome in neonate when used during third trimester. ↑fx of alcohol.

Monitor: prolactin at start, 6 months, then yearly. Regular FBC and LFTs during long-term treatment.

Interactions: ↑risk of ↓BP with atenolol, alcohol, amantadine, amitriptyline, amlodipine, aripiprazole, bendroflumethiazide, bromocriptine, candesartan, chlorpromazine, clozapine, haloperidol; CNS depressant effects with agomelatine, alcohol, alprazolam, amisulpride, aripiprazole, buprenorphine, cannabis extract, chlorphenamine, chlorpromazine, clozapine, codeine; ↓effects of amantadine, apomorphine, bromocriptine, levodopa (severe), ropinirole.

Dose: 0.25–1.5 mg po od in divided doses; elderly: initially 0.125–0.75 mg po od in divided doses.

BENZYLPENICILLIN (= PENICILLIN G)

Penicillin with poor po absorption ∴ only given im/iv: used mostly against streptococcal (esp *S. pneumoniae*) and neisserial (esp *N. gonorrhoeae*, *N. meningitidis*) infections.

Use: (usually in conjunction with other agents) severe skin infections (esp cellulitis, wound infections, gas gangrene), meningitis, endocarditis, ENT infections, pneumococcal pneumonia.

CI: penicillin hypersensitivity (*NB:* cross-reactivity with cephalosporins common).

Caution: Hx of allergy, false +ve glycosuria, R*.

SE: hypersensitivity (inc fever, arthralgia, rashes, urticaria, angioedema, anaphylaxis, serum sickness–like reactions, haemolytic ↓Hb, interstitial nephritis), **diarrhoea** (rarely AAC). Rarely blood disorders (↓Pt, ↓NØ, coagulation disorders), CNS toxicity (inc convulsions, esp at ↑doses or if RF*). ↑doses can ⇒ ↓K$^+$ (and ↑Na$^+$).

Interactions: levels ↑d by probenecid. ↑risk of rash with allopurinol. Can ↓fx of OCP.

Dose: 600 mg–1.2 g qds iv (or im/ivi). If very severe, give 2.4 g every 4 h (only as iv/ivi). *NB:* ↓**dose in RF.**

BETAMETHASONE CREAM (0.1%)/OINTMENT

'Potent' strength topical corticosteroid (rarely used as weaker 0.05% or 0.025% preparations).

Use: inflammatory skin conditions, in particular, eczema.

CI: untreated infection, rosacea, acne.

SE: skin atrophy, worsening of infections, acne.

Dose: apply thinly one to two times per day. Use 'ointment' in dry skin conditions.

BETNOVATE see Betamethasone cream 0.1% (potent strength). Available as **Betnovate RD** (moderate strength) 0.025%.

BIMATOPROST EYE DROPS/LUMIGAN

Topical PG analogue for glaucoma; see Latanoprost.

Use/CI/Caution/SE: see Latanoprost.

Dose: 1 drop od.

BISOPROLOL

β-blocker, cardioselective ($\beta_1 > \beta_2$).

Use: HTN[1], angina[2], HF[3].

CI/Caution/SE/Interactions: as propranolol, but also CI in HF needing inotropes or if SAN block; caution if psoriasis.

Dose: 10 mg od po[1,2] (maintenance 5–20 mg od); initially 1.25 mg od po[3] (↑ing slowly to max 10 mg od).[SPC/BNF] *NB:* ↓**dose in LF or RF.**

BOWEL PREPARATIONS

Bowel-cleansing solutions for preparation for GI surgery/Ix.

CI: GI obstruction/ulceration/perforation, ileus, gastric retention, toxic megacolon/colitis, dehydrated patients, **H**.
Caution: UC, DM, heart disease, reflux oesophagitis, ↑risk of regurgitation/aspiration (e.g. ↓swallow/gag reflex/GCS), **R/P**.
SE: nausea, abdo pains, vomiting, electrolyte disturbance.
Dose: see SPC/BNF.

BRICANYL see Terbutaline (inh β_2 agonist for asthma). Various delivery devices available.^{SPC/BNF}

BRIMONIDINE EYE DROPS/ALPHAGAN

Topical α_2 agonist: ↓s aqueous humour production ∴ ↓s IOP.
Use: open-angle glaucoma, ocular HTN (esp if β-blocker or PG analogue CI or fails to ↓IOP).
Caution: postural ↓BP/HR, Raynaud's, cardiovascular disease (esp IHD), cerebral insufficiency, depression*, **P/B** (avoid)/**R/L**.
SE: sedation, headache, dry mouth, HTN, blurred vision, local reactions (esp discomfort, pruritus, hyperaemia, follicular conjunctivitis). Rarely palpitations, depression*, hypersensitivity.
Interactions: ☠ MAOIs, TCAs, mianserin (or other antidepressants affecting NA transmission) are CI ☠.
Dose: 1 drop bd of 0.2% solution. Also available as od combination drop with timolol 0.5% (**Combigan**).

BRINZOLAMIDE/AZOPT

Topical carbonic anhydrase inhibitor for glaucoma. Similar to dorzolamide (↓s aqueous humour production).
CI: hyperchloraemic acidosis, **R** (GFR <30 mL/min)/**L**.
Caution: **P/B**.
Dose: 1 drop bd/tds. Also available as od combination drop with timolol 0.5% (**Azarga**).

BROMOCRIPTINE

DA agonist; ↓s pituitary release of prolactin and growth hormone.

B

Use: endocrine disorders[1] (e.g. prolactinoma, galactorrhoea, acromegaly) and NMS (unlicensed). Rarely used for parkinsonism if L-dopa insufficient/not tolerated.
CI: cardiac valvulopathy, hypersensitivity to ergot alkaloids, uncontrolled HTN. Also HTN/IHD post-partum or in puerperium.
Caution: cardiovascular disease, PU, porphyria, Raynaud's disease, serious Ψ disorders (esp psychosis, impulse control), P/B.
SE: GI upset, postural ↓BP (esp initially and if ↑alcohol intake), behavioural Δs (confusion, agitation, psychosis), ↑sleep (sudden onset/daytime). Rarely but seriously fibrosis: pulmonary, cardiac, retroperitoneal (can ⇒ AKI).
Warn: of ↑sleep. Report persistent cough or chest/abdo pain.
Monitor: BP, ESR, U&Es, CXR; pituitary size and visual fields (pregnancy and[1]); Rx > 6 m: gynaecological cytology.
Interactions: levels ↑ by ery-/clarithromycin and octreotide. Opposing action to antipsychotics.
Dose: 1–30 mg/day. *NB:* consider ↓dose in LF.

BUDESONIDE

Inh corticosteroid for asthma[1]; similar to beclometasone but stronger (approximately double the strength per microgram). Also available po or as enemas for IBD[2] (see BNF).
Caution: L.
Dose: 200–800 micrograms bd inh (aerosol or powder) or 1–2 mg bd neb[1].

BUMETANIDE

Loop diuretic: inhibits Na^+/K^+ pump in ascending loop of Henle.
Use/CI/Caution/SE/Monitor/Interactions: as furosemide; also headaches, gynaecomastia and at ↑doses can ⇒ myalgia.
Dose: 1 mg mane po (500 micrograms may suffice in elderly), ↑ing if required (5 mg/24 h usually sufficient; ↑ by adding a lunchtime dose, then ↑ing each dose). 1–2 mg im/iv (repeat after 20 min if required). 2–5 mg ivi over 30–60 min.

NB: give iv in severe oedema; bowel oedema ⇒ ↓po absorption.

BUPRENORPHINE/SUBUTEX

Partial agonist at μ-opioid receptor and antagonist at κ-opioid receptors $\Rightarrow$ $\downarrow$neuronal excitability.

Use: moderate-to-severe pain[1], adjunct in treatment of opioid dependence[2]. *NB:* Subutex is a brand of oral buprenorphine; Suboxone is a combination of buprenorphine and naloxone designed to prevent injection.

CI: acute respiratory depression, acute severe obstructive airways disease, $\uparrow$risk of paralytic ileus, delayed gastric emptying, biliary colic, acute alcoholism, $\uparrow$ICP (respiratory depression $\Rightarrow$ CO_2 retention and cerebral vasodilation $\Rightarrow$ $\uparrow$ICP), phaeo, **H** (if 2° to chronic lung disease).

Caution: $\downarrow$consciousness, $\downarrow$respiratory reserve, obstructive airways disease, $\downarrow$BP/shock, acute abdo, biliary tract disorders (*NB:* biliary colic is CI), pancreatitis, bowel obstruction, IBD, $\uparrow$prostate/urethral stricture, arrhythmias, $\downarrow$T$_4$, adrenocorticoid insufficiency, MG, **L** (can $\Rightarrow$ coma)/**R**/**P**/**B**/**E**. *For patch,* fever or external heat ($\Rightarrow$ Δs in absorption), other opioids within 24 h. *For opioid dependence,* hep B/C infection, abnormal LFTs.

SE: fatigue, sleep disorders, anxiety, $\downarrow$appetite, depression, diarrhoea, dyspnoea, GI discomfort, muscle weakness, oedema, tremor.

Warn: do not take other opioids within 24 h of patch removal (long duration of action).

Monitor: baseline and regular LFTs in[2].

Interactions: $\uparrow$risk of withdrawal if given with other opioids; $\uparrow$levels with atazanavir, clarithromycin, cobicistat, darunavir, fosamprenavir, idelalisib, itraconazole, ketoconazole, lopinavir, ritonavir, saquinavir, tipranavir, voriconazole; $\uparrow$risk of CNS excitation/depression with isocarboxazid, phenelzine, tranylcypromine; $\downarrow$fx with nalmefene.

Dose: 200–400 microgram sl every 6–8 h[1]/300–600 microgram im every 6–8 h[1]; initially 0.8–4 mg sl od, adjusted in steps of

2–4 mg sl od, usual dose 12–24 mg sl od, max 32 mg sl od[2]/initially 2 mg po od, adjusted by 2–6 mg po od, max 18 mg po od[2].

☠ Do not confuse the formulations of transdermal patches which are available as 72-hrly, 96-hrly and 7-day patches ☠.

BUPROPION/ZYBAN

NA and to lesser extent DA reuptake inhibitor (NDRI) developed as antidepressant, but also ↑s success of giving up smoking.
Use: (adjunct to) smoking cessation[1], depression (unlicensed use)[2].
CI: CNS tumour, acute alcohol/benzodiazepine withdrawal, Hx of seizures*, eating disorders, bipolar disorder, L (if severe cirrhosis)/P/B.
Caution: if ↑risk of seizures*: alcohol abuse, Hx of head trauma and DM, R/H/E.
SE: seizures*, insomnia (and other CNS reactions, e.g. anxiety, agitation, depression, fever, headaches, tremor, dizziness). Also ↑HR, AV block, ↑ or ↓BP**, chest pain, hypersensitivity (inc severe skin reactions), GI upset, ↑Wt, mild antimuscarinic fx (esp dry mouth).
Monitor: BP**.
Interactions: ↓P450 ∴ many interactions, but importantly CNS drugs, esp if ↓seizure threshold*, e.g. antidepressants (☠ MAOIs; avoid together, including <2 wk after MAOI ☠), antimalarials, antipsychotics (esp risperidone), quinolones, sedating antihistamines, systemic corticosteroids, theophyllines, tramadol; ↓tamoxifen activation. Ritonavir ⇒ ↓plasma level of bupropion. ↓dose of CYP2B6 mod antiarrhythmics.
Dose: 150 mg od for 6 days then 150 mg bd for max 9 wk (↓dose if elderly or ↑seizure risk). Start 1–2 wk before target date of stopping smoking[1]; 150 mg od, ↑ to 300 mg if no improvement after 4 wk[2]. *NB:* max 150 mg/day in LF or RF.

BUSCOPAN see Hyoscine butylbromide; GI antispasmodic.

BUSPIRONE HYDROCHLORIDE

5-HT_{1A} receptor partial agonist $\Rightarrow$ ↓firing rate of 5-HT-containing neurons in dorsal raphe.

Use: anxiety (short-term use).

CI: epilepsy.

Caution: does not assist benzodiazepine withdrawal.

SE: dizziness, headache, anxiety, GI upset, agitation, sweating.

Interactions: metab by P450 ∴ ↓dose to 2.5 mg bd when used with potent CYP3A4 inhibitors; ↑levels with atazanavir, clarithromycin, cobicistat, darunavir, fosamprenavir, idelalisib, itraconazole, ketoconazole, linezolid, lopinavir, ritonavir, saquinavir, tipranavir, voriconazole; ↓levels with carbamazepine, enzalutamide, fosphenytoin, mitotane, phenobarbital, phenytoin, primidone, rifampicin; ↑risk of ↑BP with phenelzine, isocarboxazid, tranylcypromine.

Dose: 5 mg po bd/tds, ↑ at intervals 2–3 days, usual dose 15–30 mg od in divided doses, max 45 mg od.

CACIT see Calcium carbonate.

CACIT D3 Calcium carbonate + low-dose vit D_3.

Use: Px of combined vit D and Ca^{2+} deficiency.

Caution: L.

Dose: 1 tablet od (= 12.5 mmol Ca^{2+} + 11 micrograms cholecalciferol).

CALCICHEW see Calcium carbonate.

CALCICHEW D3 Calcium carbonate + low-dose vit D_3.

Use: Px of vit D deficiency.

Dose: 1 tablet od. Each tablet = 12.5 mmol Ca^{2+} + 5 micrograms vit D_3 (cholecalciferol) or 10 micrograms vit D_3 in 'forte' preparations.

CALCIPOTRIOL OINTMENT AND CREAM

Vit D analogue for plaque psoriasis.

CI: patients with disorders of Ca^{2+} metabolism.

Caution: avoid excessive sunlight exposure use <100 g/wk, E.
SE: local skin reactions (itching, redness).
Dose: apply od or bd. Also used as ointment or gel combined with betamethasone (**Dovobet**) od ≤4 wk.

CALCIUM CARBONATE

Use: osteoporosis, ↓Ca^{2+}, ↑PO_4 (esp 2° to RF; binds PO_4 in gut ⇒ ↓absorption).
CI: conditions assoc with ↑Ca^{2+} (in serum or urine).
Caution: sarcoid, Hx of kidney stones, phenylketonuria, R.
SE: GI upset, ↑Ca^{2+} (serum or urine), ↓HR, arrhythmias.
Interactions: fx ↑ by thiazides, fx ↓ by corticosteroids, ↓s absorption of tetracyclines (give ≥2 h before or 6 h after) and bisphosphonates.
Dose: as required up to 40 mmol/day in osteoporosis if ↓dietary intake, e.g. **Calcichew** (standard 12.5 mmol or 'forte' 25 mmol tablets), **Cacit** (12.5 mmol tablets), **Calcium 500** (12.5 mmol tablets) or **Adcal** (15 mmol tablets).

CALCIUM + ERGOCALCIFEROL tablets of 2.4 mmol Ca^{2+} low-dose (10 micrograms) ergocalciferol (= calciferol = vit D_2).
Use: Px and Rx of calcium and vit D deficiency.
CI/Caution/SE: see Ergocalciferol.
Dose: 1 tablet od.[SPC/BNF]

CALPOL Paracetamol (paediatric) suspension.
Dose: according to age; all doses up to 4-hrly, max qds <3 months[BNF]: 3–5 months 60 mg, 6–23 months 120 mg, 2–3 years 180 mg, 4–5 years 240 mg, 6–7 years 250 mg, 8–9 years 375 mg, 10–11 years 500 mg, 12–15 years 480–750 mg.

NB: two strengths available: 'standard' INFANT (120 mg/5 mL) and stronger SIX Plus (250 mg/5 mL).

CANDESARTAN/AMIAS

Angiotensin II antagonist.
Use: HTN[1] or HF[2] (when ACE-i not tolerated).

CI: cholestasis, **L** (if severe)/**P/B**.

Caution/SE/Interactions: see Losartan.

Dose: initially 8 mg od[1] (4 mg if LF, 4 mg if RF/intravascular volume depletion) ↑ing at 4 wk intervals if necessary to max of 32 mg od; initially 4 mg od[2] ↑ing at intervals ≥2 wk to 'target dose' of 32 mg od (or max tolerated). *NB:* ↓**dose in LF.**

CANESTEN

Clotrimazole 1% cream: antifungal, esp for vaginal candida infections (thrush). Also available as solution and spray for hairy areas.

Dose: apply bd/tds.

CAPTOPRIL

ACE-i: short-acting; largely replaced by longer-acting drugs.

Use: HTN, HF, post-MI and diabetic nephropathy (i.e. consistent proteinuria).

CI: renovascular disease* (known or suspected bilateral RAS), angioedema/other hypersensitivity 2° to ACE-i, porphyria, **P/B**.

Caution: symptomatic aortic stenosis, Hx of idiopathic or hereditary angioedema, if taking drugs that ↑K+**, **L/R/E**.

SE: ↓BP (esp with first dose, if HF, dehydrated or on diuretics, dialysis or ↓Na+ diet ∴ *take at night*), RF*, **dry cough**, ↑K+, acidosis, **hypersensitivity** (esp rashes and **angioedema**), photosensitivity, Δ taste, upper respiratory tract symptoms (inc sore throat/sinusitis/rhinitis), GI upset, Δ LFTs (rarely cholestatic jaundice/hepatitis), pancreatitis, blood disorders, many non-specific neuro symptoms.

Monitor: U&Es, esp baseline and *2 wk after starting**.

Interactions: fx ↓d by NSAIDs (also ⇒ ↑risk RF*). **Diuretics, TCAs and antipsychotics** ⇒ risk of ↓↓BP. ↑s fx of **lithium** (and antidiabetics).

Dose: 6.25–75 mg bd po.^SPC/BNF *NB:* ↓dose in RF.

☙**Beware if on other drugs that ↑K+, e.g. amiloride, spironolactone, triamterene, ARBs and ciclosporin. Do not give with oral K+ supplements – inc dietary salt substitutes ☙

CARBAMAZEPINE/TEGRETOL

Antiepileptic, mood stabiliser, analgesic; ↓s synaptic transmission.
Use: epilepsy[1] (generalised tonic-clonic and partial seizures, but may exacerbate absence/myoclonic seizures), Px bipolar disorder[2] (if unresponsive to lithium), neuralgia[3] (esp post-herpetic, trigeminal and DM related).
CI: unpaced AV conduction dfx, Hx of BM suppression, acute porphyria.
Caution: cardiac disease, Hx of skin disorders (HLA-B*1502 in Han Chinese or Thai origin have ↑risk of SE – esp SJS), Hx of haematological drug reactions, glaucoma, L/R/P (⇒ neural tube dfx* ∴ ⇒ folate Px and screen for dfx)/B.
Dose-related SE: N&V, headache, drowsiness, dizziness, vertigo, ataxia, visual Δ (esp double vision): control by ↓ing dose, Δ dose times/spacing or use of MR preparations**.
Other SE: skin reactions (transient erythema common), blood disorders (esp ↓WCC*** – often transient, ↓Pt, aplastic anaemia), ↑γ-GT (usually not clinically relevant), oedema, ↓Na^+ (inc SIADH), HF, arrhythmias. Many rarer SEs[SPC/BNF]. including suicidal thoughts/behaviour.
Warn: watch for signs of liver/skin/haematological disease.
Monitor: U&Es, LFTs, FBC, TFTs if T_4 Rx, ± serum levels (optimum therapeutic range = 4–12 mg/L). Vit D level.
Interactions: ↑P450 – may cause failure of OCP; ↓levels of thyroid hormones if on hypothyroid Rx; fx are ↑d by ery-/clarithromycin, isoniazid, verapamil and diltiazem; and fx are ↓d by phenytoin, phenobarbitone. ☠ CI with MAOIs ☠, W−.
Dose: initially 100–200 mg od/bd (↑ slowly to max of 1.6 g/day[2,3] or 2 g/day[1]).

CEFACLOR

Oral second-generation cephalosporin.
Use: mild respiratory infections, UTIs, external infections (skin/soft tissue infections, sinusitis, otitis media), or dt *H. influenzae*.
CI: cephalosporin hypersensitivity.

Caution: if at ↑risk of **AAC** (e.g. recent other antibiotic use, ↑age, severe underlying disease, ↑hospital/nursing home stay, GI surgery, conditions/drugs that ↓gastric acidity [esp PPIs], penicillin hypersensitivity (up to 10% also allergic to cephalosporins), R/P/B (but appropriate to use*).

SE: GI upset (esp N&D, but also **AAC**), **allergy** (anaphylaxis, fever, arthralgia, skin reactions [inc severe]), **AKI, interstitial nephritis** (reversible), hepatic dysfunction, blood disorders, CNS disturbance (inc headache).

Interactions: levels ↑ by probenecid, mild **W+**.

Dose: 250 mg tds po (500 mg tds in severe infections; max 4 g/day). *NB: ↓dose in RF.*

Cephalosporins can ⇒ false-positive Coombs' and urine glucose tests.

CEFALEXIN

Oral first-generation cephalosporin.

Use/CI/Caution/SE/Interactions: see Cefaclor and AAC warning.

Dose: 250 mg qds or 500 mg bd/tds po (↑ in severe infections to max 1.5 g qds). For Px of UTI, give 125 mg po nocte. *NB: ↓dose in RF.*

CEFRADINE

Oral or parenteral first-generation cephalosporin.

Use: as cefaclor.

CI/Caution/SE/Interactions: see Cefaclor and **AAC** warning.

Dose: po: 250–500 mg qds *or* 500 mg–1 g bd (max 1 g qds). *NB: ↓dose in RF.*

CEFTRIAXONE

Parenteral third-generation cephalosporin.

Use: severe infections, esp meningitis, UTI, soft-tissue infections, gonorrhoea, pneumonia, plus pre-operative Px[1]; Lyme disease (*Borrelia burgdorferi*) with CNS[2].

CI/Caution/SE/Interactions: as cefaclor and **AAC warning**, plus L (if coexistent RF), R (if severe), caution if dehydrated, young or immobile (can precipitate in urine or gallbladder). Rarely ⇒ pancreatitis and ↑PT.

Dose: 1 g od im/iv/ivi (max 4 g/day); 1–2 g im/iv/ivi at induction[1]; 2 g iv od or 21 days[2]. *NB:* ↓dose in RF.

Max im dose = 1 g per site; if total >1 g, give at divided sites.

CEFUROXIME

Parenteral and oral second-generation cephalosporin: good for some Gram −ve infections (*H. influenzae, N. gonorrhoeae*) and better than third-generation cephalosporins for Gram +ve infections (esp *S. aureus*).

Use: po: respiratory infections[1], UTIs[2], pyelonephritis[3]; iv: severe infections[4], pre-operative Px[5].

CI/Caution/SE/Interactions: see Cefaclor and **AAC warning**.

Dose: 250–500 mg bd po[1]; 125 mg bd po[2]; 250 mg bd po[3]; 750 mg tds/qds iv/im[4] (1.5 g tds/qds iv in very severe infections and 3 g tds if meningitis); 1.5 g iv at induction (+750 mg iv/im tds for 24 h if high-risk procedure)[5]. *NB:* ↓dose in RF.

CELECOXIB/CELEBREX

NSAID which selectively inhibits COX-2 ∴ ↓GI SEs (COX-1 mediated).

Use: osteoarthritis/RA[NICE], ankylosing spondylitis.

CI: IHD, cerebrovascular disease, *active* bleeding/PU, PVD, hypersensitivity to aspirin or any other NSAID (inc asthma, angioedema, urticaria, rhinitis), *sulphonamide* hypersensitivity, IBD, L (if severe)/R (GFR <30)/H (moderate-severe)/P/B.

Caution: Hx of PU/GI bleeding, left ventricular dysfunction, HTN (monitor BP), ↑cardiovascular risk (e.g. DM, ↑lipids, smokers), oedema H (mild), asthma. R*/L (if either mild-to-moderate)/E.

SE/Interactions: as ibuprofen, but ⇒ ↓PU/GI bleeding (but only if not in combination with aspirin) and ⇒ ↑risk of MI/CVA. Very

rarely ⇒ seizures. Also, fluconazole ⇒ ↑serum levels and rifampicin ⇒ ↓serum levels. Mild **W+**.
Dose: 100–200 mg bd po. ↓**dose in RF***. Consider gastroprotective Rx.

> **COX-2 inhibitors and ↑risk of cardiovascular complications:**
> CSM advises assessment of cardiovascular risk and use in preference to other NSAIDs only if at ↑↑risk of GI ulcer, perforation or bleeding. Use lowest effective dose and duration.

CEPH- see CEF-.

CETIRIZINE
Non-sedating antihistamine: selective peripheral H_1 antagonist.
Use: symptomatic relief from allergy (esp hay fever, urticaria).
CI: acute porphyria, **P/B**.
Caution: epilepsy, ↑prostate/urinary retention, glaucoma, pyloroduodenal obstruction, **R/L**.
SE: mild antimuscarinic fx (see p. 346, refer 'Side Effect Profiles' in 'Basic Psychopharmacology' chapter), very mild rare sedation, headache.
Dose: 10 mg od po. ↓**dose in RF.**

CHARCOAL
Binds and ↓s absorption of tablets/poisons.
Use: ODs (up to 1 h post-ingestion; longer if MR/SR preparations or antimuscarinic drugs).
Caution: corrosive poisons, ↓GI motility (can ⇒ obstruction), ↓GCS (risk of aspiration, unless endotracheal tube *in situ*), may ↓absorption of prescribed drugs.
Dose: 50 g po. Give once for paracetamol and most drugs. Avoid use with alcohol and metal ions. Repeated doses (every 4 h) often needed for barbiturates, carbamazepine, phenytoin, digoxin, dapsone, paraquat, quinine, salicylates, theophylline and MR/SR preparations.

CHLORAL HYDRATE/WELLDORM

Hypnotic, short-term use.

Use: insomnia.

CI: porphyria, severe cardiac disease, gastritis, **L** (if severe)/
R (if severe)/**P/B** (⇒ infant sedation).

Caution: avoid prolonged use or contact with skin/mucous
membranes. Avoid abrupt withdrawal if long use, **E**.

SE: GI upset, dependence, hypersensitivity, headache, agitation,
ataxia, ketonuria.

Interactions: ↑fx with alcohol; delirium when used with
psychotropics or anticholinergics.

Dose: one to two tablets, alternatively 414–828 mg po od at
bedtime, max 4 tablets/2 g od.

> 💀 Can precipitate coma in hepatic impairment. 💀

CHLORAMPHENICOL EYE DROPS

Topical antibiotic, with no significant systemic fx, for superficial
bacterial eye infections (e.g. conjunctivitis), or as prophylaxis, e.g.
post-operatively or for corneal abrasions. Can rarely ⇒ aplastic
anaemia; grey baby syndrome.

Dose: 1 drop of 0.5%. Can give as 1% ointment qds (or nocte only
if using drops in daytime as well).

CHLORDIAZEPOXIDE

Long-acting benzodiazepine: GABA$_A$ receptor positive allosteric
modulator.

Use: anxiety, short-term use (esp in alcohol withdrawal).

CI/Caution/SE/Interactions: see Diazepam.

Dose: 10 mg tds po, ↑ing if required to max of 100 mg/day.
NB: ↓**dose in RF, LF and elderly**. ↑dose if benzodiazepine-resistant
or in initial Rx of alcohol withdrawal (see reducing regimen on
p. 296 ['Alcohol detoxification' heading in 'Alcohol' section in
'Substance Misuse' chapter]).

CHLORMETHIAZOLE (= CLOMETHIAZOLE)/ HEMINEVRIN

Barbiturate: binds to $GABA_A$ receptors at α/β subunits $\Rightarrow$ $\uparrow$GABA fx.

Use: severe insomnia (short-term use)[1], agitation[2], alcohol withdrawal[3].

CI: acute resp failure, alcohol dependence.

Caution: chronic resp disorder (inc sleep apnoea), drug misuse, severe personality disorder R/H/E/P/B. Avoid prolonged use and abrupt withdrawal.

SE: nasal congestion, conjunctival irritation, dependence, excessive sedation, GI upset, $\uparrow$LFTs, rash.

Interactions: 💀CNS depression with alcohol💀.

Dose: 192–384 mg po od at bedtime[1]; 192 mg po tds[2]; initially 2–4 192 mg capsules, 9–12 capsules in 3–4 divided doses in first 24 h, 6–8 capsules od in 3–4 divided doses on day 2, 4–6 capsules od in 3–4 divided doses on day 3, $\downarrow$dose gradually over days 4–6, max duration for 9 days[3].

💀Potentially fatal CNS depression with alcohol; can precipitate coma in hepatic impairment💀.

CHLORPHEN(IR)AMINE/PIRITON

Antihistamine: H_1 antagonist (peripheral *and central* $\therefore$ sedating).

Use: allergies[1] (esp drug reactions, hay fever, urticaria), anaphylaxis[2] (inc blood transfusion reaction[3]).

CI: hypersensitivity to any antihistamine.

Caution: pyloroduodenal obstruction, urinary retention/$\uparrow$prostate, thyrotoxicosis, asthma, bronchitis/bronchiectasis, severe HTN/CVD, glaucoma, epilepsy, R/L/P/B.

SE: drowsiness (rarely paradoxical stimulation), **antimuscarinic** fx (esp dry mouth; see p. 346, refer 'Side Effect Profiles' in 'Basic Psychopharmacology' chapter), GI upset, arrhythmias, $\downarrow$BP, skin and hypersensitivity reactions (inc bronchospasm, photosensitivity). If given iv can cause transient CNS stimulation.

Warn: driving may be impaired.

Interactions: can ↑phenytoin levels. ↑fx by alcohol. ↑risk serotonin syndrome. ☠ **MAOIs** can ⇒ ↑↑antimuscarinic fx (SPC says chlorphenamine CI if MAOI given within 2 wk but evidence unclear) ☠.

Dose: 4 mg 4–6 hrly po[1] (max 24 mg/24 h) ↓E; 10 mg iv over 1 min[2] (can ↑ to 20 mg, max 40 mg/24 h); 10–20 mg sc[3] (max 40 mg/24 h).

CHLORPROMAZINE/LARGACTIL

Phenothiazine ('typical') antipsychotic: dopamine antagonist (D_1 and $D_3 > D_2$ and D_4). Also blocks serotonin (5-HT_{2A}), histamine (H_1), adrenergic ($\alpha_1 > \alpha_2$) and muscarinic receptors, causing many SEs.

Use: schizophrenia, acute sedation (inc mania, severe anxiety, violent behaviour); intractable hiccups.

CI: CNS depression (inc coma), elderly patients with dementia, Hx of blood dyscrasias, **H**.

Caution: Parkinson's, drugs that ↑QTc, epilepsy, MG, phaeo, glaucoma (angle-closure), ↑prostate, severe respiratory disease, jaundice, blood disorders, predisposition to postural ↓BP, ↑ or ↓temperature. Avoid direct sunlight (⇒ photosensitivity), **L**.

SE: sedation, extrapyramidal **fx**, antimuscarinic **fx**, seizures, ↑Wt, ↓BP (esp postural), ECG Δs (↑QTc), arrhythmias, endocrine fx (menstrual Δs, galactorrhoea, gynaecomastia, sexual dysfunction), Δ LFTs/jaundice, blood disorders (inc agranulocytosis, ↓WCC), ↓ or ↑temperature (esp in elderly), rash/↑pigmentation, neuroleptic malignant syndrome. Do not crush tablets (contact hypersensitivity; also possible from iv solution).

Monitor: FBC, BP.

Interactions: may ↑sedation caused by alcohol and sedative medications. May ↑hypotension caused by other medications, fx ↑d by TCAs (esp antimuscarinic fx), lithium (esp extrapyramidal fx ± neurotoxicity), ritonavir, cimetidine and β-blockers (esp arrhythmias with sotalol; propranolol fx also ↑d by chlorpromazine). Avoid artemether/lumefantrine and drugs that ↑QTc or risk of ventricular arrhythmias (e.g. disopyramide, moxifloxacin).

Dose: 25–300 mg tds po[SPC/BNF]; 25–50 mg tds/qds im (painful, and may ⇒ ↓BP/↑HR). *NB:* ↓dose in elderly (approximately **1/3–1/2** adult dose but 10 mg od po may suffice) or if severe **RF.**

CHLOROQUINE

Antimalarial: inhibits protein synthesis and DNA/RNA polymerases.
Use: malaria Px[1] (only as Rx[2] if 'benign' spp (i.e. *P. ovale/vivax/ malariae*); *P. falciparum* often resistant. Rarely for RA, SLE.[BNF]
Caution: G6PD deficiency, severe GI disorders, can worsen psoriasis and MG, neurological disorders (esp epilepsy*), L (avoid other hepatotoxic drugs), R/P.
SE: GI upset, headache (mild, transient), **visual Δ** (rarely retinopathy**), **seizures***, hypersensitivity/skin reactions (inc pigment Δs), hair loss. Rarely **BM suppression**, cardiomyopathy. Arrhythmias common in OD.
Monitor: FBC, vision** (ophthalmology review if long-term Rx).
Interactions: absorption ↓ by antacids. ↑risk of arrhythmias with amiodarone and moxifloxacin. ↑risk of convulsions with mefloquine. ↑s levels of digoxin and ciclosporin. ↓s levels of praziquantel.
Dose: Px[1]: 310 mg once-wkly as base (*specify on prescription: do not confuse with* **salt** *doses*); start 1 wk before arrival, continue 4 wk after leaving. Used mostly in conjunction with other drugs, depending on local resistance patterns.[SPC/BNF] **Rx[2]:** see SPC/BNF. *NB:* ↓dose in RF.

CIMETIDINE

As ranitidine, but ↑↑interactions (↓**P450** and **W+**) and ↑gynaecomastia ∴ prescribed rarely.
Caution: P/B.
Dose: 400 mg bd (can ↑ to 4 hrly[SPC/BNF]). *NB:* ↓dose if LF or RF.

CIPROFLOXACIN

(Fluoro)quinolone antibiotic: inhibits DNA gyrase; 'cidal' with broad spectrum, but particularly good for Gram –ve infections.

Use: GI infections (esp salmonella, shigella, campylobacter), respiratory infections (non-pneumococcal pneumonias, esp *Pseudomonas*). Also GU infections (esp UTIs, acute uncomplicated cystitis in women, gonorrhoea), first-line initial Rx of anthrax.

CI: hypersensitivity to any quinolone, **P/B**.

Caution: seizures (inc Hx of, or predisposition to), MG (can worsen), ↑QTc (inc drugs that predispose to), G6PD deficiency, children/adolescents (theoretical risk of arthropathy), avoid ↑urine pH, DM or dehydration*, **R**.

SE: GI upset (esp N&D, sometimes AAC), pancreatitis, **neuro-Ψ fx** (esp confusion, seizures; also headache, dizziness, hallucinations, sleep and mood Δs), **tendinitis ± rupture** (esp if elderly or taking steroids), chest pain, oedema, **hypersensitivity** (rash, pruritus, fever). Rarely hepatotoxicity, RF/interstitial nephritis, crystalluria*, blood disorders, ↑glucose, skin reactions (inc photosensitivity**, SJS, TEN).

Warn: avoid UV light**, avoid ingesting Ca^{2+}-, Fe- and Zn-containing products (e.g. antacids***). May impair skilled tasks/driving.

Interactions: ↑s levels of theophyllines; NSAIDs ⇒ ↑risk of seizures; ↑s nephrotoxicity of ciclosporin; $FeSO_4$, Ca^{2+}-containing products, NB^{2+} and antacids*** ⇒ ↓po ciprofloxacin absorption (give 2 h before or 6 h after ciprofloxacin), drugs that ↑QTc, **W+**.

Dose: 250–750 mg bd po, 100–400 mg bd ivi (each dose over 1 h) according to indication[SPC/BNF] (250 mg bd po for 3 days for cystitis). *NB:* ↓dose if severe RF.

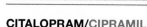 Stop if tendinitis, severe neuro-Ψ fx or hypersensitivity .

CITALOPRAM/CIPRAMIL

SSRI antidepressant.

Use: depression[1] (and panic disorder). Useful if polypharmacy, as ↓interactions and ↓cardio-/hepatotoxicity cf other SSRIs.

CI/Caution/SE/Warn: as fluoxetine, but risk of withdrawal syndrome if stopped abruptly. Can also ↑QTc (dose dependent); CI if ↑QTc (or congenital ↑QTc syndrome or taking other drugs that

can $\uparrow QT_c$) and caution if $\uparrow$risk torsades de pointes (e.g. congestive HF, recent MI, bradyarrhythmias, predisposition to $\downarrow K^+$ or $\downarrow Mg^{2+}$ dt concomitant illness or medicines), epilepsy, **P/B**.
Interaction: ☠ never give with, or <2 wk after, MAOIs ☠.
Dose: 20 mg od[1] $\uparrow$ing if necessary to max 40 mg (max 20 mg **if** elderly or **LF**).

CLARITHROMYCIN
Macrolide antibiotic: binds 50S ribosome.
Use: as erythromycin, part of triple therapy for *H. pylori*.
CI/Caution/SE/Interactions: as erythromycin, but $\Rightarrow$ $\downarrow$GI SEs.
Dose: 250–500 mg bd po or 500 mg bd iv. *NB:* $\downarrow$**dose if RF**.

CLEXANE see LMWH.

CLOBETASOL PROPIONATE 0.05% CREAM OR OINTMENT/DERMOVATE
Very-potent-strength topical corticosteroid.
Use: short-term Rx of severe inflammatory skin conditions (esp discoid lupus, lichen simplex and palmar plantar psoriasis).
CI: untreated infection including *H. zoster*, rosacea, acne.
SE: skin atrophy, worsening of infections, acne ($\uparrow$SEs cf less potent topical steroids).
Dose: apply thinly od/bd up to 4 wk, usually specialist supervision.

CLOBETASONE BUTYRATE 0.05% CREAM OR OINTMENT/EUMOVATE
Moderately potent-strength topical corticosteroid.
Use: inflammatory skin conditions, esp eczema, dermatitis.
CI: untreated infection, rosacea, acne.
SE: skin atrophy, worsening of infections, acne.
Dose: apply thinly od/bd.

L/R/H = Liver, Renal and Heart failure. E = elderly. P = pregnancy. B = breastfeeding.

CLOMIPRAMINE

TCA; blocks reuptake of 5-HT and NA, ↑extracellular concentrations in synaptic cleft, ↑serotonergic and noradrenergic neurotransmission.

Use: depression[1], phobic and obsessional states[2], adjunctive treatment of cataplexy with narcolepsy[3].

CI: mania, porphyria, arrhythmia, post-MI.

Caution: chronic constipation, DM, epilepsy, Hx of bipolar disorder/psychosis, hyperthyroidism, ↑intraocular pressure, significant risk of suicide, phaeo, prostatic hypertrophy, angle-closure glaucoma, urinary retention, cardiovascular disease H.

SE: antimuscarinic fx, cardiac fx (arrhythmias, HB, HR, postural ↓BP, dizziness, syncope: **dangerous in OD**), ↑Wt, **sedation** (often ⇒ 'hangover'), seizures, GI upset, breast enlargement, paraesthesia, sexual dysfunction. Rarely blood disorders, hypersensitivity, Δ LFTs, ↓Na+ (esp in elderly), agitation, hallucination, Δ mood, confusion, NMS, abnormal muscle tone.

Warn: withdrawal effects may occur within 5 days of stopping treatment, worse after regular administration for 8 wk+. ↓dose gradually over 4 wk+. ↑effects of alcohol.

Interactions: metab by P450; ☠↑risk of serotonin syndrome with MAOI, e.g. isocarboxazid, moclobemide, phenelzine, selegiline, tranylcypromine (avoid with/for 14 days after stopping MAOI); Δ cardiac conduction with antiarrhythmic agents; hypokalaemia and ↑risk of QT prolongation and torsades de pointes with diuretics.

Dose: initially 10 mg po od at bedtime, ↑gradually/alternatively to 30–150 mg od in divided doses, max 250 mg od[1]; initially 25 mg po od, ↑gradually to 100–150 mg od over 2 wk, max 250 mg od[2]; start at 10 mg po od, ↑gradually to 10–75 mg od[3].

☠ Overdose of TCA causes dry mouth, coma, hypotension, hypothermia, hyperreflexia, extensor plantar responses, convulsions, respiratory failure, cardiac conduction defects and arrhythmias. Dilated pupils and urinary retention also occur. ☠

CLONAZEPAM

Medium-acting benzodiazepine: $GABA_A$-receptor positive allosteric modulator.

Use: panic disorders (+/− agoraphobia) resistant to antidepressants/other anxiety disorders (unlicensed use)[1], epilepsy[2].

CI: coma, current alcohol/drug abuse, respiratory depression.

Caution: porphyrias, airway obstruction, brain damage, cerebellar ataxia, depression, spinal ataxia, suicidal ideation.

SE: alopecia, ↓concentration, ↓coordination, ↑risk of fall, ↑risk of fracture, ↓muscle tone, nystagmus, seizures, sexual dysfunction, skin reactions, speech impairment.

Warn: avoid in pregnancy (risk of neonatal withdrawal symptoms) and breastfeeding (present in milk).

Interactions: metab by P450; ↓levels of carbamazepine; ↓metabolism with ketoconazole; ↑levels of primidone, phenobarbital; Δ concentration of phenytoin.

Dose: 1–2 mg po od[1], initially 1 mg po od for 4 nights, ↑over 2–4 wk, usual dose 4–8 mg od at night, given in three to four divided doses if necessary[2].

> Overdose causes drowsiness, ataxia, dysarthria, nystagmus, respiratory depression and coma; can precipitate coma in hepatic impairment.
>
> Do not confuse with clobazam when prescribing.

CLONIDINE HYDROCHLORIDE

α_2-adrenergic receptor agonist ⇒ ↓noradrenaline release.

Use: Tourette syndrome and sedation (unlicensed)[1], HTN[2], Px of migraine/menopausal Sx[3].

CI: severe slow dysrhythmia due to second/third degree HB/SSS P/B.

Caution: depression Hx, constipation, mild-to-moderate slow dysrhythmia, neuropathy, peripheral vascular disease (inc Raynaud's), cerebrovascular disease, H.

SE: sedation, postural ↓BP, dizziness, dry mouth, depression, headache, GI upset (N, V, C), sexual dysfunction.

Monitor: ECG advised.

Interactions: ↓antihypertensive fx with amitriptyline, clomipramine, dosulepin, doxepin, imipramine, lofepramine, nortriptyline.

Dose: initially 25–50 microgram po od in divided doses, ↑ by 25 microgram per wk, usual dose 3–5 microgram/kg/day[1]; initially 50–100 microgram po tds, ↑dose every second/third day, max 1.2 mg od[2]; initially 50 microgram po bd for 2 wk, ↑ to 75 microgram bd[3].

In hypertension, must be withdrawn gradually to avoid severe rebound hypertension.

CLOPIDOGREL/PLAVIX

Antiplatelet agent: ADP receptor antagonist. ↑antiplatelet fx cf aspirin (but also ↑SEs).

Use: Px of atherothrombotic events if STEMI or NSTEMI (for 12 months in combination with aspirin, aspirin continued indefinitely), MI (within 'a few' to 35 days), ischaemic CVA (within 7 days to 6 months) or peripheral arterial disease. For use in ACS (see p. 404, refer 'Acute Coronary Syndromes' in 'Emergencies' chapter).

CI: active bleeding, **L** (if severe – otherwise caution), **P/B**.

Caution: ↑bleeding risk; trauma, surgery, drugs that ↑bleeding risk (*avoid with* warfarin), ↓fx by omeprazole, esomeprazole, **R**.

SE: haemorrhage (esp GI or intracranial), GI upset, PU, pancreatitis, headache, fatigue, dizziness, paraesthesia, rash/pruritus, hepatobiliary/respiratory/blood disorders (↓NØ, ↑EØ, very rarely, TTP).

Monitor: for signs of occult bleeding (esp after invasive procedures); FBC if suspected bleeding.

Dose: 75 mg od. If not already on clopidogrel, usually load with 300 mg for ACS, then 75 mg od starting next day. If pre-PCI, load with 300–600 mg usually on morning of procedure.

Stop 7 days before operations if antiplatelet fx not wanted (e.g. major surgery); discuss with surgeons doing operation.

CLOTRIMAZOLE/CANESTEN

Imidazole antifungal (topical).

Use: external candida infections (esp vaginal thrush).

Caution: can damage condoms and diaphragms.

Dose: two to three applications/day of 1% cream, continuing for 14 days after lesion healed. Also available as solution/spray for hairy areas, as pessary, and in 2% strength. See more.[BNF/SPC]

CLOZAPINE/CLOZARIL, ZAPONEX, DENZAPINE

Atypical antipsychotic: blocks dopamine ($D_4 > D_1 > D_2$ and D_3) and 5-HT$_{2A}$ receptors. Potent antagonist at α-adrenergic, histaminergic and muscarinic receptors.

Use: schizophrenia[1], if resistant or intolerant (e.g. severe extrapyramidal fx) to other antipsychotics, psychosis in Parkinson's[2].

CI: severe cardiac disorders (inc Hx of circulatory collapse, myocarditis, cardiomyopathy), coma/severe CNS depression, alcoholic/toxic psychosis, drug intoxication, Hx of agranulocytosis or ↓NØ, bone marrow disorders, paralytic ileus, uncontrolled epilepsy, **R/H** (if severe, otherwise caution), **L** (inc active liver disease), **B**.

Caution: Hx of epilepsy, cardiovascular disease, ↑prostate, glaucoma (angle-closure), **P/E**.

SE: ↑**salivation** (Rx with hyoscine hydrobromide), ↓BP and ↑HR (esp during initial titration), **constipation** (can ⇒ ileus/obstruction: have low threshold for giving laxatives), ↑Wt, sedation, ↓NØ* (3% of patients) and ☠ **agranulocytosis** ☠ (1%). Less commonly seizures, urinary incontinence, erectile dysfunction, **myocarditis/cardiomyopathy** (*stop immediately!*), hyperglycaemia, infections, **pneumonia** (*reduce dose/hold clozapine*), N&V, GORD, ↑BP, delirium, RF, ↓Pt. Rarely arrhythmias, hepatic dysfunction (*stop immediately!*), ↑TG, neuroleptic malignant syndrome, priapism.

Warn: to report symptoms of infection, e.g. fever, sore throat; to report changes in bowel habits, smoking habits; lifestyle advice to reduce risk of diabetes and CV disorders.

Monitor: FBC*, BP (esp during start of Rx), cardiac function (get baseline ECG/watch for persistent ↑HR).

Interactions: care with all drugs that constipate, sedate, cause hypotension, ↑QT interval or ↓leucopoiesis (e.g. cytotoxics, sulphonamides/co-trimoxazole, chloramphenicol, penicillamine, carbamazepine, phenothiazines, esp depots). **metab by P450**: Caffeine, risperidone, fluoxetine, fluvoxamine, ciprofloxacin, ritonavir, OCP, cimetidine and erythromycin ↑clozapine levels. Smoking, carbamazepine, rifampicin and phenytoin ↓clozapine levels.

Dose: initially 12.5 mg nocte, ↑ing to 200–450 mg/day[SPC/BNF] usually given bd (max 900 mg/day); slower dose titration if >60 years.[1] 12.5 mg nocte, inc in steps of 12.5 mg up to twice wkly according to response, max 50 mg daily; in exceptional circumstances, inc by 12.5 mg wkly to max 100 mg od in one to two divided doses[2].

If >2 days' doses missed, re-titration necessary. Get specialist advice.

Monitoring of WBC, NØ and PLT is done by the manufacturers: in the United Kingdom, **Clozaril** Patient Monitoring Service (tel: 0845 7698269), **Denzapine** Monitoring Service (tel: 0333 2004141) or **Zaponex** Treatment Access System (tel: 0207 3655842). Register and then authorise/monitor baseline and subsequent FBCs*. *These are very useful resources for all clozapine questions.* Report any missed doses.***

CO-AMOXICLAV/AUGMENTIN

Combination of amoxicill in + clavulanic acid (β-lactamase inhibitor) to overcome resistance.

Use: UTIs, respiratory/skin/soft-tissue (plus many other) infections. Reserve for when β-lactamase-producing strains known/strongly suspected or other Rx has failed.

CI/Caution/SE/Interactions: as ampicillin, plus caution if anticoagulated, L (↑risk of cholestasis), P.

Dose: amoxicillin 250 mg/clavulanic acid 125 mg tds po
(500 mg/125 mg tds po if severe); 1.2 g (expressed as co-amoxiclav)
tds/qds iv/ivi.

CO-BENELDOPA/MADOPAR

L-Dopa + benserazide (peripheral DOPA-decarboxylase inhibitor).
Use: parkinsonism.
CI/Caution/SE/Warn/Interactions: see Levodopa.
Dose: (*expressed as levodopa only*) initially 50 mg tds/qds, ↑ing
total dose and number of doses, according to response, to usual
maintenance of 400–800 mg/day (↓ in elderly).[BNF/SPC] Available in
dispersible form. If switching from MR levodopa to dispersible
co-beneldopa, reduce dose by 30%.

CO-CARELDOPA/SINEMET

L-Dopa + carbidopa (peripheral dopa-decarboxylase inhibitor).
Use: parkinsonism.
CI/Caution/SE/Warn/Interactions: see Levodopa.
Dose: (*expressed as levodopa only*) initially 100 mg tds, ↑ing
total dose and number of doses, according to response, to usual
maintenance of 400–800 mg/day (↓ in elderly).[BNF/SPC] Gel for enteral
tube.

CO-CODAMOL (30/500): = codeine 30 mg + paracetamol
500 mg per tablet.
Use/CI/Caution/SE/Interactions: see Paracetamol and Codeine.
Warning: prescribe by dose, as also available as 8/500 and 15/500.
Dose: 2 tablets qds prn. *NB:* ↓dose if LF, RF or elderly.

CODEINE (PHOSPHATE)

Weak opiate analgesic. Mainly metabolised to morphine.
Use: mild/moderate pain, diarrhoea, antitussive.
CI: acute respiratory depression, risk of ileus, ↑ICP/head injury/
coma.
Caution: all other conditions where morphine is either
contraindicated or cautioned.

L/R/H = Liver, Renal and Heart failure. E = elderly. P = pregnancy. B = breastfeeding.

SE: as morphine, but milder. **Constipation** is the major problem: dose and length of Rx-dependent; anticipate this and give laxative Px as appropriate, esp in elderly. Also sedation, esp if LF.

Interactions: as morphine, ☠ **MAOIs: do not give within 2 wk of ☠.**

Dose: 30–60 mg up to 4-hrly po/im (max 240 mg/24 h). Geneticultrarapid metabolisers (3% of Europeans, 8% of Americans, 40% of North Africans) risk serious toxicity, and poor metabolisers obtain little analgesia. Watch closely when initiating and adjust dose/change drug accordingly. *NB:* ↓dose if LF, RF or elderly.

CO-DYDRAMOL

Dihydrocodeine 10/20/30 mg + paracetamol 500 mg per tablet (10/500, 20/500, 30/500).

Dose: one to two tablets 4–6 hrly, max qds po. Usually prescribed 2 tablets qds (prn). *NB:* ↓dose if LF, RF or elderly.

CO-MAGALDROX antacid: (AlOH + MgOH)

Dose: 10–20 mL, 20–60 min after meals, and at bedtime or prn.

COMBIVENT Compound bronchodilator (salbutamol + ipratropium bromide).

Dose: 2.5 mL (one vial: ipratropium 500 micrograms + salbutamol 2.5 mg) tds/qds neb.[SPC/BNF]

CO-TRIMOXAZOLE/SEPTRIN

Antibiotic combination preparation: 5-to-1 mixture of sulphamethoxazole (a sulphonamide) + trimethoprim ⇒ synergistic action.

Use: PCP; other uses limited dt SEs (also rarely used for toxoplasmosis and nocardiosis).

CI: porphyria, **L/R** (if either severe, otherwise caution).

Caution: blood disorders, asthma, G6PD deficiency, risk factors for ↓folate and hyperkalaemia, **P/B/E**.

SE: skin reactions (inc SJS, TEN), **blood disorders** (↓NØ, ↓Pt, ↓glucose, BM suppression, agranulocytosis) relatively common, esp in elderly. Also N&V&D (inc AAC), ↑K+, nephrotoxicity, hepatotoxicity, hypersensitivity, anorexia, abdo pain, glossitis, stomatitis, pancreatitis, arthralgia, myalgia, SLE, pulmonary infiltrates, seizures, ataxia, myocarditis.

Interactions: ↑s phenytoin levels. ↑s risk of arrhythmias with amiodarone, crystalluria with methenamine, antifolate fx with pyrimethamine, agranulocytosis with clozapine and toxicity with ciclosporin, azathioprine, mercaptopurine and methotrexate. **W+**.

Dose: PCP Rx: 120 mg/kg/day po/ivi in two to four divided doses (PCP Px 480–960 mg od po). PCP Px.[BNF/SPC] *NB:* ↓**dose if RF.**

🔅 Stop immediately if rash or blood disorder occurs 🔅

CYCLIZINE
Antihistamine antiemetic.

Use: N&V Rx/Px (esp 2° to iv/im opioids, but not first choice in angina/MI/LVF*), vertigo, motion sickness, labyrinthine disorders.

CI/Caution/SE/Warn: as chlorphenamine, but also avoid in severe HF* (may undo haemodynamic benefits of opioids). Antimuscarinic fx (see p. 346, refer 'Cholinoceptors' in 'Side Effect Profiles' in 'Basic Psychopharmacology' chapter) are most prominent SEs.

Dose: 50 mg po/im/iv tds.

CYPROHEPTADINE HYDROCHLORIDE
Potent histamine H_1-receptor and 5-HT_2-receptor antagonist; competes with serotonin and histamine for receptor binding.

Use: allergy[1], adjunct in treatment of moderate serotonin syndrome (unlicensed)[2].

CI: porphyria, **L**.

Caution: ↑prostate/urinary retention, obstruction at pyloric junction, ↑risk of angle-closure glaucoma, seizures.

SE: drowsiness, insomnia, dizziness, **antimuscarinic fx** (see p. 346, refer 'Cholinoceptors' in 'Side Effect Profiles' in 'Basic Psychopharmacology' chapter), ataxia, GI upset, ↑Wt, paraesthesia, hyperhidrosis, Ψ fx (agitation, hallucination), cytopoenias, hypersensitivity reactions (inc bronchospasm, photosensitivity), arrhythmias, epistaxis, hepatic disorders, ↓BP, labyrinthitis, irregular menstruation, oedema, seizure, tinnitus, tremor.
Warn: ↑sedation with alcohol.
Interactions: ↓fx of citalopram, dapoxetine, escitalopram, fluoxetine, fluvoxamine, metyrapone, paroxetine, sertraline, and other antidepressants (opposes action); ↓absorption of levodopa.
Dose: 4 mg po tds, usual dose 4–20 mg od, max 32 mg od[1]; 12 mg po as a single dose, repeated once if necessary, for longer-acting serotonergic agents (e.g. fluoxetine) regular lower doses (e.g. 4 mg tds) should be used (BMJ Best Practice)[2].

DABIGATRAN (ETEXILATE)/PRADAXA

Oral anticoagulant; direct thrombin inhibitor. Rapid onset and does not require therapeutic monitoring (unlike warfarin).
Use: Px of VTE (after THR/TKR)[1]; Rx of DVT or PE and Px of recurrent DVT or recurrent PE[2]; non-valve AF embolism Px[3].BNF
CI: active bleeding, impaired haemostasis, L (if severe), P/B.
Caution: bleeding disorders, active GI ulceration, recent surgery, bacterial endocarditis, anaesthesia with post-operative indwelling epidural catheter (risk of paralysis; give initial dose ≥2 h after catheter removal and monitor for neurological signs), Wt <50 kg, R (avoid if creatinine clearance <30 mL/min), H/E.
SE: **haemorrhage**, hepatobiliary disorders.
Monitor: for ↓Hb or signs of bleeding (stop drug if severe). Assess RF before initiating Rx and annually for patients and elderly with renal failure.

Interactions: P-gp inducers and inhibitors[SPC/BNF] **NSAIDs** ↑risk of bleeding. Levels ↑ by amiodarone*.

Dose: 110 mg (75 mg if >75 years old) 1–4 h after surgery, then 220 mg od (150 mg if >75 years old) for 10 days, to be taken from first day after knee replacement or 28–35 days from first day after hip replacement[1]; 150 mg po bd after at least 5 days parenteral anticoagulant[2] (>74 years old see BNF for dose); 150 mg po bd[3]. *NB:* ↓**dose in RF, elderly or if taking amiodarone or verapamil.***

DANTROLENE SODIUM

Postsynaptic muscle relaxant; ↓excitation-contraction coupling in skeletal muscle by binding to ryanodine receptor, ↓intracellular calcium concentration.

Use: chronic severe spasticity of voluntary muscle (malignant hyperthermia by rapid iv injection).

CI: acute muscle spasm.

Caution: ↑risk of hepatotoxicity if female, age >30 or daily dose >400 mg. H/P/B.

SE: ↓appetite, Ψ fx (depression, anxiety), ↓sleep, seizure, visual disturbance, pericarditis, pleural effusion with ↑eosinophils, resp depression, GI upset (N, V, abdo pain), hepatotoxicity, rash, fever.

Warn: may cause severe liver damage, discontinue if no response within 6–8 wk.

Monitor: LFTs at initiation and regularly during Rx.

Interactions: ↑neuromuscular blockade with vecuronium bromide; ↑sedation with CNS depressants; ↑muscle weakness with benzodiazepines; hepatoxicity with combined oral contraceptive pill (COCP) and hormone replacement therapy in females.

Dose: initially 25 mg po od, ↑dose at wkly intervals; usual dose 75 mg tds od, max 100 mg qds od.

DAPAGLIFLOZIN/FORXIGA

Antidiabetic (reversible sodium glucose cotransporter 2 [SGLT2] inhibitor): ↓renal reabsorption of glucose and ↑urinary excretion of excess glucose.

Use: type 2 DM – reserved for combination therapy when other treatment options have failed. Combined with metformin or a sulphonylurea, or both, or with pioglitazone, or with both metformin and pioglitazone, in patients who have not achieved adequate glycaemic control with these drugs alone or in combination.

CI: ketoacidosis, P/B.

Caution: risk factors for DKA (including ↓β-cell reserve, conditions leading to restricted food intake or severe dehydration, sudden ↓ in insulin, ↑insulin requirements due to acute illness, surgery or alcohol abuse); cardiovascular disease (risk of ↓BP); E (risk of ↓BP); electrolyte disturbances; ↓BP; ↑Hct. Correct hypovolaemia before starting Rx. L/R.

SE: GI upset, back pain, dizziness, dyslipidaemia, hypoglycaemia (in combination with insulin or sulphonylurea), ↑risk of infection, rash, urinary disorders, thirst hypovolaemia, RF, balanitis, genital pruritus, ↓Wt. Rarely DKA.

Dose: 10 mg od. Dose of concomitant sulfonylurea or insulin may need to be ↓d. ↓dose and caution in severe LF – ↑exposure risk. Not recommended if >75 yrs old.

> ☠ DKA on SGLT2 inhibitors may be atypical with only moderately ↑blood glucose. Warn patients of risk factors and signs and symptoms of DKA. Advise patients to seek immediate medical advice if they develop any. Test for ↑ketones if signs or symptoms of DKA, even if plasma glucose near normal. Stop SGLT2 inhibitor Rx if DKA is suspected or diagnosed. Do not restart Rx with any SGLT2 inhibitor in patients with DKA during use, unless another cause for DKA is identified and resolved. Interrupt SGLT2 inhibitor treatment in patients in hospital for major surgery or acute, serious illness. Rx may be restarted once condition stabilised ☠.

DERMOVATE see Clobetasol propionate (steroid) cream 0.05%.

DESFERRIOXAMINE

Chelating agent; binds Fe (and Al) in gut ↓ing absorption/↑ing clearance.

Use: ↑Fe: acute (OD/poisoning[1]), chronic (e.g. xs transfusions for blood disorders, haemochromatosis when venesection CI). Also for ↑Al (e.g. 2° to dialysis).

CI: **P** (first trimester).

Caution: Al-induced encephalopathy (may worsen), ↑risk of *Yersinia*/mucormycosis infection **R/P/B**.

SE: ↓BP (related to rate of ivi), lens opacities, retinopathy, GI upset, blood disorders, hypersensitivity. Also neurological/respiratory/renal dysfunction. ↑doses can ⇒ ↓growth and bone Δs.

Monitor: vision and hearing during chronic **Rx**.

Dose: sc infusion or iv/im if issues with sc: acutely up to 15 mg/kg/h ivi (max 80 mg/kg/day)[1]. Otherwise according to degree of Fe or Al overload.[SPC/BNF]

▼ DEXAMFETAMINE SULPHATE (= DEXAMFETAMINE)

CNS stimulant; stimulates release of DA > NA and 5-HT from pre-synaptic nerve terminals.

Use: refractory ADHD (unlicensed use in adults)[1] if response to lisdexamfetamine but cannot tolerate prolonged fx[NICE], narcolepsy[2].

CI: agitation, cardiac/vascular disorders, Hx of alcohol/drug misuse, ↑thyroid, moderate-to-severe HTN, **H/P/B**.

Caution: some Ψ disorders (psychosis, BPAD, anorexia), seizures, mild HTN, tics, ↑risk of angle-closure glaucoma.

SE: ↓appetite, ↓Wt, ↓sleep, agitation, **cardiac fx** (↑HR, ↑BP, arrhythmia), GI upset, dry mouth, arthralgia, dizziness, headache.

Monitor: aggression early in Rx (↓dose or stop); pulse, BP, Wt, Ht at start of Rx, after dose Δ and at intervals ≤6 months.

Interactions: ☠ ↑risk of hypertensive crisis with isocarboxazid, phenelzine, tranylcypromine, moclobemide, rasagiline, safinamide, selegiline (avoid with/for 14 days after stopping MAOI) ☠; ↓fx of

apraclonidine, guanethidine; ↑level with fluoxetine, paroxetine, ritonavir, tipranavir; ↑risk of SE with atomoxetine, nabilone.
Dose: initially 5 mg po bd, ↑dose at wkly intervals, maintenance dose given in two to four divided doses, max 60 mg od[1]; initially 10 mg po od in divided doses, ↑ in steps of 10 mg every wk, maintenance dose given in two to four divided doses, max 60 mg od[2].

> Overdose causes wakefulness, excessive activity, paranoia, hallucinations, hypertension followed by exhaustion, convulsions, hyperthermia and coma.

DIAMORPHINE (HEROIN HYDROCHLORIDE)
Strong opiate (1.5× strength of morphine if both given iv).
Use: severe pain (acute and chronic)[1], AMI[2], acute LVF[3].
CI/Caution/SE/Interactions: as morphine, but less nausea/↓BP and does not interact with baclofen, gabapentin and ritonavir.
Respiratory depression (esp elderly).
Dose: 5–10 mg sc/im (or 1/4–1/2 this dose iv) up to 4 hrly[1]; 5 mg iv (at 1 mg/min) followed by further 2.5–5 mg if necessary[2]; 2.5–5 mg iv (at 1 mg/min)[3]. Can give via sc pump in chronic pain/palliative care. *NB:* ↓**dose if elderly, LF or RF.**[BNF/SPC]

DIAZEMULS iv diazepam emulsion: ⇒ ↓venous irritation.

DIAZEPAM
Long-acting benzodiazepine: GABA$_A$-receptor positive allosteric modulator.
Use: seizures (esp status epilepticus[1], febrile convulsions), *short-term* Rx of acute alcohol withdrawal[2], anxiety[3], insomnia[4] (if also anxiety; if not, then shorter-acting forms preferred, as ⇒ ↓hangover sedation). Also used for muscle spasm[5].
CI: respiratory depression, marked neuromuscular respiratory weakness inc unstable myasthenia gravis, sleep apnoea, acute pulmonary insufficiency, chronic psychosis, depression (do not give diazepam alone), L (if severe).

Caution: respiratory disease, muscle weakness (inc MG), Hx of drug/alcohol abuse, personality disorder, porphyria, L/R/P/B/E.

SE: respiratory depression (rarely apnoea), drowsiness, dependence. Also ataxia, amnesia, headache, vertigo, GI upset, jaundice, ↓BP, ↓HR, visual/libido/urinary disturbances, blood disorders, paradoxical disinhibition in Ψ disorder.

Warn: sedation ↑ by alcohol. Do not stop suddenly, as can ⇒ withdrawal.

Interactions: metab by P450 ∴ many: ery-/clari-/telithromycin, quinu-/dalfopristin and flu-/itra-/keto-/posaconazole can ↑levels. Sedative fx ↑ by antipsychotics, antidepressants, antiepileptics and antiretrovirals. Can ↑fx of zidovudine and sodium oxybate. ↑risk of ↓HR/BP and respiratory depression with im olanzapine.

Dose: 10 mg iv, then 10 mg after 10 min if required, at rate of 1 mL (5 mg)/min for status epilepticus[1]; 10 mg im, then 10 mg after at least 4 h if required for acute alcohol withdrawal[2]; 2 mg tds po (↑ up to 30 mg/day)[3,5]; 5–15 mg nocte po[4]. *NB:* ↓dose if elderly, LF or RF. If chronic exposure to benzodiazepines, ↑doses may be needed; do not stop suddenly, as can ⇒ withdrawal – taper cautiously, speed depending on duration of use and indication. If giving IV, use Diazemuls, an emulsion, to avoid venous irritation.

> ☠ **Respiratory depression:** if ↑doses used (esp iv/im), monitor O_2 sats and have O_2 (± intubation equipment) at hand, caution with flumazenil – see p. 382, refer 'Benzodiazepine Overdose' in 'Drug Toxicity Syndromes' in 'Emergencies' chapter ☠.

DICLOFENAC

Medium-strength NSAID; non-selective COX inhibitor.

Use: pain/inflammation, esp musculoskeletal; RA, osteoarthritis, acute gout, migraine, post-op and dental pain.

CI/Caution/SE/Interactions: as ibuprofen, but ↑risk of PU/GI bleeds and thrombotic events (↓risk of PU/GI bleeds if given with misoprostol as Arthrotec). Avoid in IHD, CVD, CCF, peripheral artery disease, acute porphyria. Ciclosporin ⇒ ↑serum levels.

No known interaction with baclofen. Mild **W+**.

Dose: 25–50 mg tds po or 75 mg bd po (or im, but for max of 2 days); 75–150 mg/day pr (**divided doses**). Rarely used iv.[BNF/SPC] MR and top preparations available.[BNF/SPC] *NB:* **avoid/↓dose in RF and consider gastroprotective Rx**.

DIFFLAM Benzydamine: topical NSAID for painful inflammatory conditions of oropharynx (e.g. mouth ulcers, radio-/chemotherapy-induced mucositis). Available as spray (4–8 sprays 1.5–3 hrly) or oral rinse (15 mL, 1.5–3 hrly, diluting in 15 mL water if stinging). Rarely ⇒ hypersensitivity reactions.

DIGIFAB Antidigoxin Ab for digoxin toxicity/OD unresponsive to supportive Rx. See SPC for dose.

DIGOXIN

Cardiac glycoside: ↓s HR by slowing AVN conduction and ↑ing vagal tone. Also weak inotrope.

Use: AF (and other SVTs), HF.

CI: HB (intermittent complete), second-degree AV block, VF, VT, HOCM (can use with care if also AF and HF), SVTs 2° to WPW.

Caution: recent MI, ↓K+*/↓T_4 (both ⇒ ↑digoxin sensitivity*), SSS, rhythms resembling AF (e.g. atrial tachycardia with variable AV block), R/E (↓dose), P.

SE: generally mild unless rapid ivi, xs Rx or OD: GI upset (esp nausea), **arrhythmias/HB**, neuro-Ψ disturbances (inc visual Δs, esp blurred vision and yellow/green halos), fatigue, weakness, confusion, hallucinations, mood Δs. Also gynaecomastia (if chronic Rx), rarely ↓Pt, rash, ↑EØ. See DigiFab for treating serious toxicity.

Monitor: U&Es, digoxin levels (take blood at least 6 h post-dose: therapeutic range = 1–2 micrograms/L).

Interactions: digoxin fx/toxicity ↑d by Ca^{2+} antagonists (esp verapamil), amiodarone, propafenone, quinidine, antimalarials, itraconazole, amphotericin, ciclosporin, St John's wort and diuretics (mostly via ↓K+*), but also ACE-i/ARBs and spironolactone (despite potential ↑K+). Cholestyramine and antacids can ↓digoxin absorption.

Dose: *non-acute AF/SVTs:* load with 125–250 micrograms bd po (maintenance dose 62.5–250 micrograms od). For HF: 62.5–125 micrograms od. *NB:* ↓**dose if RF, elderly or digoxin given <2 wk ago.**

Digoxin loading for acute AF/SVTs: *either* 750 micrograms–1 mg as ivi over 2 h *or* 500 micrograms po repeated 12 h later. Then follow non-acute schedule.

DIHYDROCODEINE see Codeine: similar-strength opioid.
Dose: 30 mg 4–6 hrly po (or up to 50 mg 4–6 hrly im/sc) with or after food. Maximum 240 mg in 24 h. ↑doses can be given under close supervision. ↓**dose if RF.**

DILATING EYE DROPS (for funduscopy). Generally safe but rarely ⇒ angle-closure glaucoma (suspect if develops red painful eye with ↓vision and nausea; *ophthalmic emergency*). Dilation blurs vision. Driving unsafe for at least 4 h when both eyes dilated. Apply one drop and allow 15 min for effect.

1 **Tropicamide 1%:** Most common; CI in children <1 year old (use 0.5%)
2 **Phenylephrine 2.5% or 10%:** Frequently used in combination with tropicamide. 2.5% most common. 10% ↑s systemic SEs. CI if cardiac disease, HTN, ↑HR, aneurysms, ↑T_4

Consider cycloplegic forms (e.g. cyclopentolate 1%) for refraction in children or if analgesia required, e.g. corneal abrasions and uveitis (↓s ciliary spasm).

DILTIAZEM
Rate-limiting benzothiazepine Ca^{2+} channel blocker: ↓s HR and contractility* (but < verapamil) and ↓s BP. Also dilates peripheral/coronary arteries.
Use: Rx/Px of angina[1] (esp if β-blockers CI) and HTN[2].
CI: LVF* with pulmonary congestion, ↓↓HR, second/third-degree AV block (without pacemaker), SSS, acute porphyria **P/B**.

Caution: first-degree AV block, ↓HR, ↑PR interval, L/R/H.

SE: headache, flushing, GI upset (esp N&C), oedema (esp ankle), ↓HR, ↓BP, gum hyperplasia. Rarely SAN/AVN block, arrhythmias, rash, hepatotoxicity, gynaecomastia.

Interactions: β-blockers and verapamil (can ⇒ asystole, AV block, ↓↓HR, HF). ↑s fx of digoxin, ciclosporin, theophyllines, carbamazepine and phenytoin. ☠ ↑risk of VF with iv dantrolene ☠.

Dose: 60 mg tds (↑ing to max of 360 mg/day)[1]; 180–480 mg/day in one or two doses[2] (suitable for HTN only as MR preparation: no non-proprietary forms exist and brands vary in clinical fx ∴ specify which is required[SPC/BNF]). *NB:* consider ↓ing doses if LF or RF.

DIPROBASE Paraffin-based emollient cream/ointment for dry skin conditions (e.g. eczema, psoriasis).

DISODIUM ETIDRONATE see Pamidronate.

DISODIUM PAMIDRONATE see Pamidronate.

DISULFIRAM/ANTABUSE

Alcohol dehydrogenase inhibitor: ⇒ ↑systemic acetaldehyde ⇒ unpleasant SE when alcohol ingested (inc small amounts ∴ care with alcohol-containing medications, foods, toiletries).

Use: maintenance of abstinence in alcohol dependence.

CI: Hx of IHD or CVA, HTN, psychosis, ↑suicide risk, severe personality disorder, H/P/B.

Caution: DM, epilepsy, respiratory disease, L/R.

SE: only if alcohol ingested – N&V, flushing, headache, ↑HR, ↓BP (± collapse if xs alcohol intake).

Interactions: ↑s fx of phenytoin, ↑toxicity with paraldehyde, W+.

Dose: initially 200 mg od, ↑dose if needed: max 500 mg po od. Review patient on Rx every 2 wk for first 2 months, then monthly for next 4 months and then 6 monthly thereafter.

NB: must have consumed no alcohol within at least 24 h of first dose. Prescribe under specialist supervision.

DOCUSATE SODIUM

Stimulant laxative: $\Rightarrow$ ↑GI motility (also a softening agent).
Use/Caution/SE: see Senna (CI if GI obstruction).
Dose: 50–100 mg up to tds po (max 500 mg/day). Also available as enemas.[SPC/BNF]

▼ DOMPERIDONE

Antiemetic: D_2 antagonist – inhibits central nausea chemoreceptor trigger zone. Poor blood-brain barrier penetration ∴ ↓central SEs (extrapyramidal fx, sedation) cf other dopamine antagonists.
Use: N&V, esp 2° to chemotherapy, and in Parkinson's disease or migraine, **H**.
CI: prolactinoma, cardiac disease (inc conditions where cardiac conduction is, or could be, impaired), GI obstruction, drugs that ↓CYP3A4 or ↑QTc, **H/L**.
Caution: GI obstruction, **R/P/B/E**.
SE: ↑QTc, rash, allergy, ↑prolactin (can $\Rightarrow$ gynaecomastia, galactorrhoea and hyperprolactinoma). Rarely ↓libido, dystonia and extrapyramidal fx.
Dose: 10 mg tds po, not available im/iv. *NB:* ↓**dose if RF**.

DONEPEZIL/ARICEPT

Acetylcholinesterase inhibitor (reversible).
Use: mild to moderately severe dementia in Alzheimer's disease.
CI: **P/B**.
Caution: supraventricular conduction dfx (esp SSS), ↑risk of PU (e.g. Hx of PU or NSAID), COPD/asthma, **L**.
Class SE: cholinergic fx, GI upset (esp initially), **insomnia** (if occurs, change dose to mane), **headache**, fatigue, dizziness, syncope, rash, Ψ disturbances. Rarely ↓ or ↑BP, seizures, PU/GI bleeds, SAN/AVN block, hepatotoxicity, extrapyramidal symptoms can worsen.

Interactions: metab by P450 ∴ inhibitors and inducers could ↑ or ↓levels, respectively.
Dose: 5 mg nocte (↑ to 10 mg after 1 month if necessary); specialist use only – need review for clinical response and tolerance.

DORZOLAMIDE/TRUSOPT

Topical carbonic anhydrase inhibitor: as acetazolamide (oral preparation, which is more potent but has ↑SEs*).
Use: glaucoma (esp if β-blocker or PG analogue CI or fails to ↓OP).
CI: ↑Cl⁻ acidosis, **R** (severe only), **P/B**.
Caution: Hx of renal stones†, **L**.
SE: local irritation and allergic reactions, blurred vision, bitter taste, rash. Rarely* systemic SEs (esp urolithiasis†) and interactions
Dose: apply 2% drop tds (bd with topical β-blocker). Available as combination drop with timolol 0.5% (**Cosopt**).

DOSULEPIN HYDROCHLORIDE

TCA: blocks reuptake of NA (and 5-HT) through binding to noradrenaline transporter (NAT) and serotonin transport (SERT).
Use: depression (less suitable for prescribing).
CI: as for amitriptyline **L/H**.
Caution: as for amitriptyline **P/E**.
Class SE: antimuscarinic fx (constipation, dry mouth, blurred vision), **cardiac fx** (arrhythmias, HB↑, HR, postural ↓BP, dizziness, syncope: **dangerous in OD**), ↑Wt, **sedation** (often ⇒ 'hangover'), seizures, Δ LFTs, ↓Na⁺ (esp in elderly), agitation, confusion, neuroleptic malignant syndrome.
Warn: discontinuation symptoms if stopped abruptly.
Monitor: elderly patients for cardiac and Ψ SE and electrolytes.
Interactions: ☠ Never give with, or ≤2 wk after, MAOIs; do not give MAOIs within 2 wk of stopping dosulepin ☠; ↑risk of neurotoxicity with lithium; ↑levels with bupropion, cinacalcet, dronedarone, fluoxetine, paroxetine, terbinafine; ↑fx of adrenaline, noradrenaline, phenylephrine; ↓fx of ephedrine.

Dose: initially 75 mg po od at bedtime (or in divided doses), ↑ gradually to 150 mg od.

> 🕱 Overdose is associated with high rate of fatality. TCA overdose ⇒ dilated pupils, arrhythmias, ↓BP, hypothermia, hyperreflexia, extensor plantar responses, seizures, respiratory depression and coma. 🕱

DOXAZOSIN/CARDURA

α_1-Blocker ⇒ systemic vasodilation and relaxation of internal urethral sphincter ∴ ⇒ ↓TPR[1] and ↑bladder outflow[2].

Use: HTN[1], BPH[2].

CI: postural ↓BP, anuria, **B**.

Caution: postural ↓BP, micturition syncope, pulmonary oedema due to aortic or mitral stenosis **L/H/P/E**.

SE: postural ↓BP (esp after first dose*), dizziness, headache, urinary incontinence (esp women), GI upset (esp N&V), drowsiness/fatigue, syncope, mood Δs, dry mouth, oedema, somnolence, blurred vision, rhinitis. Rarely erectile dysfunction, ↑HR, arrhythmias, hypersensitivity/rash.

Interactions: ↑s hypotensive fx of diuretics, β-blockers, Ca^{2+} antagonists, silden-/tadal-/vardenafil, general anaesthetics, moxisylyte and antidepressants.

Dose: initially 1 mg od (give first dose before bed*), then slowly ↑ according to response (max 16 mg/day[1] or 8 mg/day[2]). 4 mg or 8 mg od if MR preparation, as **Cardura XL**.

DOXEPIN HYDROCHLORIDE/SINEPIN

TCA: blocks reuptake of NA and 5-HT through binding to noradrenaline transporter (NAT) and serotonin transport (SERT).

Use: depression (less suitable for prescribing).

CI: as for amitriptyline **L/H**.

Caution: as for amitriptyline **P/E**.

Class SE: **antimuscarinic fx** (constipation, dry mouth, blurred vision), **cardiac fx** (arrhythmias, HB, ↑HR, postural ↓BP, dizziness,

syncope: **dangerous in OD**), ↑Wt, **sedation** (often ⇒ 'hangover'),
seizures, Δ LFTs, ↓Na⁺ (esp in elderly), agitation, confusion,
neuroleptic malignant syndrome.

Warn: discontinuation symptoms if stopped abruptly.

Monitor: elderly patients for cardiac and Ψ SE and electrolytes.

Interactions: ☠ Never give with, or ≤2 wk after, MAOIs; do
not give MAOIs within 2 wk of stopping doxepin ☠; ↑risk of
neurotoxicity with lithium; ↑levels with bupropion, cinacalcet,
dronedarone, fluoxetine, paroxetine, terbinafine; ↑fx of adrenaline,
noradrenaline, phenylephrine; ↓fx of ephedrine.

Dose: initially 75 mg po od at bedtime (or in divided doses),
maintenance 25–300 mg od, doses >100 mg given in three divided
doses.

> ☠ Overdose is associated with high rate of fatality. TCA overdose ⇒
> dilated pupils, arrhythmias, ↓BP, hypothermia, hyperreflexia,
> extensor plantar responses, seizures, respiratory depression and
> coma. ☠

DOXYCYCLINE

Tetracycline antibiotic: inhibits ribosomal (30S) subunit.

Use: genital infections, esp syphilis, chlamydia, PID, salpingitis,
urethritis (non-gonococcal). Also *Rickettsia* (inc Q fever), *Brucella,*
Lyme disease (*Borrelia burgdorferi*), malaria (Px/Rx, not first
line), mycoplasma (genital/respiratory), COPD infective exac
(H. influenzae), MRSA infection (if mild, sensitive strain).

CI/Caution/SE/Interactions: as tetracycline, but can give with
caution if RF; also CI in SLE and achlorhydria. Can ⇒ anorexia,
flushing, tinnitus, oesophageal ulceration and ↑ciclosporin levels.

Warn: avoid UV light and products containing Zn/Fe/Ca²⁺ (e.g.
antacids). Swallow whole with plenty of fluid, while sitting or
standing.

Dose: 100–200 mg od/bd.^SPC/BNF *NB:* ↓**dose in RF.**

DROPERIDOL

Butyrophenone: blocks dopamine receptors in chemoreceptor trigger zone.

Use: post-operative N&V[1]; acute behavioural disturbance (unlicensed)[2].

CI: ↓HR, ↓GCS, electrolyte Δs (↓K^+, ↓Mg^{2+}), phaeo, ↑QTc.

Caution: Parkinson's, drugs that ↑QTc, epilepsy, MG, glaucoma (angle-closure), ↑prostate, jaundice, blood disorders, electrolyte Δs, alcohol misuse, respiratory disease.

SE: see Haloperidol, but concerns about ↑QTc.

Warn: avoid direct sunlight (photosensitisation) with ↑doses, ↑fx of alcohol.

Monitor: prolactin at initiation, 6 months, then annually. Continuous SpO_2 if ventricular arrhythmia risk; ECG if cardiovascular risk factors identified.

Interactions: metab by P450; ↑levels with CYP1A2/3A4 inhibitors, e.g. ciprofloxacin, diltiazem, erythromycin, fluconazole, indinavir, verapamil, cimetidine; ↑risks of torsades de pointes/QT prolongation with antiarrhythmics (quinidine, disopyramide, procainamide, amiodarone, sotalol), antibiotics (erythromycin, clarithromycin, sparfloxacin), antihistamines (astemizole, terfenadine), antipsychotics (chlorpromazine, haloperidol, pimozide, thioridazine), antimalarial agents (chloroquine, halofantrine), cisapride, domperidone, methadone, pentamidine; ↑EPSE with metoclopramide, neuroleptics; avoid alcohol.

Dose: 0.625–1.25 mg iv, dose to be given 30 min before end of surgery, then 0.625–1.25 mg every 6 h as required[1], up to 10 mg im as required[2].

DULOXETINE/CYMBALTA

5-HT and noradrenaline reuptake inhibitor.

Use: depression[1], generalised anxiety disorder[2], diabetic neuropathy[3] (review need ≤3 monthly and stop if inadequate response after 2 months), stress urinary incontinence[4] (assess benefit/tolerability after 2–4 wk).

CI: R (if eGFR <30 mL/min/1.73 m^2), **L**.

Caution: cardiac disease, Hx mania, epilepsy, ↑IOP, ↑risk of glaucoma (angle-closure), bleeding disorder/on drugs ↑ing bleeding risk, **H/P/B/E**.

SE: GI upset (N&V&C), abdo pain, Wt Δ, ↓appetite, palpitations, hot flushes, insomnia, sexual dysfunction, suicidal behaviour.

Warn: patient not to stop suddenly.

Interactions: metabolism ↓ by ciprofloxacin, fluvoxamine. ↑5-HT fx with St John's wort and antidepressants (esp moclobemide and MAOIs; avoid concomitant use and do not start for 1 wk after stopping duloxetine). Avoid with artemether/lumefantrine. ↑risk CNS toxicity with sibutramine.

Dose: 60 mg od[1]; initially 30 mg od (↑ to max 120 mg/day if required)[2]; 60 mg od (↑ to bd if required)[3]; 40 mg bd[4]. *NB:* stop gradually over 1–2 wk to ↓risk of withdrawal fx.

EMPAGLIFLOZIN/JARDIANCE

Oral antidiabetic (reversible sodium glucose cotransporter 2 [SGLT2] inhibitor): ↓renal reabsorption of glucose and ↑urinary excretion of excess glucose.

Use: type 2 DM – reserved for monotherapy (if metformin inappropriate) or combination Rx with insulin or other antidiabetic drugs (if existing Rx fails to achieve adequate glycaemic control: for adults 18–84 years of age).

CI: ketoacidosis, **R** (if severe), **L** (if severe), **P/B**.

Caution: monitor renal function before Rx, then risk factors for DKA (including ↓β-cell reserve; conditions leading to restricted food intake or volume depletion/severe dehydration including GI illness; sudden ↓ in insulin; ↑insulin requirements due to acute illness, surgery or alcohol abuse), CVD (risk of ↓BP); **E** > 75 years of age (risk of ↓BP); electrolyte disturbances; ↓BP, concomitant antihypertensive Rx (increased risk of ↓volume), HF and other concomitant use of diuretics, ↑Hct; complicated UTI – consider temporarily interrupting Rx. Correct hypovolaemia before starting Rx and at least annually on Rx.

SE: balanitis; hypoglycaemia (in combination with insulin or sulphonylurea); ↑risk of infection, pruritus, thirst, urinary disorders, hypovolaemia. Rarely DKA.

Dose: 10 mg od po, increased to 25 mg od if necessary and if tolerated. Doses of concomitant insulin or drugs that stimulate insulin secretion may need to be ↓. ↓dose in mild RF. Avoid in severe RF or LF.

> ☠ DKA on SGLT2 inhibitors may be atypical with only moderately ↑blood glucose. Warn patients of risk factors and signs and symptoms of DKA. Advise patients to seek immediate medical advice if they develop any. Test for ↑ketones if signs or symptoms of DKA, even if plasma glucose near normal. Stop SGLT2 inhibitor Rx if DKA is suspected or diagnosed. Do not restart Rx with any SGLT2 inhibitor in patients with DKA during use, unless another cause for DKA is identified and resolved. Interrupt SGLT2 inhibitor treatment in patients in hospital for major surgery or acute serious illness. Rx may be restarted once condition stabilised ☠.

ENALAPRIL/INNOVACE

ACE-i.

Use: HTN[1], LVF[2].

CI/Caution/SE/Interactions: as captopril, plus L.

Dose: initially 5 mg od[1] (2.5 mg od[2]) ↑ing according to response, max 40 mg/day. *NB:* ↓dose if elderly, taking diuretics or RF.

ENSURE Protein and calorie supplement drinks.

EPADERM Paraffin-based emollient ointment for very dry skin (and as soap substitute).

▼ **EPILIM** see Valproate.

EPROSARTAN/TEVETEN
Angiotensin II antagonist; see Losartan.
Use: HTN.
CI: L (if severe), P/B.
Caution/SE/Interactions: see Losartan.
Dose: 600 mg od. ↓ if elderly, RF or LF.

ERGOCALCIFEROL (= CALCIFEROL)
Vit D_2: needs renal (1) and hepatic (25) hydroxylation for activation.
Use: vit D deficiency.
CI: ↑Ca^{2+}, metastatic calcification. P (only high doses).
Caution: R (if high 'pharmacological'* doses used), B.
SE: ↑Ca^{2+}. If over-Rx: GI upset, weakness, headache, polydipsia/polyuria, anorexia, RF, arrhythmias.
Monitor: Ca^{2+} (esp if N&V develops or ↑doses in RF*).
Interactions: fx ↓ by anticonvulsants and ↑ by thiazides.
Dose: 10–20 micrograms (400–800 units) od as part of multivitamin preparations or combined with calcium lactate or phosphate as 'calcium + ergocalciferol': non-proprietary preparations available but is often prescribed by trade name (e.g. Adcal D3, Accrete D3 or Calcichew D3). ↑doses of 250 micrograms–1 mg od (of 'pharmacological strength' preparations*) used for GI malabsorption and chronic liver disease (up to 5 mg daily for ↓PTH or renal osteodystrophy).

*Specify strength of tablet required to avoid confusion.SPC/BNF

ERYTHROMYCIN

Macrolide antibiotic: binds 50S ribosome.

Use: atypical pneumonias (with other agents)[1], rarely *Chlamydia/* other GU infections, *Campylobacter* enteritis. Often used if allergy to penicillin. GI stasis (unlicensed)[2].

CI: macrolide hypersensitivity or if taking simvastatin, terfenadine, pimozide, ergotamine or dihydroergotamine (see SPC for other drug CI).

Caution: ↑QTc (inc drugs that predispose to), porphyria, MG, L/R/P/B.

SE: GI upset (rarely AAC), **dry itchy skin**, hypersensitivity (inc SJS, TEN), arrhythmias (esp VT), chest pain, reversible hearing loss (dose-related, esp if RF), cholestatic jaundice.

Interactions: ↓P450 ∴ many; most importantly ↑s levels of ciclosporin, digoxin, theophyllines and carbamazepine, other drugs that ↑QTc, **W+**.

Dose: 500 mg qds po (250 mg qds if mild infection, 1 g qds if severe)[1]; 50 mg/kg daily iv in four divided doses[1]. 250–500 mg tds for up to 4 wk, to be taken before food[2].

NB: venous irritant ∴ give po if possible.

ERYTHROPOIETIN

Recombinant erythropoietin.

Use: ↓Hb 2° to CRF or chemotherapy (AZT or platinum containing). Also unlicensed use for myeloma, lymphoma and certain myelodysplasias. Three types: α (**Eprex**), β (**NeoRecormon**) and longer-acting darbepoetin (**Aranesp**).

SE: ↑BP (monitor – interrupt Rx if BP uncontrolled), ↑K+, headache, arthralgia, oedema, TE. ☠ Rarely ⇒ severe rash; red cell aplasia (esp subcutaneous **Eprex** if RF, which is now CI) ☠.

CI/Caution/Dose: specialist use only[SPC/BNF]; given subcutaneously (self-administered) or iv (as inpatient). ↓Fe/folate (monitor), ↑Al, infections and inflammatory disease can ↓response. *NB: transfusion is first-line Rx for ↓Hb 2° to cancer chemotherapy.*

E

ESCITALOPRAM/CIPRALEX
SSRI (active enantiomer of citalopram).
Use: depression, OCD, anxiety disorders.
CI/Caution/SE/Warn/Interactions: as citalopram.
Dose: initially 10 mg od, ↑ing if necessary to 20 mg od. *NB:* **max dose 10 mg in elderly and halve doses in LF and for most anxiety disorders.**

ESOMEPRAZOLE/NEXIUM
PPI; as omeprazole, plus CI **R** (if severe).
Dose: 20 mg od po (40 mg od for first 4 wk, if for gastro-oesophageal reflux); 20–40 mg/day iv[SPC/BNF]. *NB:* max 20 mg/day if severe LF.

ETORICOXIB/ARCOXIA
NSAID which selectively inhibits COX-2 ∴ ⇒ GI SEs (COX-1 mediated). *Provides no Px against IHD/CVA* (unlike aspirin).
Use: osteo-[1]/rheumatoid[2] arthritis[NICE], ankylosing spondylitis[2], acute gout[3].
CI/Caution/SE/Interactions: as celecoxib (except fluconazole interaction), plus CI in uncontrolled HTN (persistently >140/90 mm Hg) – monitor BP within 2 wk of starting and regularly thereafter. Also ↑s ethinylestradiol levels. *Not* CI in *sulphonamide* hypersensitivity. Mild **W+**.
Dose: 30–60 mg od[1]; 90 mg od[2]; 120 mg od[3] for max 8 days. *NB:* ↓dose if LF.

EUMOVATE see Clobetasone butyrate 0.05%; steroid cream.

EXENATIDE/BYETTA
Sc antidiabetic (glucagon-like peptide-1 receptor agonist): ⇒ ↑insulin secretion and ↓glucagon secretion and ↓gastric emptying.
Use: type 2 DM – reserved for combination therapy when other treatment options have failed. Combined with metformin or a sulphonylurea, or both, or with pioglitazone, or with both

metformin and pioglitazone, in patients who have not achieved adequate glycaemic control with these drugs alone or in combination.

CI: ketoacidosis; severe gastrointestinal disease, **B/P**.

Caution/Interactions: may cause $\downarrow$Wt >1.5 kg/wk, pancreatitis, **R/E**. With standard-release exenatide some po drugs should be taken >1 h before, or 4 h after exenatide injection.[BNF]

SE: GI upset, $\downarrow$appetite, asthenia, dizziness, headache, skin reactions. Less common: alopecia, burping, drowsiness, hyperhidrosis, RF, altered taste, angioedema. Rarely severe pancreatitis (discontinue permanently if occurs).

Dose: sc using immediate- or modified-release medicines. See BNF for dosing. Dose of concomitant sulphonylurea may need to be $\downarrow$.

FELODIPINE/PLENDIL

Ca^{2+} channel blocker (dihydropyridine): as amlodipine but $\Rightarrow$ $\downarrow$HF/–ve inotropic fx.

Use: HTN[1], angina Px[2].

CI: IHD (if unstable angina or within 1 month of MI), significant aortic stenosis, **H** (if uncontrolled)/**P**.

Caution: stop drug if angina/HF worsen, **L/B**.

SE: as nifedipine but $\uparrow$ankle swelling and possibly $\downarrow$vasodilator fx (headache, flushing and dizziness).

Interactions: metab by **P450** $\therefore$ levels $\uparrow$ by cimetidine, erythromycin, ketoconazole and grapefruit juice. Hypotensive fx $\uparrow$ by α-blockers. Levels $\downarrow$ by primidone. $\uparrow$s fx of tacrolimus.

Dose: initially 5 mg od, $\uparrow$ if required to 10 mg (max 20 mg[1]).

NB: $\downarrow$**dose if LF or elderly.**

FENTANYL

Strong opioid; used in severe chronic/palliative pain (top/sl/buccal/nasal spray) and in anaesthesia (iv).

CI: acute respiratory depression, risk of ileus, $\uparrow$ICP/head injury/coma.

Caution: all other conditions where morphine is CI or cautioned, but better tolerated in RF. Also DM, cerebral tumour.

SE: as morphine but generally ↓N&V/constipation.

Warn: patients/carers of signs/symptoms of opiate toxicity; 💀 serious opioid toxicity from accidental exposure to patches 💀.

Interactions: as morphine but levels ↑ (not ↓) by ritonavir, levels ↑ by itra-/fluconazole and no known interaction with gabapentin. May ↑levels of midazolam.

Dose: patches (do not cut): last 72 h and come in six strengths: 12, 25, 37.5, 50, 75 and 100, which denote release of microgram/h (to calculate initial dose, these are approximately equivalent to daily oral morphine salt requirement of 30, 60, 90, 120, 180 and 240 mg, respectively). **Lozenges (buccal)** for 'breakthrough' pain as Actiq: initially 200 micrograms over 15 min, repeating after 15 min if needed and adjusting dose to give max 4 lozenges daily (available as 200, 400, 600, 800, 1200 or 1600 micrograms).

Tablets: for 'breakthrough' pain as Effentora (buccal) or Abstral (sl) 100, 200, 400, 600 and 800 micrograms.SPC/BNF *Only use if taking regular opioids (fatalities reported otherwise). If >4 doses/day needed, adjust background analgesia.* **Nasal spray:** for 'breakthrough' pain as Instanyl or PecFent.SPC/BNF *NB:* ↓dose if LF or elderly. No initial ↓dose needed in RF, but may accumulate over time. Unless given iv has prolonged onset/offset; use only when opioid requirements stable and cover first 12 h after initial Rx with prn short-acting opioid. Only for use if have previously tolerated opioids. If serious adverse reactions, remove patch immediately and monitor for up to 24 h. Fever/external heat can ⇒ ↑absorption (∴ ↑fx) from patches.

FERROUS FUMARATE

As ferrous sulphate, but ↓GI upset; available in United Kingdom as Fersaday (322 mg tablet od as Px or bd as Rx) (1 tablet of 210 mg od/bd Px; tds Rx) or Galfer (305 mg capsule od as Px/bd as Rx).

FERROUS GLUCONATE

As ferrous sulphate, but ↓GI upset. Px: 600 mg od; Rx: 1.2–1.8 g/ day in two to three divided doses before food.

FERROUS SULPHATE

Oral Fe preparation.

Use: Fe-deficient $\downarrow$Hb Rx/Px.

Caution: P.

SE: dark stools (can confuse with melaena, which smells worse), **GI upset** (esp nausea; consider switching to ferrous gluconate/fumarate or take with food, but latter can $\Rightarrow$ $\downarrow$absorption), Δ bowel habit (dose dependent).

Dose: Rx: 200 mg/tds[BNF]. Px: 200 mg od/bd.

FINASTERIDE

Antiandrogen: 5-α-reductase inhibitor; prevents conversion of testosterone to more potent dihydrotestosterone.

Use: BPH[1] ($\downarrow$s prostate size and symptoms), male-pattern baldness[2].

Caution: Ca prostate (can $\Rightarrow$ $\downarrow$PSA and $\therefore$ mask), obstructive uropathy, P (teratogenic; although not taken by women, partners of those on the drug can absorb it from handling crushed tablets and from semen, in which it is excreted $\therefore$ *females must avoid handling crushed or broken tablets, and sexual partners of those on the drug must use condoms if, or likely to become, pregnant*).

SE: sexual dysfunction, testicular pain, gynaecomastia, hypersensitivity (inc swelling of lips/face), male breast cancer. Rare reports of depression and suicidal thoughts.[MHRA]

Dose: 5 mg od[1] (**Proscar**), 1 mg od[2] (**Propecia**).

FLAGYL see Metronidazole; antibiotic for anaerobes.

FLIXOTIDE see Fluticasone (inh steroid). 50, 100, 250 or 500 micrograms/blister as powder. 50, 125 or 250 micrograms/blister as aerosol.

Dose: 100–2000 micrograms/day[SPC/BNF] in two divided doses.

FLOMAXTRA XL see Tamsulosin; α_1-blocker for $\uparrow$prostate.

FLUCLOXACILLIN

Penicillin (penicillinase-resistant).

Use: penicillin-resistant (β-lactamase-producing) staphylococcal and streptococcal infections, esp skin[1] (surgical wounds, iv sites, cellulitis, impetigo, otitis externa), rarely as adjunct in pneumonia[1]. Also osteomyelitis[2], endocarditis[3].

CI/Caution/SE/Interactions: as benzylpenicillin, plus CI if Hx of flucloxacillin-assoc jaundice/hepatic dysfunction and caution if LF, as rarely ⇒ hepatitis or **cholestatic jaundice** (may develop up to 2 months after Rx stopped).

Dose: 250–500 mg qds po/im (or up to 2 g qds iv)[1]; up to 2 g qds iv[2]; 2 g qds (4 hrly if Wt >85 kg) iv[3]. *NB:* ↓dose in severe RF.

FLUCONAZOLE

Triazole antifungal: good po absorption and CSF penetration.
Use: fungal meningitis (esp cryptococcal), candidiasis (mucosal, vaginal, systemic), other fungal infections (esp tinea, pityriasis).
CI: acute porphyria.
Caution: susceptibility to ↑QTc, L/R/P/B.
SE: GI upset, hypersensitivity (can ⇒ angioedema, TEN, SJS, anaphylaxis: if develops rash, stop drug or monitor closely), hepatotoxicity, headache. Rarely blood/metabolic (↑lipids, ↓K^+) disorders, dizziness, seizures, alopecia.
Monitor: LFTs; stop drug if features of liver disease develop.
Interactions: ↓P450 ∴ many; most importantly, ↑s fx of theophyllines, ciclosporin, phenytoin and tacrolimus. Hepatotoxic drugs. Also ↓clopidogrel fx. W+.
Dose: 50–400 mg/day po or iv according to indication.[SPC/BNF] *NB:* ↓dose in RF.

FLUDROCORTISONE

Mineralocorticoid (also has glucocorticoid actions).
Use: adrenocortical insufficiency esp Addison's disease[1], neuropathic postural ↓BP (unlicensed)[2].
CI/Caution/Interactions: see Prednisolone.
SE: H_2O/Na^+ retention, ↓K^+ (monitor U&Es). Also can ⇒ immunosuppression (and other SEs of corticosteroids – see Hydrocortisone iv/po).

Dose: 50–300 micrograms/day po[1]; 100–400 micrograms daily[2].

FLUMAZENIL

Benzodiazepine antagonist (competitive).

Use: benzodiazepine OD/toxicity (only if respiratory depression and ventilatory support not immediately available).

CI: life-threatening conditions controlled by benzodiazepines (e.g. ↑ICP, status epilepticus).

Caution: mixed ODs (esp TCAs), benzodiazepine dependence (may ⇒ withdrawal fx), Hx of panic disorder (can ⇒ relapse), head injury, epileptics on long-term benzodiazepine Rx (may ⇒ fits), L/P/B/E.

SE: N&V, dizziness, flushing, rebound anxiety/agitation, transient ↑BP/HR. Very rarely anaphylaxis.

Dose: initially 200 micrograms iv over 15 sec, then, if required, further doses of 100 micrograms at 1 min intervals. *Max total dose 1 mg (2 mg in ITU).* Can also give as ivi at 100–400 micrograms/h adjusting to response. *NB:* see p. 382, refer 'Benzodiazepine Overdose' in 'Emergencies' chapter – TOXBASE recommends higher doses.

NB: short $t_{1/2}$ (40–80 min); observe closely after Rx and consider further doses or ivi (at 100–400 micrograms/h adjusted to response).

> ☠ *Flumazenil is not recommended as a diagnostic test and should not be given routinely in overdoses, as risk of inducing:*
>
> * fits (esp if epileptic, or if co-ingested drugs that predispose to fits)
> * withdrawal syndrome (if habituated to benzodiazepines)
> * arrhythmias (esp if co-ingested TCA or amphetamine-like drug)
>
>   If in any doubt get senior opinion, exclude habituation to benzodiazepines and get ECG before giving unless life-threatening respiratory depression and benzodiazepine known to be cause ☠.

L/R/H = Liver, Renal and Heart failure. E = elderly. P = pregnancy. B = breastfeeding.

F

FLUOXETINE/PROZAC

SSRI antidepressant: long $t_{1/2}$ compared with others.

Use: depression[1], bulimia[2], OCD[3].

CI: mania, poorly controlled epilepsy.

Caution: epilepsy, receiving ECT, Hx of mania or bleeding disorder (esp GI), DM[†], glaucoma (angle-closure), ↑risk of bleeding, age <18 years, H.

Class SE: GI upset, ↓Wt, insomnia, agitation, headache, hypersensitivity. Can ⇒ withdrawal fx when stopped. ∴ *stop slowly*; more important for SSRIs with ↓$t_{1/2}$. Rarely extrapyramidal and antimuscarinic fx, sexual dysfunction, convulsions, ↓Na^+ (inc SIADH), bleeding disorders, GI bleed, serotonin syndrome and suicidal thoughts/behaviour, ↑risk of bone fracture, glaucoma.

Specific SE: rarely hypoglycaemia[†], **vasculitis** (rash may be first sign).

Warn: may cause discontinuation symptoms if stopped suddenly.

Interactions: ↓P450 ∴ many, but most importantly ↑s levels of TCAs, benzodiazepines, clozapine and haloperidol. ↑s lithium toxicity and ⇒ HTN and ↑CNS fx with sele-/rasagiline (and other dopaminergics). ↑risk of CNS toxicity (serotonin syndrome; see p. 389, refer 'Serotonin Syndrome' in 'Emergencies' chapter) with drugs that ↑5-HT (e.g. tramadol, sibutramine, sumatriptan, St John's wort). Risk of bleeding with anticoagulants, aspirin and NSAIDs. Levels ↑ by ritonavir. Antagonises antiepileptics (but ↑s levels of carbamazepine and phenytoin). Avoid with artemether/lumefantrine and tamoxifen. ☠ **Never give with, or ≤2 wk after, MAOIs; do not give MAOIs within 5 wk of stopping fluoxetine.** (Mild **W+**.) ☠

Dose: initially, 20 mg od[1,3] ↑ to max 60 mg od or divided doses; 60 mg od[2] – give mane, as can ↓sleep. *NB:* long half-life. ↓dose in LF.

FLUPENTIXOL/DEPIXOL/FLUANXOL

Typical antipsychotic: D_1/D_2 dopamine receptor antagonist; weak $5-HT_2$ antagonist.

Use: psychosis[1], depression[2].

CI: CNS depression, overactivity, phaeo, circulatory collapse.
Caution: as for other antipsychotics, and agitated states, thyroid disease, E.
Class SE: EPSE, ↑prolactin and assoc Sx, sedation, ↑Wt, QT prolongation, VTE, blood dyscrasias, ↓seizure threshold, NMS.
Specific SE: ↑salivation, appetite changes, impaired glucose tolerance, urinary disorder.
Warn: photosensitivity at higher doses.
Monitor: as for all antipsychotics – baseline ECG, BMI, FBC, lipids, HbA1c, prolactin; frequently at the start of treatment and at least annually when stable.
Interactions: ↑risk of QT prolongation with 5-HT$_3$ antagonists and TCAs; ↑risk of lithium toxicity and NMS with lithium; ↓fx of amantadine, apomorphine, bromocriptine, cabergoline, pergolide, pramipexole, quinagolide, ropinirole, rotigotine.
Dose: 18–65 years: 3–9 mg od/bd, up to max 18 mg/day[1]; >65 years: 0.75–4.5 mg od/bd, up to max 18 mg/day[2]. ≥18 years: 1 mg mane, ↑ to max 3 mg in divided doses at wkly intervals, stop if no benefit; last dose to be given before 4 p.m.

FLUPENTIXOL DECANOATE/DEPIXOL

Typical antipsychotic: D$_1$/D$_2$ dopamine receptor antagonist; weak 5-HT$_2$ antagonist. Long-acting injection (t$_{1/2}$ ~ 21 days).
Use: maintenance treatment psychosis for patients stabilised on oral therapy.
CI/Caution/SE/Warn/Monitor/Interactions: as for flupentixol.
Dose: initial test dose 20 mg im (administered into upper outer buttock/lateral thigh), then 20–40 mg after 7 days, and 20–40 mg every 2–4 wk, doses above 80 mg every 4 wk should rarely be exceeded , ↓dose in elderly.

FLUPHENAZINE DECANOATE/MODECATE

Typical antipsychotic: D$_1$/D$_2$ dopamine receptor antagonist. Long-acting injection (t$_{1/2}$ ~ 2–16 wk).

Use: maintenance in psychosis.

CI: CNS depression, cerebrovascular disease, phaeo, blood dyscrasias, hypersensitivity to **sesame oil, L/R/H**.

Caution: as for other antipsychotics, and thyroid disease, **L/R/H** disease.

Class SE: EPSE, ↑prolactin and assoc Sx, sedation, ↑Wt, QT prolongation, VTE, blood dyscrasias, ↓seizure threshold, NMS.

Specific SE: jaundice, abnormal skin pigmentation, lens opacities, impaired body temperature regulation.

Monitor: as for all antipsychotics – baseline ECG, BMI, FBC, lipids, HbA1c, prolactin; frequently at the start of treatment and at least annually when stable.

Interactions: metab by P450; ↑risk of QT prolongation with concurrent use of other medications that also prolong QT – anti-arrhythmics, quinidine, disopyramide, procainamide, amiodarone, sotalol, TCAs (e.g. amitriptyline), antipsychotics (e.g. phenothiazines, pimozide), antihistamines (e.g. terfenadine), lithium, quinine, pentamidine, sparfloxacin; ↑risk of ↓K+ (↑risk of torsade de pointes) with amiodarone (and other anti-arrhythmics), amino-/theophylline, corticosteroids, diuretics, amphotericin, fludrocortisone, salbutamol, terbutaline; ↑risk of NMS with MAOIs.

Dose: initial test dose 12.5 mg im (administered into the gluteal muscle), then 12.5–100 mg after 4–7 days, and 12.5–100 mg every 14–35 days.

FLUTICASONE/FLIXOTIDE (various delivery devices available[BNF])
Inhaled corticosteroid for asthma: see Beclometasone.

Dose: 100–2000 micrograms/day inh (or 500 micrograms–2 mg bd as nebs).

1 microgram equivalent to 2 micrograms of beclometasone or budesonide.

FLUVOXAMINE

SSRI antidepressant; potent P450 enzyme inhibitor.

Use: depression[1], obsessive-compulsive disorder[2].

CI: poorly controlled epilepsy, mania.

Caution: ECT, DM, epilepsy, bleeding disorders, Hx mania, glaucoma (angle-closure) H/P/B.

Class SE: GI upset, ↓Wt, insomnia, agitation, headache, hypersensitivity. Can ⇒ withdrawal fx when stopped ∴ *stop slowly.* Rarely extrapyramidal and antimuscarinic fx, sexual dysfunction, convulsions, ↓Na+ (inc SIADH), bleeding disorders, GI bleed, serotonin syndrome and suicidal thoughts/behaviour, ↑risk of fracture, glaucoma.

Specific SE: impaired liver function.

Warn: withdrawal fx may occur within 5 days of stopping treatment, worse after regular administration for 8 wk+; ↓dose gradually over 4 wk+.

Interactions: ↓P450 ∴ ↓fx of clopidogrel; ↑levels of drugs primarily metabolised by CYP1A2/2C19 (e.g. caffeine, some TCAs, some antipsychotics, some benzodiazepines, ropinirole, propranolol, W+); ☠ ↑levels of drugs with narrow TI (e.g. warfarin, tacrine, theophylline, methadone, phenytoin, carbamazepine and ciclosporin)☠; ↑risk of bleeding with anticoagulants, antiplatelets, fibrinolytics; ↑risk of serotonin syndrome with drugs that ↑5-HT; never give with, or ≤2 wk after, MAOIs; do not give MAOIs within 1 wk of stopping fluvoxamine.

Dose: 50–100 mg in evening, ↑dose gradually if necessary to 300 mg[1,2]; maintenance dose: 100 mg[1], 100–300 mg[2]; if daily dose >150 mg, give in 2–3 divided doses.

☠Poisoning by SSRIs causes N&V, agitation, tremor, nystagmus, drowsiness , seizure, ↑HR. Severe poisoning may result in serotonin syndrome.☠

FOLIC ACID (= FOLATE)

Vitamin: building block of nucleic acids. Essential co-factor for DNA synthesis ⇒ normal erythropoiesis.

Use: folate-deficient megaloblastic ↓Hb Rx/Px if haemolysis/dialysis[1] (or GI malabsorption where ↑doses may be needed), Px against neural-tube dfx in pregnancy[2] (esp if on antiepileptics), Px of methotrexate-induced side effects such as mucositis and GI upset (do not give folic acid on same day as methotrexate)[3].

CI: malignancy (unless megaloblastic ↓Hb due to ↓folate is an important complication).

Caution: undiagnosed megaloblastic ↓Hb (i.e. ↓B_{12}, as found in pernicious anaemia) – never give alone if B_{12} *deficiency, as can precipitate subacute combined degeneration of spinal cord.*

SE: GI disturbance (rare).

Dose: 5 mg od[1] (in maintenance, ↓frequency of dose, often to wkly); 400 micrograms od from before conception until wk 12 of pregnancy[2] (unless mother has neural-tube defect herself or has previously had or has risk of a child with a neural-tube defect, when 5 mg od needed[BNF]); 5 mg once wkly[3].

FOMEPIZOLE Antidote for ethylene glycol and methanol.[BNF]

FONDAPARINUX/ARIXTRA

Synthetic anticoagulant; activated factor X inhibitor.

Use: ACS (UA, NSTEMI or STEMI), Px of VTE, Rx of DVT/PE.

CI: active bleeding, bacterial endocarditis, B.

Caution: bleeding disorders, active PU, other drugs that ↑risk of bleeding, recent intracranial haemorrhage, recent brain/ophthalmic/spinal surgery, spinal/epidural anaesthesia (avoid Rx doses), Wt <50 kg. R (avoid or ↓dose according to indication and creatinine clearance[SPC/BNF]), L/P/E.

SE: bleeding, ↓Hb, ↓(or ↑)Pt, coagulopathy, purpura, oedema, LFT Δs, GI upset. Rarely ↓K⁺, ↓BP, hypersensitivity.

Dose: UA/NSTEMI/Px of VTE 2.5 mg sc od (start 6 h post-op); STEMI 2.5 mg iv/ivi od for first day then sc; Rx of PE/DVT by Wt (<50 kg = 5 mg sc od, 50–100 kg = 7.5 mg sc od, >100 kg = 10 mg sc od). *NB:* length of Rx depends on indication[SPC/BNF], timing of doses post-op critical if Wt <50 kg or elderly. Consider ↓**dose in RF**.

Specialist use only: get senior advice or contact on-call cardiology/ haematology.

FORMOTEROL (= EFORMOTEROL)/FORADIL, OXIS, ATIMOS

Long-acting β₂ agonist 'LABA'; as Salmeterol plus **L**.

Dose: 6–48 micrograms daily (mostly bd regime)[SPC/BNF] inh (min/ max doses vary with preparations[SPC/BNF]).

FOSPHENYTOIN

Antiepileptic: prodrug of phenytoin; allows safer rapid loading.

Use: epilepsy (esp 'status' and seizures assoc with neurosurgery/ head injury) if oral phenytoin not possible/CI.

CI/Caution/SE/Warn/Monitor/Interactions: as phenytoin, but ↓SEs (esp ↓arrhythmias and 'purple glove syndrome').

Dose: as phenytoin, but prescribe as 'phenytoin sodium equivalent' and note ☠ **fosphenytoin sodium 1.5 mg = phenytoin sodium 1 mg** ☠. *NB:* consider ↓dose: L/R/E.

FOSTAIR

Combination asthma inhaler: each puff contains 100 or 200* micrograms beclometasone (steroid) + 6 micrograms formoterol (long-acting β₂-agonist) in a metered dose inhaler.

Dose: 1–2 puffs bd inh. Specify inhaler strength (100 or 200).*

FRAGMIN see LMWH.

FRUSEMIDE now called Furosemide.

FUROSEMIDE (previously FRUSEMIDE)

Loop diuretic: inhibits Na^+/K^+ co-transport in ascending loop of Henle $\Rightarrow$ $\downarrow$reabsorption and $\therefore$ $\uparrow$loss of $Na^+/K^+/Cl/H_2O$.

Use: LVF (esp in acute pulmonary oedema, but also in chronic LVF/CCF or as Px during blood transfusion), resistant HTN, oliguria secondary to AKI (after correcting hypovolaemia first).

CI: $\downarrow\downarrow K^+$, $\downarrow Na^+$, Addison's, cirrhosis (if pre-comatose or comatose), **R** (if anuria).

Caution: $\downarrow$BP, $\uparrow$prostate, porphyria, diabetes, L/P/B.

SE: $\downarrow$BP (inc postural), $\downarrow K^+$, $\downarrow Na^+$, $\downarrow Ca^{2+}$, $\downarrow Mg^{2+}$, $\downarrow$Cl alkalosis, $\downarrow$proteinaemia. Also $\uparrow$urate/gout, GI upset, $\uparrow$glucose/impaired glucose tolerance, $\uparrow$cholesterol/TGs (temporary). Rarely **BM** suppression (stop drug), RF, skin reactions, pancreatitis, tinnitus/deafness (if $\uparrow$doses or RF or rapid administration: reversible).

Monitor: U&Es, glucose; if $\downarrow K^+$, add po K^+ supplements/K^+-sparing diuretic or change to combination tablet (e.g. co-amilofruse).

Interactions: $\uparrow$s toxicity of digoxin, flecainide, sotalol, NSAIDs, vancomycin, gentamicin and lithium. $\downarrow$s fx of antidiabetics. NSAIDs may $\downarrow$diuretic response.

Dose: usually 20–80 mg po/im/iv daily in divided doses. $\uparrow$doses used in acute LVF and oliguria. If HF or RF, ivi (max 4 mg/min) can $\Rightarrow$ smoother control of fluid balance.^SPC/BNF For blood transfusions, a rough guide is to give 20 mg with every unit if *existing LVF,* and with every second unit if *at risk of LVF.* NB: may need $\uparrow$dose in RF.

Give iv if severe oedema, as bowel oedema $\Rightarrow$ $\downarrow$po absorption.

FUSIDIC ACID/FUCIDIN

Antibiotic; good bone penetration and activity against *S. aureus.*

Use: osteomyelitis, endocarditis (2° to penicillin-resistant staphylococci) – needs second antibiotic to prevent resistance.

Caution: biliary disease or obstruction (⇒ ↓elimination), L/P/B.
SE: GI upset, hepatitis*. Rarely skin/blood disorders, AKI.
Monitor: LFTs* (esp if chronic Rx, ↑doses or LF).
Dose: 500 mg tds po (equivalent to 750 mg tds if using suspension) – in severe infection ↑ to 1 g tds po. Skin infection: 250 mg bd.
NB: ↓dose in LF.

FYBOGEL

Laxative: bulking agent (ispaghula husk) for constipation (inc IBS).
CI: ↓swallow, GI obstruction, faecal impaction, colonic atony.
Dose: 1 sachet after meals with water.

GABAPENTIN

Antiepileptic: binds to voltage-gated Ca^{2+} channels in the CNS; modulates GABA and glutamate synthesis.
Use: neuropathic pain, epilepsy (adjunctive Rx of focal seizures ± 2° generalisation).
Caution: Hx psychosis or DM, mixed seizures.
SE: fatigue/somnolence, **dizziness**, **cerebellar fx** (esp ataxia), dipl-/amblyopia, headache, rhinitis, ↓WCC, GI upset, arthra-/myalgia, skin reactions, suicidal ideation. Rarely ⇒ severe respiratory depression.
Interactions: fx ↓ by antidepressants and antimalarials (esp mefloquine). Antipsychotics ↓seizure threshold.
Dose: initially 300 mg od, ↑ing by 300 mg/day to max 3.6 g daily in three divided doses (*NB: stop drug over ≥1 wk*).[BNF] *NB:* ↓dose in RF.[BNF]

Can give false-positive urinary dipstick results for proteinuria.

GALANTAMINE

Acetylcholinesterase inhibitor (reversible); also ↑fx of ACh at nicotinic receptors.
Use: mild-to-moderate Alzheimer's disease.
CI: GI obstruction/post-GI surgery, urinary obstruction/post-bladder surgery, **R** (CrCl < 9 mL/min), **L** (if severe, Child-Pugh > 9).

Caution: as for donepezil, and electrolyte disturbances, Hx of seizures, lower respiratory tract infection, **H**.

SE: as for Donepezil, and asthenia.

Warn: take with food. Stop if rash appears.

Interactions: metab by P450; ↑levels with CYP2D6/3A4 inhibitors, e.g. bupropion, cinacalcet, clarithromycin, cobicistat, darunavir, fluoxetine, itra-/ketoconazole, paroxetine; ↓fx of neuromuscular blocking agents (atracurium, cisatracurium, mivacurium, pancuronium) and anticholinergic agents (atropine, procyclidine, trihexyphenidyl); ↑risk of bradycardia with amiodarone, β-blockers, diltiazem, digoxin, ivabradine.

Dose: immediate-release: initially 4 mg bd for 4 wk, ↑ to 8 mg bd for 4 wk+, maintenance 8–12 mg bd; modified-release: initially 8 mg od for 4 wk, ↑ to 16 mg od for 4 wk+, maintenance 16–24 mg od; halve dose in moderate LF.

> ☠ Serious skin hypersensitivity may occur (inc SJS and acute generalised exanthematous pustulosis). ☠

GASTROCOTE Compound alginate for acid reflux.

Dose: 5–15 mL or 1–2 tablets after meals and at bedtime (*NB:* 2.13 mmol Na^+/5 mL and 1 mmol Na^+/tablet).

GAVISCON (ADVANCE) Alginate raft-forming oral suspension for acid reflux.

Dose: 5–10 mL or 1–2 tablets after meals and at bedtime. (*NB:* 2.3 mmol Na^+ and 1 mmol K^+/5 mL and 2.25 mmol Na^+ and 1 mmol K^+/tablet.)

> Ensure good hydration, esp if elderly, GI narrowing or ↓GI motility.

GENTAMICIN

Aminoglycoside: broad-spectrum 'cidal' antibiotic; inhibits ribosomal 30S subunit. Good Gram –ve aerobe/staphylococci cover; other organisms often need concurrent penicillin ± metronidazole.

Use: severe infections, esp sepsis, meningitis, endocarditis. Also pyelonephritis/prostatitis, biliary tract infections, pneumonia.

CI: MG*.

Caution: obesity, R/P/B/E.

SE: ototoxic, nephrotoxic (dose and Rx length dependent), hypersensitivity, rash. Rarely AAC, N&V, seizures, encephalopathy, blood disorders, myasthenia-like syndrome* (at ↑doses; reversible), ↓Mg^{2+} (if prolonged Rx).

Monitor: U&Es before and during Rx; serum levels** after three or four doses of multiple daily dosing, or 48 h of once-daily dosing or after dose change (earlier if RF).

Interactions: fx (esp toxicity) ↑ by loop diuretics (esp furosemide), cephalosporins, vancomycin, amphotericin, ciclosporin, tacrolimus and cytotoxics; if these drugs must be given, space doses as far from time of gentamicin dose as possible. ↑s fx of muscle relaxants and anticholinesterases, **W+**.

Dose: refer to local protocol if available, otherwise: once-daily regimen: initially, 5–7 mg/kg ivi (ideal Wt for Ht) adjusting to levels (*NB:* consult local protocol; od regimen not suitable if endocarditis, >20% total body surface burns or creatinine clearance <20 mL/ min). Multiple daily regimen: 3–5 mg/kg/day in three divided doses im/iv/ivi (if endocarditis, give 1 mg/kg bd iv).

NB: ↓doses if RF (and consider if elderly or ↑↑BMI), otherwise adjust according to serum levels*: call microbiology department if unsure.

Gentamicin levels: Measure peak at 1 h post-dose (ideally = 5–10 mg/L) and trough immediately pre-dose (multi-dosing ≤2 mg/L; od dosing <1 mg/L). Halve ideal peak levels if for endocarditis. If levels high, can ↑*spacing* of doses (as well as ↓ing *amount* of dose); as ⇒ ↑risk of ototoxicity, monitor auditory/vestibular function. *NB: od regimens usually only require* **pre-dose *level.*

GLIBENCLAMIDE

Oral antidiabetic (long-acting sulphonylurea): ↑s pancreatic insulin release – stimulates β-islet cell receptors (and inhibits gluconeogenesis).

G

Use: type 2 DM; requires endogenous insulin to work. Not recommended for obese* (use metformin) or elderly** (use short-acting preparations, e.g. gliclazide). Gestational diabetes: second and third trimesters (unlicensed[BNF]).

CI: ketoacidosis, porphyria, **L/R** (if either severe, otherwise caution), **P/B**.

Caution: may need to replace with insulin during intercurrent illness/surgery, porphyria, G6PD deficiency, **E**.

SE: hypoglycaemia (esp in elderly**), GI upset, ↑Wt*. Rarely hypersensitivity (inc skin) reactions, blood disorders, hepatotoxicity and transient visual Δs (esp initially).

Interactions: fx ↑d by chloramphenicol, sulphonamides (inc co-trimoxazole), sulfinpyrazone, antifungals (esp flu-/miconazole), warfarin, fibrates and NSAIDs. Levels ↓ by rifampicin/rifabutin. ↑risk of hepatotoxicity with bosentan.

Dose: initially 5 mg mane (with food), ↑ing as necessary (max 15 mg/day). *NB:* ↓dose in severe LF.

GLICLAZIDE

Oral antidiabetic (short-acting sulphonylurea).

Use/Caution/SE/Interactions: as glibenclamide, but shorter action* and hepatic metabolism** mean ↓d risk of hypoglycaemia (esp in elderly* and RF**).

CI: ketoacidosis.

Dose: initially 40–80 mg mane (with breakfast), ↑ing as necessary (max 320 mg/day). MR tablets available (**Diamicron MR, also Vitile XL, Dacadis MR**) of which 30 mg has equivalent effect to 80 mg of normal release (dose initially is 30 mg od, ↑ing if necessary to max 120 mg od). *NB:* ↓dose in RF or severe LF.

GLIMEPIRIDE

Oral antidiabetic (short-acting sulphonylurea).

Use/CI/Caution/SE/Interactions: as gliclazide, (also SE: ↓Na+). Manufacturer recommends monitoring of FBC and LFTs. CI in severe LF and ketoacidosis. Not CI in acute porphyria. May need to substitute with insulin; seek specialist advice.

Dose: initially 1 mg mane with food, ↑ as necessary[BNF] (max 6 mg/day).

GLIPIZIDE

Oral antidiabetic (short-acting sulphonylurea).
Use/CI/Caution/SE/Interactions: as gliclazide, plus avoid if both **L** and **R**. Not CI in acute porphyria. CI in ketoacidosis.
Dose: initially 2.5–5 mg mane (with food), ↑ing as necessary (max single dose 15 mg; max daily dose 20 mg). *NB:* ↓**dose in severe LF and RF.**

GLUCAGON

Polypeptide hormone: ↑s hepatic glycogen conversion to glucose.
Use: hypoglycaemia: if acute and severe, esp if no iv access or if 2° to xs insulin (see p. 414, refer '↓Glucose' in 'Emergencies' chapter).
CI: phaeo.
Caution: glucagonomas/insulinomas. Will not work if hypoglycaemia is chronic (inc starvation) or 2° to adrenal insufficiency.
SE: N&V, ↓ or ↑BP, ↓K+, ↑HR, rarely hypersensitivity, **W+**.
Dose: 1 mg (= 1 unit) im (or sc/iv)[SPC/BNF]; if no response in 10 min, iv glucose must be given.

Often stocked in cardiac arrest ('crash') trolleys. Good option in psych units, where iv access often limited.

GLYCEROL (= GLYCERIN) SUPPOSITORIES

Rectal irritant bowel stimulant.
Use: constipation: first-line suppository if oral methods such as lactulose and senna fail.
Dose: <1 year 1 g; 1–12 years 2 g; >12 years and adult 4 g pr prn.

GLYCERYL TRINITRATE see GTN.

GTN (= GLYCERYL TRINITRATE)

Nitrate: ⇒ coronary artery + systemic vein dilation ⇒ ↑O_2 supply to myocardium and ↓preload, ∴ ↓O_2 demand of myocardium.

G

Use: angina[1], unstable angina/acute MI[2], HF[2], anal fissure[3].
CI: ↓BP, ↓↓Hb, aortic/mitral stenosis, constrictive pericarditis, tamponade, HOCM, hypovolaemia, ↑ICP, toxic pulmonary oedema.
Caution: recent MI, ↓T_4, hypothermia, head trauma, cerebral haemorrhage, malnutrition, glaucoma (closed-angle), L/R (if either severe).
SE: ↓BP (inc postural), headache, dizziness, flushing, ↑HR.
Warn: may develop tolerance with ↓therapeutic effect (esp if long-term transdermal patch use) and do not stop abruptly.
Interactions: ☠ sildenafil, tadalafil and vardenafil (are CI as ⇒ ↓↓BP) ☠. ↓s fx of heparins (if given iv).
Dose: 1–2 sprays or 1–2 tablets sl prn (also available as transdermal SR patches[SPC/BNF])[1]. 10–200 micrograms/min ivi, titrating to clinical response and BP max 400 micrograms/min ivi[2]. 2.5 cm of ointment pr bd for up to 8 wk[3].

▼ GUANFACINE/INTUNIV

α_2-adrenergic receptor agonist ⇒ ↓noradrenaline release.
Use: ADHD in children if stimulants not suitable (initiated under specialist).
CI: hypersensitivity.
Caution: ↓HR/HB/↓K^+ (↑risk of torsade de pointes), Hx CVD/↑QTc, lactose intolerance.
SE: sedation, ↓BP, ↓HR, headache, GI upset, fatigue, ↓appetite, Δ mood, anxiety, ↓sleep, dizziness, rash, enuresis, ↑Wt.
Warn: If >1 dose missed, inform prescriber ⇒ consider re-titration. On discontinuation, rebound ↑BP/HR.
Monitor: assess at baseline to identify cardiac status (risks of ↓BP/HR, ↑QTc, arrhythmias), BMI and potential for sedation. Monitor wkly during titration, 3-monthly in first year, then 6-monthly. Check BP/HR when weaning down and after cessation.
Interactions: metab by P450; ↑levels with CYP3A4/3A5 inhibitors (e.g. ketoconazole, clarithromycin, indinavir),

↓levels with CYP3A4 inducers (e.g. rifampicin, carbamazepine, phenobarbital, phenytoin); also ↑levels of valproic acid; ↑risks of hypotension/syncope with antihypertensives; ↑risks of sedation/somnolence with CNS depressants.

Dose: 6–12 years (≥25 kg): initially 1 mg po od, adjusted by 1 mg/wk, maintenance 0.05–0.12 mg/kg od (max 4 mg); 13–17 years (34–41.4 kg): same as previous; 13–17 years (41.5–49.4 kg): same as previous – max 5 mg; 13–17 years (49.5–58.4 kg): same as previous – max 6 mg; 13–17 years (≥58.5 kg): same as previous – max 7 mg).

NB: ↓dose by half with concurrent use of moderate/potent CYP3A4 inhibitors; ↑dose up to max 7 mg od with concurrent use of potent CYP3A4 inducers.

☠ Overdose ⇒ ↑ then ↓BP, ↓HR, resp depression, lethargy. If lethargy develops, observe for up to 24 h. ☠

HALOPERIDOL/HALDOL

Typical antipsychotic: D_2 dopamine receptor antagonist.

Use: schizophrenia and schizoaffective disorder[1], mania in bipolar disorder[2], acute agitation[3]; where other treatments have failed: delirium, tic disorders, Huntington's; in palliative care: N&V, restlessness, confusion.

CI: CNS depression, ↑QTc, Hx ventricular arrhythmia, recent acute myocardial infarction, ↓K+, Parkinson's & related disorders, H.

Caution: as for other antipsychotics, **baseline and follow-up ECG needed,** L.

Class SE: EPSE, ↑prolactin and assoc Sx, sedation, ↑Wt, ↑QTc, VTE, blood dyscrasias, ↓seizure threshold, NMS.

Interactions: metab by P450; levels ↑ by fluoxetine, venlafaxine, quinidine, buspirone and ritonavir. Levels ↓ by carbamazepine, phenytoin, rifampicin. ↑risk of arrhythmias with amiodarone and ↓s fx of anticonvulsants.

Dose: 2–10 mg po daily in one to two divided doses (max 20 mg/day)[1]; 2–10 mg po daily in one to two divided doses (max 15 mg/day)[2]; 5–10 mg po, repeated after 12 h if necessary (max 20 mg/day) or 5 mg im, repeated hrly if necessary (max 12 mg but some sources, e.g. BNF & some SPCs, give max dose as 20 mg im)[3]; use quarter to half adult doses in elderly; bioavailability varies by route: 5 mg po = 3 mg im.

☠ Start at bottom of dose range if naive to antipsychotics, esp if elderly. See p. 373, refer 'Rapid Tranquilisation' section in 'Emergencies' chapter for rapid tranquilisation guidelines.

HALOPERIDOL DECANOATE/HALDOL DECANOATE

Typical antipsychotic: D_2 dopamine receptor antagonist. Long-acting injection ($t_{1/2} \sim 21$ days).

Use: maintenance treatment of schizophrenia and schizoaffective disorder in patients stabilised on po haloperidol.

CI/Caution/SE/Warn/Monitor: as for haloperidol.

Interactions: metab by P450; levels ↑ by fluoxetine, venlafaxine, quinidine, buspirone and ritonavir. Levels ↓ by carbamazepine, phenytoin, rifampicin. ↑risk of arrhythmias with amiodarone and ↓s fx of anticonvulsants.

Dose: 10–15 times the daily dose of po haloperidol given every 4 wk im (administered into upper outer buttock/lateral thigh), adjusted if necessary in steps of 50 mg every 4 wk; usual maintenance dose 50–200 mg every 4 wk, max 300 mg every 4 wk. Elderly: initially 12.5–25 mg every 4 wk; usual maintenance dose 25–75 mg every 4 wk, max 75 mg every 4 wk.

HUMALOG short-acting recombinant insulin. Also available as biphasic preparations (Mix 25, Mix 50), are combined with longer-acting isophane suspension.

HUMULIN Recombinant insulin available in various forms:

1 HUMULIN S soluble, short-acting for iv/acute use.
2 HUMULIN I isophane (with protamine), intermediate acting.

3 HUMULIN M 'biphasic' preparations, combination of short-acting (S) and intermediate-acting (I) forms to give smoother control throughout the day. Numbers denote 1/10% of soluble insulin (i.e. M3 = 30% soluble insulin).

HYDROCORTISONE BUTYRATE CREAM (0.1%)

Potent-strength topical corticosteroid. *NB*: much stronger than 'standard' (i.e. non-butyrate) hydrocortisone cream; see next entry.

HYDROCORTISONE CREAM/OINTMENT (1%)

Mild-strength topical corticosteroid (rarely used as weaker 0.5%, 0.25% and 0.1% preparations).
Use: inflammatory skin conditions, in particular, eczema.
CI: untreated infection, rosacea, acne.
SE: rare compared to more potent steroids: skin atrophy, worsening of infections, acne.
Dose: apply thinly to affected area(s) one or two times per day.

HYDROCORTISONE IV/PO

Glucocorticoid (with significant mineralocorticoid activity).
Use: acute hypersensitivity (esp anaphylaxis, angioedema), Addisonian crisis, asthma, COPD, $\downarrow T_4$ (and $\uparrow T_4$), IBD. Also used po in chronic adrenocortical insufficiency.
CI: systemic infection (unless appropriate antibiotics prescribed), live vaccines, cerebral oedema due to head injury/CVA.
Caution: DM, epilepsy, HTN, glaucoma, osteoporosis, PU, TB, severe mood disorders, L/R.
SE: ↑infections, metabolic (fluid retention, ↑lipids, ↑Wt, DM, ↑Na^+, ↓K^+), adrenal suppression, bruising, cardiac (HTN, CCF, myocardial rupture post-MI, TE), musculoskeletal (proximal myopathy, osteoporosis), worsening of seizures, Ψ fx (anxiety, depression, psychosis), ocular (cataract, glaucoma, corneal/scleral thinning), GI (peptic/duodenal ulcer – give PPI if on ↑doses, pancreatitis).
Warn: avoid contact with chickenpox if not infected previously.
☠Risk of Addisonian crisis if abrupt withdrawal – must ↓ slowly if >3 wk Rx ☠.

L/R/H = Liver, Renal and Heart failure. E = elderly. P = pregnancy. B = breastfeeding.

Interactions: fx can be ↓d by rifampicin, carbamazepine, phenytoin and phenobarbital. fx (and risk of adrenal suppression) can be ↑d by erythromycin, ritonavir, ketoconazole, itraconazole and ciclosporin (whose own fx are ↑d by methylprednisolone). ↑risk of ↓K^+ with amphotericin and digoxin. Risk of ↑ or ↓anticoagulant effect of coumarins.

Dose: *acutely:* 100–500 mg im or slowly iv up to qds if required. Exact dose recommendations vary: consult local protocol if unsure. *Chronic replacement:* usually 20–30 mg po daily in divided doses (usually 2/3 in morning and 1/3 nocte), often together with fludrocortisone.

HYDROXOCOBALAMIN

Vit B_{12} replacement.
Use: pernicious anaemia (also macrocytic anaemias with neurological involvement, tobacco amblyopia, Leber's optic atrophy). Cyanide poisoning.
SE: skin reactions, nausea, flu-like symptoms, ↓K^+(initially), rarely anaphylaxis.
Interactions: fx ↓ by OCP and chloramphenicol.
Dose: 1 mg im injection: frequently at first for Rx (2–3/wk: exact number depends on indication[SPC/BNF]) until no further improvement, then ↓frequency (to once every 1–3 months) for maintenance. For cyanide poisoning, see BNF.

HYOSCINE BUTYLBROMIDE/BUSCOPAN

Antimuscarinic: ↓s GI motility. Does not cross blood-brain barrier (unlike hyoscine *hydrobromide*): less sedative.
Use: GI (or GU) smooth-muscle spasm; esp biliary colic, diverticulitis and IBS. Also xs respiratory secretions and rarely dysmenorrhoea.
CI: glaucoma (closed-angle), MG, megacolon, ↑prostate.
Caution: GI obstruction, ↑prostate/urinary retention, ↑HR (inc ↑T_4), H/P/E.
SE: antimuscarinic fx (see p. 346, refer 'Cholinoceptors' in 'Basic Psychopharmacology' chapter), drowsiness, confusion.

Interactions: ↓s fx of metoclopramide (and vice versa) and sublingual nitrates. ↑s tachycardic fx of β-agonists.

Dose: 20 mg qds po (for IBS, start at 10 mg tds) or 20 mg im/iv (repeating once after 30 min, if necessary; max 100 mg/day).

Do not confuse with hyoscine *hydrobromide*: different fx and doses.

HYOSCINE HYDROBROMIDE (= SCOPOLAMINE)

Antimuscarinic: predominant fx on CNS (↓s vestibular activity[1]). Also ↓s respiratory/oral secretions[2,3].

Use: motion sickness[1], terminal care/chronic ↓swallow[2] (e.g. CVA), hypersalivation 2° to antipsychotics[3] (unlicensed use).

CI: GI obstruction, severe UC, pyloric stenosis, ↑prostate/urinary retention, glaucoma (closed-angle).

Caution: cardiovascular disease, HTN, porphyria, Down syndrome, MG, diarrhoea, GORD, UC, ↑thyroid, glaucoma, fever L/R/P/B/E.

SE: antimuscarinic fx, generally sedative (although rarely ⇒ paradoxical agitation when given as sc infusion).

Interactions: ↓s fx of sublingual nitrates (e.g. GTN).

Dose: 150–300 micrograms 6-hrly po (max 900 micrograms/24 h)[1] (or as transdermal patches; release 1 mg over 72 h); 600 micrograms–2.4 mg/24 h as sc infusion[2]; 300 micrograms bd po[3] (can ↑ to tds).

Do not confuse with hyoscine butylbromide with different fx and doses.

HYPROMELLOSE 0.3% EYE DROPS

Artificial tears for treatment of dry eyes.

Dose: 1–2 drops prn.

IBUGEL see Ibuprofen; topical gel for musculoskeletal pain.

IBUPROFEN

Mild-to-moderate strength NSAID. Non-selective COX inhibitor; analgesic, anti-inflammatory and antipyrexial† properties.

L/R/H = Liver, Renal and Heart failure. E = elderly. P = pregnancy. B = breastfeeding.

Use: mild-to-moderate pain[1] (inc musculoskeletal, headache, migraine, dysmenorrhoea, dental, post-op; not first choice for gout/RA, as ↓anti-inflammatory fx compared to other NSAIDs), mild local inflammation[2].

CI: Hx of hypersensitivity to aspirin or any other NSAID (inc asthma/angioedema/urticaria/rhinitis). **Active/Hx of PU/GI bleeding/perforation, L/R/H** (if any of these three are severe)/**P** (third trimester). Topical: do not use on broken skin.

Caution: asthma, allergic disorders, uncontrolled HTN, IHD, PVD, cerebrovascular disease, cardiovascular risk factors, connective tissue disorders, coagulopathy, IBD. *Can mask signs of infection*† **L/R/H/P** (first/second trimester: preferably avoid)/**B/E**.

SE: GI upset/bleeding/PU (*less than other NSAIDs*). AKI, hypersensitivity reactions (esp bronchospasm and skin reactions, inc, very rarely, SJS/TEN), fluid retention/oedema, headache, dizziness, nervousness, depression, drowsiness, insomnia, tinnitus, photosensitivity, haematuria. >1.2 g/day ⇒ small ↑risk of thrombotic events. Reversible ↓female fertility if long-term use. Very rarely, blood disorders, ↑BP, ↑K⁺.

Interactions: ↑risk GI bleeding with aspirin, clopidogrel, anti-coagulants, corticosteroids, SSRIs, venlafaxine and erlotinib. ↑s (toxic) fx of digoxin, quinolones, lithium, phenytoin, baclofen, methotrexate, zidovudine and sulphonylureas. ↑risk of RF with ACE-i, ARB, diuretics, tacrolimus and ciclosporin. ↑risk of ↑K⁺ with K-sparing diuretics and aldosterone antagonists. ↓s fx of antihypertensives and diuretics. ↑levels with ritonavir and triazoles. Mild **W+**.

Dose: initially 200–400 mg tds po[1] (max 2.4 g/day); topically as gel: apply to affected areas up to tds[2].

NB: avoid/↓dose in RF and consider gastroprotective Rx.

IMIPRAMINE

TCA: blocks reuptake of NA and 5-HT through binding to noradrenaline transporter (NAT) and serotonin transport (SERT).
Use: depression[1], nocturnal enuresis in children, ADHD in children (unlicensed).

CI: as for amitriptyline, **L/H**.

Caution: as for amitriptyline, **L/H/P/E**.

Class SE: antimuscarinic fx (constipation, dry mouth, blurred vision), **cardiac fx** (arrhythmias, HB, ↑HR, postural ↓BP, dizziness, syncope: **dangerous in OD**), ↑**Wt, sedation** (often ⇒ 'hangover'), seizures, Δ LFTs, ↓Na⁺ (esp in elderly), agitation, confusion, NMS.

Warn: may cause discontinuation symptoms if stopped abruptly.

Monitor: elderly patients for cardiac and psychiatric SE and electrolytes.

Interactions: ☠ never give with, or ≤3 wk after, MAOIs; do not give MAOIs within 3 wk of stopping imipramine.☠

Dose: initially 75 mg po in divided doses, increasing to 150–200 mg daily; determine maintenance dose (usually 50–100 mg) once in remission[1],[SPC]

☠ Overdose is associated with high rate of fatality. TCA overdose ⇒ dilated pupils, arrhythmias, ↓BP, hypothermia, hyperreflexia, extensor plantar responses, seizures, respiratory depression and coma. ☠

INDAPAMIDE

Thiazide derivative diuretic; see Bendroflumethiazide.

Use: HTN.

CI: Hx of sulphonamide derivative allergy, ↓K⁺, ↓Na⁺, ↑Ca²⁺, **L/R** (if either severe).

Caution: ↑PTH (stop if ↑Ca²⁺), ↑aldosterone, gout, nephrotic syndrome, porphyria, previous photosensitivity with other thiazide and related diuretics, **R/P/B/E**.

SE: as bendroflumethiazide, but reportedly fewer metabolic disturbances (esp less hyperglycaemia).

Monitor: U&Es, urate.

Interactions: as bendroflumethiazide (*NB:* ↑s lithium levels).

Dose: 2.5 mg od mane (or 1.5 mg od of MR preparation).

INFLIXIMAB/REMICADE/ERELZI

Monoclonal Ab against TNF-α (inflammatory cytokine).
Use: Crohn's/UC[NICE], RA[NICE], psoriasis (for skin or arthritis)[NICE] or ankylosing spondylitis.[NICE]
CI: TB or other severe infections, **H** (unless mild when only caution), **P/B**.
Caution: infections, demyelinating CNS disorders, malignancy (inc Hx of), **L/R**.
SE: severe infections, TB (inc extrapulmonary), CCF (exac of), CNS demyelination. Also GI upset, flu-like symptoms, cough, fatigue, headache. ↑incidence of hypersensitivity (esp transfusion) reactions.
Dose: specialist use only. Often prescribed concurrently with methotrexate.

INSULATARD Intermediate-acting (isophane) insulin, either recombinant human or porcine/bovine.

INSULIN see under brand name.

IPRATROPIUM

Inh short-acting muscarinic antagonist; bronchodilator and ↓s bronchial secretions.
Use: chronic[1] and acute[2] bronchospasm (COPD > asthma). Rarely used topically for rhinitis.
SE: antimuscarinic fx (see p. 346, refer 'Cholinoceptors' in 'Basic Psychopharmacology' chapter), usually minimal.
Caution: glaucoma (angle-closure only; protect patient's eyes from drug, esp if giving nebs: use tight-fitting mask), bladder outflow obstruction (e.g. ↑prostate), cystic fibrosis, **P/B**.
Dose: 20–40 micrograms tds/qds inh[1] (max 80 micrograms qds); 250–500 micrograms qds neb[2] (↑ing up to 4 hrly if severe).

IRBESARTAN/APROVEL

Angiotensin II antagonist.
Use: HTN, type 2 DM nephropathy.
CI: **P/B**.

Caution/SE/Interactions: see Losartan.
Dose: initially 150 mg od, ↑ing to 300 mg od if required (halve initial dose if age >75 years or on haemodialysis).

IRON TABLETS see Ferrous sulphate/fumarate/gluconate.

ISMN see Isosorbide mononitrate.

ISMO see Isosorbide mononitrate.

ISOCARBOXAZID

MAOI; non-selective and irreversible inhibitor of monoamine oxidase, ↑5-HT, NA and DA in CNS.
Use: depression.
CI: cerebrovascular disease, mania, phaeo, **L**.
Caution: porphyria, agitation, blood disorders, concurrent ECT, DM, epilepsy, severe hypertensive reaction, surgery.
SE: postural ↓BP, arrhythmia, oedema, dizziness, dry mouth, GI upset (N&V&C), ↓sleep, blurred vision, drowsiness.
Warn: Avoid tyramine-/dopa-rich food/drinks during Rx/for 2–3 wk after stopping MAOI, withdrawal fx may occur within 5 days of stopping treatment, ↑symptoms after regular administration for 8 wk+, dose reduction gradually over 4 wk+.
Monitor: BP (↑risk of postural hypotension and hypertensive responses).
Interactions: ☠↑risk of severe toxic reaction with serotonergics, dopaminergics and noradrenergics: SSRIs, SNRIs, NARIs, TCAs (and related drugs), other MAOIs (inc for Parkinson's disease), carbamazepine, linezolid, triptans, pethidine, tramadol.☠

- Do not start isocarboxazid until these drugs have been stopped and they have cleared: 5 wk for fluoxetine, 3 wk for clomipramine/imipramine, at least 7–14 days for other drugs.
- Wait 2 wk after stopping isocarboxazid before starting any of these medicines.

↑risk of hypertensive crisis with sympathomimetics, dopamine agonists, CNS stimulants, buspirone. ↑fx of CNS depressants, antimuscarinics, antidiabetics, antihypertensives.

Dose: initially 30 mg po od, in single/divided doses, ↑ after 4 wk to 60 mg od for 4–6 wk, then ↓ to maintenance dose 10–20 mg od up to 40 mg od.

🙋 Hypertensive crisis may develop if taken with food high in tyramine or DOPA. See p. 236, refer 'MAOI tyramine effect' heading in 'Depression' section of 'Disorders' chapter. 🙋

ISOSORBIDE MONONITRATE (ISMN)

Nitrate; as GTN, but po rather than sl delivery. GTN usually treatment, but ISMN generally prophylaxis.
Use/CI/Caution/SE/Interactions: as GTN, but ⇒ ↓headache.
Dose: 10–40 mg bd po (od MR preparations available^SPC/BNF).

ISTIN see Amlodipine; Ca²⁺ channel blocker for HTN/IHD.

ITRACONAZOLE/SPORANOX

Triazole antifungal: needs acidic pH for good po absorption*.
Use: fungal infections (candida, tinea, cryptococcus, aspergillosis, histoplasmosis, onychomycosis, pityriasis versicolor).
Caution: risk of HF: Hx of cardiac disease or if on negative inotropic drugs (risk ↑s with dose, length of Rx and age), L/R/P/B.
SE: HF, hepatotoxicity**, GI upset, headache, dizziness, peripheral neuropathy (if occurs, stop drug), cholestasis, menstrual Δs, skin reactions (inc angioedema, SJS). With prolonged Rx can ⇒ ↓K⁺, oedema, hair loss.
Monitor: LFTs** if Rx >1 month or Hx of (or develop clinical features of) liver disease: stop drug if become abnormal.
Interactions: ↓P450 ∴ many; most importantly ↑s risk of myopathy with statins (avoid together) and ↑s risk of HF with negative inotropes (esp Ca²⁺ blockers). ↑s fx of 🙋 midazolam, quinidine, pimozide 🙋, ciclosporin, digoxin, indinavir and siro-/tacrolimus. fx ↓d by rifampicin, phenytoin and antacids*, W+.
Dose: dependent on indication.^SPC/BNF *Take capsules with food (or water on empty stomach). NB:* consider ↓dose in LF.

IVABRADINE/PROCORALAN

↓s HR by selective cardiac pacemaker I_f channel current blockade ⇒ ↓SAN myocyte Na^+ and K^+ entry.

Use: angina[1] (if sinus rhythm and β-blockers CI/not tolerated), HF[2].

CI: ↓HR (<70 bpm[1] or <75 bpm[2]) or ↓BP, cardiogenic shock, ACS (inc acute MI), acute CVA, second- or third-degree HB, SSS, pacemaker dependent, SAN block congenital ↑QT syndrome, strong **P450 3A4** inhibitors/diltiazem/verapamil**, **L** (if severe)/**H** (if moderate/severe)/**P/B**.

Caution: retinitis pigmentosa, galactose intolerance*/Lapp lactase deficiency*/glucose-galactose malabsorption*, **R/E**.

SE: visual Δs (esp luminous phenomena*), ↓HR, HB, ectopics, VF, headaches, dizziness. Less commonly GI upset, cramps, dyspnoea, ↑EØ, ↑uric acid, ↓GFR.

Warn: tablets contain lactose*, may ↓vision if night driving/using machinery with rapid light intensity Δs.

Monitor: HR (maintain resting ventricular rate >50 bpm) and rhythm, BP.

Interactions: ☠ metab by P450 3A4; inhibitors ↑levels and strong inhibitors** (clari-/ery-/josa-/telithromycin, itra-/ketoconazole, nelfi-/ritonavir, nefazodone) are CI but ↓doses can be given with fluconazole. Inducers ↓levels (inc rifampicin, barbiturates, phenytoin, St John's wort). Levels also ↑ by diltiazem and verapamil. ↑risk of VF with drugs that ↑QTc (inc amiodarone, disopyramide, mefloquine, pentamidine, pimozide, sertindole, sotalol) ☠.

Dose: initially 5 mg bd po; ↑ing if required after 3–4 wk[1] or 2 wk[2] to max 7.5 mg bd po. *NB:* consider ↓dose if not tolerated, elderly or severe RF.^SPC/BNF

KAY-CEE-L

KCl syrup (1 mmol/mL) for ↓K^+; see **Sando-K**.

Dose: according to serum K^+: average 25–50 mL/day in divided doses if diet normal. Caution if taking other drugs that ↑K^+. Give after food. *NB:* ↓dose if **RF**.

L

KEPPRA see Levetiracetam.

LABETALOL

β-blocker with arteriolar vasodilatory properties ∴ also ⇒ ↓TPR.
Use: uncontrolled/severe HTN (inc during pregnancy[1] or post-MI[2] or with angina).
CI/Caution/SE/Interactions: as propranolol, plus can ⇒
☠ severe/postural ↓BP ☠ and hepatotoxicity* (L).
Monitor: LFTs* (if deteriorate stop drug).
Dose: initially 100 mg bd po (halve dose in elderly), ↑ing every fortnight if necessary to max of 600 mg qds po; if essential to ↓BP rapidly give 50 mg iv over ≥1 min repeating after 5 min if necessary (or can give 2 mg/min ivi), up to max total dose 200 mg; 20 mg/h ivi[1], doubling every 30 min to max of 160 mg/h; 15 mg/h ivi[2], ↑ing slowly to max of 120 mg/h. *NB:* consider ↓dose in RF and elderly.

LACRI-LUBE

Artificial tears for dry eyes.
SE: blurred vision ∴ usually used at bedtime (or if vision secondary consideration, e.g. Bell's palsy or blind eye).
Dose: one application prn.

LACTULOSE

Osmotic laxative[1]. Also ↓s growth of NH_4-producing bacteria[2].
Use: constipation[1], hepatic encephalopathy[2].
CI: GI obstruction, digestive perforation (or risk of) or galactosaemia.
Caution: lactose intolerance.
SE: flatulence, distension, abdo pains.
Dose: 15 mL od/bd[1] (↑dose according to response; *NB: can take 2 days to work*); 30–45 mL tds-qds[2]. *Take with plenty of water.*

LAMISIL see Terbinafine.

LAMOTRIGINE/LAMICTAL

Antiepileptic: ↓s release of excitatory amino acids (esp glutamate) via action on voltage-sensitive Na^+ channels.

Use: epilepsy (esp focal and 1° or 2° generalised tonic-clonic), Px depressive episode in bipolar disorder.

Caution: avoid abrupt withdrawal† (rebound seizure risk; taper off over ≥2 wk unless stopping due to serious skin reaction). Myoclonic seizures and Parkinson's can be exacerbated. L/R/P/B/E.

SE: cerebellar symptoms, skin reactions (often severe, e.g. SJS, TEN, lupus, esp in children, if on valproate, or high initial doses), blood disorders (↓Hb, ↓WCC, ↓Pt), N&V. Rarely, ↓memory, sedation, aggression, irritability, sleep Δ, pretibial ulcers, alopecia, worsening of seizures, poly-/anuria, **hepatotoxicity.**

Warn: report rash plus any flu-like symptoms, signs of infection/↓Hb or bruising. Do not stop tablets suddenly†. Risk of suicidal ideation.

Monitor: U&Es, FBC, LFTs, clotting.

Interactions: fx are ↓d by OCP, phenytoin, carbamazepine fx ↑d by valproate.

Dose: 25–500 mg daily; ↑dose slowly to ↓risk of skin reactions (also need to restart at low dose; repeat dose titration if >5 days missed); standard titration in bipolar disorder: 25 mg od for 14 days, then 50 mg in 1–2 divided doses for 14 days, then 100 mg in 1–2 divided doses for 7 days, then 200 mg maintenance in 1–2 divided doses; titration speed and final dose need adjustment if co-prescribed with valproate or enzyme inducers[BNF,SPC]. *NB:* ↓**dose in LF.**

LANSOPRAZOLE/ZOTON

PPI. As omeprazole, but ↓interactions.

Dose: 15–30 mg od po (↓ to 15 mg od for maintenance). For *H. pylori* eradication: 30 mg bd for 7 days.

LASIX see Furosemide; loop diuretic.

LATANOPROST 0.005%/XALATAN

Topical PG analogue: ↑s uveoscleral outflow.

Use: ↑IOP in glaucoma and *ocular* HTN (first-line agent).

CI: herpetic keratitis (inc recurrent Hx of).

Caution: asthma (if severe), aphakia, pseudophakia, uveitis, macular oedema, P/B.

SE: iris colour Δ* (can $\Rightarrow$ permanent ↑brown pigmentation, esp if uniocular use), blurred vision, local reactions (e.g. conjunctival hyperaemia in up to 30% initially). Also darkening of periocular skin and ↑eyelash length (both reversible). Rarely cystoid macular oedema (if aphakia), uveitis, angina.

Warn: can Δ iris colour*.

Dose: 1 drop od 50 microgram/mL (=0.005%) (preferably in the evening).

LEVETIRACETAM/KEPPRA

Antiepileptic: Δs intraneuronal Ca^{2+} levels/inhibits pre-synaptic Ca^{2+} channels. Binds to synaptic vesicle glycoprotein 2A.

Use: focal seizures (monotherapy[1] or adjunctive[2]), myoclonic/tonic-clonic seizures[3].

Caution: avoid abrupt withdrawal, suicidal ideation, R/P/B.

SE: nasopharyngitis, headache, somnolence, anorexia (uncommonly $\Rightarrow$ ↓Wt), N&V&D, abdo pain, dyspepsia, tremor, dizziness, vertigo, convulsion, lethargy, drowsiness, fatigue, agitation, Ψ disturbance (depression, anxiety, personality disorder). Uncommonly visual Δ (blurred/diplopia), thrombocyto-/leukopenia, rash, alopecia, suicidal ideation, confusion, amnesia, paraesthesia, Δ LFTs. Rarely pancreatitis, LF, movement disorders, neutro-/pancytopenia, SJS/TEN.

Warn: to seek medical advice if depression/suicidality develop and not to discontinue drug abruptly against medical advice (risk of withdrawal syndrome).

Monitor: for signs of depression and/or suicidality.

Interactions: levels may be ↑ by probenecid (and other drugs affecting tubular secretion). fx potentially ↓ if taken <1 h after macrogol. Can ↑ methotrexate levels.

Dose: initially 250 mg od[1] or 250 mg bd[2,3] po/ivi, ↑ing slowly[BNF/SPC] to max 1.5 g bd po/iv. *NB:* consider ↓dose in elderly or if LF or RF.[BNF/SPC]

LEVOBUNOLOL

β-blocker eye drops: similar to timolol ⇒ ↓aqueous humour production. *Significant systemic absorption can occur.*
Use: chronic simple (wide-/open-angle) glaucoma.
CI/Caution/Interactions: as propranolol; interactions less likely; corneal disease is caution.
SE: local reactions. Rarely anterior uveitis and anaphylaxis. Can ⇒ systemic fx, esp bronchoconstriction/cardiac fx; see Propranolol.
Dose: 1 drop of 0.5% solution od/bd.

LEVODOPA (= L-DOPA)

Precursor of dopamine: needs concomitant peripheral dopa decarboxylase inhibitor such as benserazide (see Co-beneldopa) or carbidopa (see Co-careldopa) to limit SEs.
Use: parkinsonism.
CI: glaucoma (closed-angle), taking MAO-A inhibitors, melanoma[†], severe psychosis, **P/B**.
Caution: pulmonary/cardiovascular/Ψ disease, endocrine disorder, glaucoma (open-angle), osteomalacia, Hx of PU or seizures, ventricular arrhythmias, **L/R**.
SE: dyskinesias, abdo upset, postural ↓BP, arrhythmias, drowsiness, **aggression**, Ψ **disorders** (confusion, depression, suicide, hallucinations, psychosis, hypomania, impulse control disorders), seizures, dizziness, headache, flushing, sweating, peripheral neuropathy, taste Δs, rash/pruritus, can reactivate melanoma,[†] Δ LFTs, GI bleeding, blood disorders, dark body fluids (inc sweat).
Warn: can ⇒ daytime sleepiness (inc sudden-onset sleep).
Interactions: fx ↓d by neuroleptics, SEs ↑d by bupropion, **risk of ↑BP crisis with MAOIs** (but can give with MAO-B inhibitors), iron ↓s absorption, risk of arrhythmias with halothane.
Dose: 150–800 mg daily (expressed as levodopa), *after food,* ↑ing according to response.

Abrupt withdrawal can ⇒ neuroleptic malignant-like syndrome.

L/R/H = Liver, Renal and Heart failure. E = elderly. P = pregnancy. B = breastfeeding.

L

LEVOMEPROMAZINE (= METHOTRIMEPRAZINE)

Phenothiazine antipsychotic; as chlorpromazine, but used in palliative care, as has good antiemetic[1] and sedative[2] fx but little respiratory depression.

Use: refractory N&V[1] or restlessness/distress[2] in the terminally ill.

CI/Caution/SE/Interactions: as chlorpromazine, but ↑risk of postural ↓BP (esp in elderly: do not give if age >50 years and ambulant) and ↑risk of seizures (caution if epilepsy/brain tumour). Also caution if FHx of ↑QTc.

Dose: 6.25–25 mg po/sc/im/iv od/bd (can ↑ to tds/qds), or 25–200 mg/24 h sc infusion. **Parenteral dose is half equivalent oral dose.** *NB: for N&V low doses may be effective and ⇒ ↓sedation. Doses >25 mg sc/24 h rarely needed unless sedation required and >100 mg sc/24 h require specialist supervision. NB: ↓dose in RF and elderly.*

LEVOTHYROXINE see Thyroxine.

LIBRIUM see Chlordiazepoxide; long-acting benzodiazepine.

LIDOCAINE (previously LIGNOCAINE)

Class Ib antiarrhythmic (↓s conduction in Purkinje and ventricular muscle fibres), local anaesthetic (blocks axonal Na+ channels).

Use: ventricular arrhythmias (esp post-MI), local anaesthesia.

CI: myocardial depression (if severe), SAN disorders, atrioventricular block (all grades).

Caution: epilepsy, severe hypoxia/hypovolaemia/↓HR, porphyria, L/H/P/E.

SE: dizziness, drowsiness, confusion, tinnitus, blurred vision, paraesthesia, GI upset, arrhythmias, ↓BP, ↓HR. Rarely respiratory depression, seizures, anaphylaxis.

Monitor: ECG during iv administration.

Interactions: ↑risk of arrhythmias with antipsychotics, dolasetron and quinu-/dalfopristin. ↑myocardial depression with other antiarrhythmics and β-blockers. Levels ↑ by propranolol, ataza-/lopinavir and cimetidine. Prolongs action of suxamethonium.

Dose (for ventricular arrhythmias): 50–100 mg iv at rate of 25–30 mg/min followed immediately by ivi at 4 mg/min for 30 min then 2 mg/min for 2 h and 1 mg/min thereafter (↓dose further if drug needed for >24 h). *NB:* short $t_{1/2}$ ∴ if 15 min delay in setting up ivi, can give max two further doses of 50–100 mg iv ≥10 min apart. In emergencies, can often be found stocked in crash trolleys as Minijet syringes of 1% (10 mg/mL) or 2% (20 mg/mL) solutions.

☠ Local anaesthetic preparations must never be injected into veins or inflamed tissue, as can ⇒ systemic fx (esp arrhythmias) ☠.

LIGNOCAINE see Lidocaine.

LIOTHYRONINE (= L-TRI-IODOTHYRONINE) SODIUM

Synthetic T_3: quicker and more potent action than thyroxine (T_4).
Use: severe hypothyroidism (e.g. myxoedema coma*)[1] Treatment-resistant depression (off-license)[2].
CI/Caution/SE/Interactions: see Thyroxine.
Dose: 5–20 micrograms iv slowly. Repeat every 4–12 h as necessary; seek expert help[1] 25–50 microgram/day po[2].
NB: 20 micrograms liothyronine =100 micrograms (levo)thyroxine.

Concurrent hydrocortisone iv is often also needed*

LISINOPRIL

ACE-i; see Captopril.
Use: HTN[1], HF[2], Px of IHD post-MI[3], DM nephropathy[4].
CI/Caution/SE/Interactions: as captopril.
Dose: initially 10 mg od[1] (2.5–5 mg if RF or used with diuretic), ↑ing if necessary to max 80 mg/day; initially 2.5–5 mg od[2,4] adjusted to response to usual maintenance of 5–20 mg/day (max 35 mg/day[2]). Doses post-MI[3] depend on BP.[SPC/BNF] *NB:* ↓dose in LF or RF.

LITHIUM

Mood stabiliser: modulates intracellular signalling; blocks neuronal Ca^{2+} channels and changes GABA pathways.

L

Use: mania Rx/Px, bipolar disorder Px. Rarely for recurrent depression Px and aggressive/self-mutilating behaviour Rx.

CI: ↓T$_4$ (if untreated), Addison's, SSS, dehydration, cardiovascular disease, **R/H/B**.
(*NB:* manufacturers do not agree on definitive list and all CI are relative – decisions should be made in clinical context and expert help sought if unsure.)

Caution: thyroid disease, MG, epilepsy, ↑QTc, psoriasis (risk of exacerbation), **P** (⇒ Ebstein's anomaly: esp in first trimester) **E**.

SE: thirst, polyuria, GI upset (↑Wt, N&V&D), *fine tremor**.
(*NB:* in toxicity ⇒ *coarse* tremor), tardive dyskinesia, muscular weakness, acne, psoriasis exacerbation, ↑WCC, ↑Pt. Rarer but serious: ↓ (or ↑) T$_4$ ± goitre (esp in females), renal impairment (diabetes insipidus, interstitial nephritis), arrhythmias. Very rarely can ⇒ neuroleptic malignant syndrome.

Warn: report symptoms of ↓T$_4$, avoid dehydration/salt depletion/abrupt withdrawal.

Monitor: serum levels *12 h post-dose:* keep at 0.6–1 mmol/L (>1.5 mmol/L may ⇒ toxicity, esp if elderly), U&Es, TFTs, cardiac function.

Interactions: toxicity (± levels) ↑d by **NSAIDs, diuretics**** (esp thiazides), SSRIs, ACE-i, ARBs, amiodarone, methyldopa, carbamazepine and haloperidol. Theophyllines, caffeine and antacids may ↓lithium levels.

Dose: see SPC/BNF: two *types* (salts) available with different doses ('carbonate' 200 mg = 'citrate' 509 mg) and bioavailabilities of particular *brands* vary ∴ *must specify salt and brand required.* For 'carbonate', starting dose usually 200 mg nocte, adjusting to plasma levels (maintenance usually 600 mg–1 g nocte).
NB: ↓dose in RF.

Consider stopping 24 h before major surgery or ECT; restart once e'lytes return to normal. Discuss with anaesthetist ± psychiatrist.

!!

> *Lithium toxicity*
> *Features:* D&V, coarse tremor*, cerebellar signs, renal
> impairment/oliguria, ↓BP, ↑reflexes, convulsions, drowsiness
> ⇒ coma, arrhythmia. *Rx:* stop drug, control seizures, correct
> electrolytes (normally need saline ivi; high risk if ↑Na⁺: avoid
> low-salt diets and diuretics**). Consider haemodialysis if RF.

LOCOID see Hydrocortisone butyrate 0.1% (potent steroid) cream.

LOFEPRAMINE
Second-generation TCA.
Use: depression.
CI/Caution/SE/Warn/Monitor/Interactions: as amitriptyline but
also **R** (if severe). Also ⇒ ↓sedation (sometimes alerting – do not give
nocte if occurs) and ↓anticholinergic and cardiac SEs ∴ ↓*danger in OD*.
Dose: 140–210 mg daily in divided (bd/tds) doses (consider ↓dose
in elderly).

LOFEXIDINE HYDROCHLORIDE
α_2-adrenergic receptor agonist ⇒ ↓noradrenaline release.
Use: symptomatic relief of opioid withdrawal.
Caution: ↓BP/HR, Hx of ↑QTc, coronary artery disease,
cerebrovascular disease, depression, metabolic Δs.
SE: drowsiness, cardiac fx (↓BP, ↓HR), mucosal dryness, ↑QTc.
Warn: withdraw gradually over 2–4 days+ to ↓risk of rebound
HTN.
Monitor: pulse, BP at initiation, for at least 72 h/until stable dose
achieved, and on discontinuation.
Interactions: ↑risk of ↑QTc with amifampridine, amiodarone,
amisulpride, apomorphine, clari-/erythromycin, clopamide,
(es)citalopram, fluconazole, haloperidol; ↑risk of ↓K⁺ (↑risk
of torsade de pointes) with aminophylline, corticosteroids,
bendroflumethiazide, fludrocortisone, furosemide, ↑CNS
depressive fx of alcohol, barbiturates, other sedatives; ↑fx of
antihypertensives; ↓fx with TCA.

Dose: initially 800 microgram po od in divided doses, ↑ in steps of 400–800 microgram od, max 800 microgram per dose, max 2.4 mg od, duration of 7–10 days if no opioid use.

LOPERAMIDE/IMODIUM
Antimotility agent: synthetic opioid analogue; binds to receptors in GI muscle ⇒ ↓peristalsis, ↑transit time, ↑H_2O/electrolyte resorption, ↓gut secretions, ↑sphincter tone. Extensive first-pass metabolism ⇒ minimal systemic opioid fx.
Use: acute diarrhoea[1], chronic diarrhoea[2], pain in bowel colic in palliative care[3].
CI: constipation, ileus, megacolon, bacterial enterocolitis 2° to invasive organisms (e.g. salmonella, *Shigella, Campylobacter*), abdo distension, active UC/AAC, pseudomembranous colitis.
Caution: in young (can ⇒ fluid + electrolyte depletion). *Reports of serious cardiovascular events (such as ↑QTc, torsades de pointes, and cardiac arrest), including fatalities, with ↑doses of loperamide associated with abuse or misuse.* L/P/B.
SE: headache, constipation, nausea, flatulence, abdo cramps, bloating, dizziness, drowsiness, fatigue. Rarely hypersensitivity (esp skin reactions), paralytic ileus.
Dose: initially 4 mg, then 2 mg after each loose stool (max 16 mg/day for 5 days[1]), 4–8 mg in divided doses, up to 8 mg bd[2], 2–4 mg qds[3]. *NB: can mask serious GI conditions.*

LORATADINE
Non-sedating antihistamine: see Cetirizine.
Caution: L/P/B.
Dose: 10 mg od. Non-proprietary or as Clarityn.

LORAZEPAM
Benzodiazepine, short-acting.
Use: sedation[1] (esp acute behavioural disturbance/Ψ disorders, e.g. acute psychosis), status epilepticus[2].
CI/Caution/SE/Interactions: see Diazepam. Do not give im within 1 h of im olanzapine.

Dose: 500 micrograms–2 mg po/im/iv prn (bottom of this range if elderly/respiratory disease/naive to benzodiazepines; top of range if young/recent exposure to benzodiazepines; max 4 mg/day)[1]; 100 micrograms/kg ivi at 2 mg/min (max 4 mg repeated once after 10 min if necessary)[2]. *NB:* ↓dose in RF/LF and use im route only when po/iv not available.

Beware respiratory depression: have O_2 (± resuscitation trolley) at hand, esp if respiratory disease or giving high doses im/iv .

LOSARTAN/COZAAR

Angiotensin II receptor antagonist: specifically blocks renin-angiotensin system ∴ does not inhibit bradykinin and ⇒ dry cough.
Use: HTN[1], type 2 DM nephropathy[2] (if ACE-i not tolerated*), chronic HF when ACE-i unsuitable/CI[3].
CI: L(if severe)/H (if severe)/P/B, combination with aliskiren in eGFR <60 mL/min/1.73 m^2 or in DM.
Caution: RAS, HOCM, mitral/aortic stenosis, if taking drugs that ↑K$^+$**, 1° hyperaldosteronism (may not benefit), L/R/E.
SE/Interactions: as captopril, but ↓dry cough (major reason for ACE-i intolerance*). As with ACE-i, can ⇒ ↑K$^+$ (esp if taking ↑K$^+$-sparing diuretics/salt substitutes or if RF).
Dose: initially 25–50 mg od (↑ing to max 100 mg od)[1,2]; 12.5 mg od (↑ing to max 150 mg od)[3]. *NB:* ↓dose in LF or RF.

**Beware if on other drugs that ↑K$^+$, e.g. amiloride, spironolactone, triamterene, ACE-i and ciclosporin. Do not give with oral K$^+$ supplements (inc dietary salt substitutes) .

LOSEC see Omeprazole; PPI (ulcer-healing drug).

LYMECYCLINE

Tetracycline, broad-spectrum antibiotic (see Tetracycline).
Use: acne vulgaris, rosacea.

CI/Caution/SE/Interactions: as tetracycline.
Dose: 408 mg od for ≥8 wk (can ↑ to bd for other indications).

MADOPAR see Co-beneldopa; L-dopa for Parkinson's.

MAXOLON see Metoclopramide; antiemetic (DA antagonist).

MEBEVERINE
Antispasmodic: direct action on GI muscle.
Use: GI smooth-muscle cramps (esp IBS, diverticulitis).
CI: ileus (paralytic).
Caution: porphyria, P/B.
SE: hypersensitivity/skin reactions.
Dose: 135 mg tds (20 min before food) or 200 mg bd of SR
preparation (Colofac MR).

MEFENAMIC ACID/PONSTAN
Mild NSAID; non-selective COX inhibitor.
Use: musculoskeletal pain (RA/OA), post-op pain, dysmenorrhoea,
menorrhagia.
CI/Caution/SE/Interactions: as ibuprofen, but also CI if IBD,
caution if epilepsy or acute porphyria. Can ⇒ severe diarrhoea,
skin reactions, stomatitis, paraesthesia, fatigue, haemolytic/aplastic
↓Hb, ↓Pt. No known interaction with baclofen or triazoles.
Mild **W+**.
Dose: 500 mg tds.

MELATONIN
Tryptophan derivative; binds to melatonin receptors MT_1/MT_2
involved in regulation of circadian rhythms and sleep regulation.
Use: insomnia (short-term use).
Caution: autoimmune disease.
SE: arthralgia, headaches, ↑risk of infection, pain.
Interactions: ↑levels with fluvoxamine.
Dose: 2 mg po od taken with food 1–2 h before bedtime, for up to
13 wk.

MEMANTINE

Glutamatergic NMDA receptor antagonist $\Rightarrow$ ↓prolonged influx of Ca^{2+}, ↓neuronal excitotoxicity.

Use: moderate-to-severe Alzheimer's disease.

CI: L(if severe)/R (if eGFR <5 mL/min/1.73 m²).

Caution: seizures, epilepsy risk factors.

SE: dizziness, headache, constipation, somnolence, ↑BP, hypersensitivity, impaired balance.

Interactions: ↑risk of CNS toxicity/SE with amantadine, ketamine.

Dose: initially 5 mg po od, ↑ in steps of 5 mg every wk, maintenance dose 20 mg od, max 20 mg od.

METFORMIN

Oral antidiabetic (biguanide): $\Rightarrow$ ↑insulin sensitivity without affecting levels ($\Rightarrow$ ↓gluconeogenesis and ↓GI absorption of glucose and ↑peripheral use of glucose). Only active in presence of endogenous insulin (i.e. functional islet cells).

Use: type 2 DM[1]: usually first line if diet and exercise control unsuccessful (esp if obese, as $\Rightarrow$ less ↑Wt than sulphonylureas). Also used in PCOS[2] (unlicensed; specialist use).

CI: DKA, ↑risk of lactic acidosis (e.g. RF, severe dehydration/infection/peripheral vascular disease, shock, major trauma, respiratory failure, alcohol dependence, recent MI*), L/R/P/B.

Caution: general anaesthetic** or iodine-containing radiology contrast media*, H.

SE: GI upset (esp initially or if ↑doses), taste disturbance. Rarely ↓vit B_{12} absorption, lactic acidosis† (stop drug).

Dose: initially 500 mg mane, ↑ing as required to max 3 g/day in divided doses. For MR tablets initially 500 mg daily, ↑ing as required to max 2 g daily in 1 dose[1]. 500 mg od up to 1.5–1.7 g/day in two to three divided doses[2]. *Take with meals.* NB: ↓dose in mild RF, avoid in **severe RF**.

M

☠ *Both often coexist in coronary angiography: stop drug on day of procedure (giving insulin if necessary) and restart 48 h later, having checked that renal function has not deteriorated. Stop on day of surgery ahead of general anaesthetic** and restart when renal function normal ☠.

METHADONE

Opioid agonist: ↓euphoria and long $t_{1/2}$ ($\Rightarrow$ ↓withdrawal symptoms) compared with other opioids.

Use: opioid dependence as aid to withdrawal.

CI/Caution/SE/Interactions: as morphine, but levels ↓ by ritonavir, but are ↑ by voriconazole and cimetidine, and ↑risk of ventricular arrhythmias with atomoxetine and amisulpride. Can ↑QTc (caution if FHx of sudden death); ECG monitoring if risk factors for ↑QTc or dose >100 mg/day.

Dose: *individual requirements vary widely according to level of previous abuse:* sensible starting dose is 10–20 mg/day po, ↑ing by 10–20 mg every day until no signs or symptoms of withdrawal – which usually stop at 60–120 mg/day. Then aim to wean off gradually. Available as non-proprietary solutions (1 mg/mL) or as Methadose (10 or 20 mg/mL). Can give sc/im for severe pain. *NB:* ↓dose if LF, RF or elderly.

☠ Do not confuse solutions of different strengths ☠.

METHYLDOPA

Centrally acting α_2-adrenergic agonist.

Use: HTN, esp pregnancy induced and 1° HTN during pregnancy.

CI: depression, phaeo, porphyria, L (if active liver disease).

Caution: Hx of depression/L, R.

SE: (minimal if dose <1 g/day) dry mouth, sedation, dizziness, weakness, headache, GI upset, postural ↓BP, ↓HR. Rarely blood disorders, hepatotoxicity, pancreatitis, Ψ disorders, parkinsonism, lupus-like syndrome, false +ve direct Coombs' test.

Monitor: FBC, LFTs.

Interactions: ↑s neurotoxicity of lithium. Hypotensive fx ↑d by antidepressants, anaesthetics and salbutamol ivi. ☠ **Avoid with, or within 2 wk of, MAOIs** ☠.
Dose: initially 250 mg bd/tds (125 mg bd in elderly), ↑ing gradually at intervals ≥2 days to max of 3 g/day (max 2 g/day in elderly).
NB: ↓**dose in RF.**

METHYLPHENIDATE HYDROCHLORIDE/
CONCERTA XL

CNS stimulant; noradrenaline–dopamine reuptake inhibitor
Use: ADHD[1], narcolepsy[2].
CI: cardiac disease (but see p. 279, refer 'Physical Health Problems' heading in 'Prescribing in Special Groups' section of 'ADHD' part of 'Disorders' chapter), severe HTN, vasculitis, cerebrovascular disease, ↑thyroid, phaeo, some Ψ disorders (psychosis, severe depression, suicidal ideation, uncontrolled BPAD, anorexia), **H**.
Caution: tic disorder (or FHx), substance misuse, agitation, epilepsy dysphagia, restricted GI lumen, glaucoma (angle-closure).
SE: ↓sleep, anxiety, headache, nasopharyngitis, ↓appetite, ↓growth in Ht and Wt, agitation, Δ mood, movement disorder, paraesthesia, visual problems, dizziness, **cardiac fx** (arrhythmia, ↑HR, ↑BP), GI upset, ↑LFTs, alopecia, rash, arthralgia, muscle spasm, sexual dysfunction, pyrexia, fatigue.
Warn: avoid abrupt withdrawal.
Monitor: pulse, BP, psychiatric symptoms, appetite, Wt and Ht at initiation of therapy, following each dose adjustment and every 6 months thereafter.
Interactions: ☠ ↑**risk of hypertensive crisis with MAOIs & linezolid;** ↑risk of dyskinesias with risperidone; ↓fx of apraclonidine.
Dose: specify brand on prescription, as MR preparations can have different fx and $t_{1/2}$. Initially 18 mg po od in morning, adjusted at wkly intervals, max 108 mg od (>54 mg od not licensed)[1]; 10–60 mg po od in divided doses; usual dose 20–30 mg od in divided doses before meals[2].

METHYLPREDNISOLONE

Glucocorticoid (mild mineralocorticoid activity).

Use: acute flares of inflammatory diseases[1] (esp rheumatoid arthritis, MS), cerebral oedema, Rx of graft rejection.

CI/Caution/SE/Interactions: see Prednisolone.

Dose: acutely, 10–500 mg ivi[1]; up to 1 g ivi od for up to 3 days[2]. Also available po and as im depot.[BNF]

METOCLOPRAMIDE/MAXOLON

Antiemetic: D_2 antagonist: acts on central chemoreceptor trigger zone and directly stimulates GI tract (⇒ ↑motility).

Use: N&V (indications now restricted due to risk of extrapyramidal fx[BNF/SPC]).

CI: GI obstruction/perforation/haemorrhage (inc 3–4 days post-GI surgery), phaeo, **B**.

Caution: epilepsy, porphyria, 15–19 years old, L/R/P/E.

SE: extrapyramidal fx (see p. 348, refer 'Extrapyramidal Effects' in 'Basic Psychopharmacology' chapter – esp in elderly and young females: potentially reversible if drug stopped within 24 h or with procyclidine), drowsiness, restlessness, GI upset, behavioural/mood Δs, ↑prolactin. Rarely skin reactions, NMS.

Interactions: ↑s risk of extrapyramidal fx of antipsychotics, SSRIs and TCAs.

Dose: 10 mg tds po/im/iv (max 500 micrograms/kg/day in three divided doses if Wt <60 kg* for 5 days). *NB:* ↓dose if RF, LF, **15–19 years old** or Wt <60 kg*. Give iv doses over >3 min.

METRONIDAZOLE/FLAGYL

Antibiotic, 'cidal': binds DNA of anaerobic (and microaerophilic) bacteria/protozoa.

Use: anaerobic and protozoal infections, abdo sepsis (esp *Bacteroides),* aspiration pneumonia, *C. difficile* (AAC), *H. pylori* eradication, *Giardia/Entamoeba* infections, Px during GI surgery. Also dental/gynaecological infections, bacterial vaginosis (*Gardnerella*), PID.

Caution: avoid with alcohol: drug metabolised to acetaldehyde and other toxins ⇒ flushing, abdo pain, ↓BP ('disulfiram-like' reaction), acute porphyria, avoid xs sun/UV light, L/P/B.

SE: GI upset (esp N&V), taste disturbed, skin reactions. Rarely drowsiness, headache, dizziness, dark urine, hepatotoxicity, blood disorders, myalgia, arthralgia, seizures (transient), ataxia, **peripheral and central neuropathy** (if prolonged Rx).

Interactions: can ↑busulfan, lithium, 5-fluorouracil, ciclosporin and phenytoin levels, W+.

Dose: 500 mg tds ivi/400 mg tds po for severe infections. Lower doses can be given po or higher doses pr (1 g bd/tds) according to indication.[SPC/BNF] *NB:* ↓dose in LF.

MIANSERIN HYDROCHLORIDE

Tetracyclic antidepressant; blocks presynaptic α-adrenoceptors, ↑NA release.

Use: depression.

CI: cardiac arrhythmia, post-MI, porphyria, mania, L/P.

Caution: some Ψ states (Hx BPAD/psychosis, ↑suicide risk), epilepsy, ↑prostatic/urinary retention, chronic constipation, DM, ↑thyroid, glaucoma (angle-closure)/↑IOP, phaeo, R/H.

SE: drowsiness, headache, tremor, blood dyscrasias, Ψ fx (Δ mood, psychosis, suicidality), breast abnormalities, postural ↓BP, rash, seizure, sexual dysfunction, withdrawal Sx, oedema, ↓Na⁺, arthralgia, jaundice.

Warn: withdrawal fx, worse after use for ≥8 wk. ↓dose gradually over ≥4 wk. If signs of infection, obtain urgent medical assistance.

Monitor: full blood count every 4 wk during first 3 months of treatment; monitor for signs of infection (e.g. fever, sore throat, stomatitis).

Interactions: ☠ ↑risk of toxicity with isocarboxazid, moclobemide, phenelzine, tranylcypromine (avoid with/for 14 days after stopping MAOI)☠; ↓fx of ephedrine.

Dose: initially 30–40 mg po od at bedtime/in divided doses; ↑ gradually, usual dose 30–90 mg.

M

MICONAZOLE

Imidazole antifungal (topical) but *systemic absorption can occur.*
Use: oral fungal infections (give po), cutaneous fungal infections (give topically).
CI: L.
Caution: acute porphyria, P/B.
SE: GI upset. Rarely hypersensitivity, hepatotoxicity.
Interactions: as ketoconazole, but less commonly significant. W+.
Dose: po oral gel (Daktarin) 2.5 mL qds after food or buccal tablets (Loramyc) 50 mg od mane. *NB:* with oral gel treat for 48 h after lesions healed. top: apply 1–2 times/day and treat for 10 days after lesions healed.

MIDAZOLAM

Very short-acting benzodiazepine: $GABA_A$ receptor positive allosteric modulator.
Use: sedation for stressful/painful procedures[1] (esp if amnesia desirable) and for agitation/distress in palliative care[2].
CI/Caution/SE/Warn/Interactions: see Diazepam.
Dose: 1–7.5 mg iv[1]; initially 2 mg (500 micrograms–1 mg if elderly) over 60 sec, then titrate up slowly until desired sedation achieved using 500 micrograms–1 mg boluses over 30 sec (can also give im); 2.5–5 mg sc prn[2] (or via sc pump). Also available as buccal liquid (10 mg/mL, special preparation) – unlicensed use. *NB:* ↓dose in RF or elderly.

☠ Beware respiratory depression: have flumazenil and O_2 (± resuscitation trolley) at hand, esp if respiratory disease or giving high doses im/iv ☠.

MINOCYCLINE

Tetracycline antibiotic: inhibits ribosomal (30S subunit) protein synthesis; broadest spectrum of tetracyclines.

Use: acne[1], rosacea.

CI/Caution/SE/Interactions: as tetracycline, but ↓bacterial resistance, although ↑risk of SLE and irreversible skin/body fluid discoloration. Can also use (with caution) in RF. Check hepatic toxicity every 3 months – discontinue if develops.

Dose: 100 mg od po[1] (can ↑ to bd for other indications). Use for ≥6 wk in acne.

MIRTAZAPINE/ZISPIN

Antidepressant: noradrenaline and specific serotonergic antagonist (NASSA); specifically stimulates 5-HT_1 receptors, antagonises $5\text{-HT}_{2C}/5\text{-HT}_3$ and central presynaptic α_2 receptors.

Use: depression, esp in elderly* or if insomnia†.

CI/Caution/SE: as fluoxetine, but ⇒ ↓**sexual dysfunction**/GI upset, ↑sedation† (esp during titration) and ↑**appetite/Wt** (can be beneficial in elderly*). Rarely, blood disorders (inc agranulocytosis), Δ LFTs, convulsions, myoclonus, oedema.

Warn: of initial sedation, to not stop suddenly (risk of withdrawal) and to report signs of infection (esp sore throat, fever): stop drug and check FBC if concerned.

Interactions: avoid with other sedatives (inc alcohol), artemether/lumefantrine and methylthioninium. ☠ Never give with, or ≤2 wk after, MAOIs ☠.

Dose: initially 15 mg nocte, ↑ing to 30 mg after 1–2 wk (max 45 mg/day). *NB: lower doses may be more sedating than higher doses.*

MOCLOBEMIDE

MAOI; selective, reversible inhibitor of monoamine oxidase A (MAO-A), ↓metabolism of monoamines, ↑NA, DA and 5-HT.

Use: depression[1], social anxiety disorder[2].

CI: delirium, phaeo.

Caution: ↑thyroid state, agitation, BPAD.

SE: Δ sleep, dizziness, headache, GI upset (N&D&C&V), dry mouth, agitation, paraesthesia, cardiac fx (↑QTc, ↓BP), rash. Rarely serotonin syndrome.

Warn: avoid large quantities of tyramine-rich foods (e.g. mature cheese, salami, pickled herring); withdrawal fx, worse if used for 8 wk+; ↓dose gradually over 4 wk+.

Interactions: ↑risk of severe toxic reaction with TCAs and mianserin; ↑risk of severe HTN with bupropion, ephedrine, isometheptene, lisdexamfetamine, methylphenidate, phenylephrine, reboxetine.

Dose: initially 300 mg po od taken after food in divided doses, usual dose 150–600 mg od[1]; initially 300 mg po od for 3 days, ↑ to 600 mg od in two divided doses continued for 8–12 wk[2].

MODAFINIL
Stimulant; dopamine reuptake inhibitor.

Use: excessive daytime sleepiness in narcolepsy.

CI: cardiac disease, moderate-to-severe HTN (if uncontrolled), P/B.

Caution: Hx of substance misuse/psychosis/mania/depression.

SE: headache, ↓appetite, ↓sleep, Ψ Sx (agitation, depression, confusion), paraesthesia, visual problems, cardiac fx (↑HR, arrhythmia, vasodilatation, chest pain), GI upset (N&D&C&abdo pain), ↑LFTs.

Monitor: ECG before initiation; monitor BP & HR if known HTN.

Interactions: ↑P450 (CYP1A2, CYP3A4, CYP2B6), ↓P450 (CYP2C9, CYP2C19); ↓fx of COCP, desogestrel, etonogestrel, levonorgestrel, norethisterone, ulipristal; ↓levels of bosutinib, voxilaprevir.

Dose: initially 200 mg po od taken in the morning/in two divided doses taken in the morning and at noon, ↑ to 200–400 mg od/in two divided doses.

MOMETASONE (FUROATE) CREAM OR OINTMENT/ELOCON

Potent topical corticosteroid.

Use: inflammatory skin conditions, esp eczema.

CI: untreated infection, rosacea, acne, widespread plaque psoriasis (rebound relapse).

SE: skin atrophy, worsening of infections, acne.

Dose: apply thinly od top (use 'ointment' in dry skin conditions).

MONTELUKAST/SINGULAIR

Leukotriene receptor antagonist: ↓s Ag-induced bronchoconstriction.

Use: *non-acute* asthma, esp if large exercise-induced component or assoc seasonal allergic rhinitis.

Caution: acute asthma, Churg-Strauss syndrome, P/B.

SE: headache, GI upset, myalgia, URTI, dry mouth/thirst. Rarely Churg-Strauss syndrome: asthma (± rhin-/sinusitis) with systemic vasculitis and ↑EØ*.

Monitor: FBC* and for development of vasculitic (purpuric/non-blanching) rash, peripheral neuropathy, ↑respiratory/cardiac symptoms: all signs of possible Churg-Strauss syndrome.

Dose: 10 mg nocte (↓doses if <15 years old[SPC/BNF]).

MORPHGESIC SR Morphine (sulphate) SR (10, 30, 60 or 100 mg). Given bd. See Morphine.

MORPHINE (SULPHATE)

Opiate analgesic.

Use: severe pain (inc post-op), palliative care (pain and cough), AMI and acute LVF.

CI: acute respiratory depression, acute severe obstructive airways disease, ↑risk of paralytic ileus, delayed gastric emptying, biliary colic, acute alcoholism, ↑ICP/head injury (respiratory depression ⇒ CO_2 retention and cerebral vasodilation ⇒ ↑ICP), phaeo, H (if 2° to chronic lung disease).

Caution: ↓respiratory reserve, obstructive airways disease, ↓BP/shock, acute abdo, biliary tract disorders (*NB:* biliary colic is CI), pancreatitis, bowel obstruction, IBD, ↑prostate/urethral stricture, arrhythmias, ↓T₄, adrenocorticoid insufficiency, MG, L (can ⇒ coma), R/P/B/E.

SE: N&V (and other GI disturbance), constipation* (can ⇒ ileus), respiratory depression, ↓BP (inc orthostatic. *NB:* rarely ⇒ ↑BP), ↓/↑HR, pulmonary oedema, oedema, bronchospasm, ↓cough reflex, sedation, urinary retention, RF, biliary tract spasm, ↑pancreatitis, Δ LFTs, hypothermia, muscle rigidity/fasciculation/myoclonus, ↑ICP, dry mouth, vertigo, syncope, headache, miosis, sensory disturbance, pruritis, anorexia, allodynia, mood Δs (↑ or ↓), delirium, hallucinations, restlessness, seizures (at ↑doses), rhabdomyolysis, amenorrhoea, ↓libido, dependence. Rarely skin reactions.

Interactions: ☠ MAOIs (do not give within 2 wk of discontinuing) ☠. Levels ↓ by ritonavir and rifampicin. ↓s levels of ciprofloxacin. ↑sedative fx with antihistamines, baclofen, alcohol (also ⇒ ↓BP), TCAs, antipsychotics (also ↓BP), anxiolytics, hypnotics, barbiturates and moclobemide (also ⇒ ↑/↓BP). ↑s fx of sodium oxybate, gabapentin.

Dose: acute pain: 5–10 mg po or 5–20 mg sc/im 4 hrly; 2.5–15 mg iv up to 4 hrly (2 mg/min). *NB:* iv doses are generally 1/4–1/2 im doses.

AMI: 5–10 mg iv (1–2 mg/min), repeated if necessary.

Acute LVF: 5–10 mg iv (2 mg/min). **Chronic pain:** use po as Oramorph solution or as MST Continus, Morphgesic, MXL, Sevredol or Zomorph tablets. Dose adjustment may be required when switching brands. Also available pr as suppositories of 10, 15, 20 and 30 mg giving 15–30 mg up to 4 hrly. *Unless short-term Rx, always consider laxative Px*.* **Cough in palliative care:** 5 mg po 4 hrly. Can ↑doses and frequency with expert supervision. Always adjust dose to response. *NB:* ↓dose if LF, RF or elderly.

☠ If ↓BMI or elderly, titrate dose up slowly, monitor O₂ sats and have naloxone ± resuscitation trolley at hand ☠.

MST CONTINUS Oral morphine (sulphate), equivalent in efficacy to **Oramorph** but SR: dose every 12 h. Need to specify if *tablets* (5, 10, 15, 30, 60, 100 or 200 mg) or *suspension* (sachets of 20, 30, 60, 100 or 200 mg to be mixed with water). prn doses for 'breakthrough pain' often needed.

MUPIROCIN/BACTROBAN
Topical antibiotic for bacterial infections (esp eradication of nasal MRSA carriage); available as nasal ointment (applied bd/tds) or as cream/ointment (tds for up to 10 days).

Local MRSA eradication protocols often exist; if not, then a sensible regimen is to give for 5 days and then swab 2 days later, repeating regimen if culture still positive.

MXL CAPSULES Morphine (sulphate) capsules (30, 60, 90, 120, 150 or 200 mg), equivalent in efficacy to **Oramorph** but SR: dose od. *NB*: ↓dose if LF, RF or elderly.

MYCOPHENOLATE MOFETIL (MMF)
Immunosuppressant: ↓s B-/T-cell lymphocytes (and ↓s Ab production by B cells).
Use: transplant rejection Px, autoimmune diseases, vasculitis.
CI: P/B.
Caution: active serious GI diseases[†], E.
SE: GI upset, **blood disorders** (esp ↓NØ, ↓Pt), weakness, tremor, taste Δ, headache, ↑cholesterol, ↑ or ↓K⁺. Rarely GI ulceration/bleeding/perforation[†], hepatotoxicity, skin neoplasms*.
Warn: patient to report unexplained bruises/bleeding/signs of infection. Avoid strong sunlight*. Male patients or female partner should use effective contraception during Rx and for 90 days after stopping Rx.[MHRA]
Monitor: FBC and LFTs (wkly for first 4 wk, 2-wkly for 2 months, then monthly for first year).
Interactions: levels ↓ by rifampicin.
Dose: specialist use only.[SPC/BNF]

L/R/H = Liver, Renal and Heart failure. E = elderly. P = pregnancy. B = breastfeeding.

N-ACETYLCYSTEINE

see Acetylcysteine; paracetamol antidote.

NALOXONE/NARCAN

Opioid receptor antagonist for opioid reversal if OD or over-Rx.
Caution: cardiovascular disease, if taking cardiotoxic drugs,
physical dependence on opioids, H.
Dose: 400 micrograms–2 mg iv (or sc/im), much larger doses may
be needed for certain opioids (e.g. tramadol), repeating after 2 min
if no response (or ↑ing if severe poisoning). *NB: short-acting: may
need repeating every 2–3 min (to total 10 mg) then review and
consider ivi (10 mg made up to 50 mL with 5% dextrose; useful
start rate is 60% of initial dose over 1 h, then adjusted to response).*

NALTREXONE

Opioid antagonist: ↓s euphoria of opioids if dependence and ↓s
craving and relapse rate in both opioid and alcohol dependence.
Use: opioid and alcohol dependence relapse prevention.
CI: if still taking opioids (can precipitate withdrawal), L (inc acute
hepatitis), severe R/B.
Caution: P.
SE: GI upset, hepatotoxicity, sleep and Δ mood.
Warn: patient trying to overcome opiate blockade by overdosing
can ⇒ acute intoxication.
Monitor: LFTs.
Dose: initial dose 25 mg od po, thereafter, 50 mg od (or 350 mg per
wk split into 2 × 100 mg and 1 × 150 mg doses); specialist use only.

NB: also ↓s fx of opioid analgesics.

NAPROXEN

Moderate-strength NSAID; non-selective COX inhibitor.
Use: rheumatic disease[1]; acute musculoskeletal pain and
dysmenorrhoea[2]; acute gout[3].
CI/Caution/SE/Interactions: as ibuprofen, but somewhat ↑SEs,
notably, ↑risk PU/GI bleeds. Lowest thrombotic risk of any NSAID.

Probenecid ⇒ ↑serum levels. No known interaction with baclofen or triazoles. Mild **W+**.

Dose: 500 mg–1 g daily in one to two divided doses[1]; 500 mg initially then 250 mg 6–8 hrly (max 1.25 g/day)[2]; 750 mg initially then 250 mg 8 hrly until attack passed[3]. Also available with esomeprazole as Px against PU (as **Vimovo**). *NB:* **avoid or ↓dose in RF and consider gastroprotective Rx.**

NARATRIPTAN/NARAMIG

5-HT$_{1B/1D}$ agonist for acute migraine.

CI/Caution/SE: see Sumatriptan. Not recommended if >65 years.

Interactions: Ergotamine; increased risk of vasospasms: avoid ergotamine for 24 h after naratriptan, avoid naratriptan for 24 h after ergotamine.

Dose: 2.5 mg po (can repeat after ≥4 h if responded then recurs). Max 5 mg/24 h (2.5 mg if LF or RF, avoid if severe).

NICOTINE/NICORETTE, NICOTINELL, NIQUITIN

Nicotinic acetylcholine receptor (nAChR) agonist.

Use: nicotine replacement therapy (NRT).

Caution: **haemodynamically unstable** with CVA/MI/arrhythmia, uncontrolled ↑thyroid, phaeo; **inhalation:** obstructive airway disease, bronchospasm; **intranasal:** asthma; **oral:** dentures, GORD; **transdermal:** skin disease, avoid placing on damaged skin.

SE: dizziness, headache, GI upset (N, gastritis), skin reactions; **inhalation:** cough, throat irritation, dry mouth; **intranasal:** nasal irritation (short-lived); **oral:** jaw ache, ↑saliva, throat irritation, denture damage (rare); **sublingual:** irritation to mouth/throat; **transdermal:** local skin reactions.

Warn: acidic beverages (coffee, fruit juice) ↓absorption of nicotine through buccal mucosa (avoid for 15 min before use of oral NRT).

Monitor: diabetes – blood glucose when initiating.

Dose: *NRT in those who smoke <20 cigarettes/day* – 2 mg strength chewing gum, chew one piece when urge to smoke occurs/prevent cravings, continue for 3 months before ↓dose; 1 sublingual

tablet every hour, ↑ to 2 tablets every hour, continue for up to
3 months before ↓dose, max 40 tablets/day; *NRT in those who
smoke >20 cigarettes/day or require >15 pieces of 2 mg strength
gum/day* – 4 mg strength chewing gum, chew one piece when urge
to smoke occurs/prevent cravings, should not exceed 15 pieces
of 4 mg strength gum/day, continue for 3 months before ↓dose;
2 sublingual tablets every 1 h, continue for up to 3 months before
↓dose, maximum 40 tablets/day.

Inhalation: should not exceed 12 cartridges of 10 mg strength/day
or 6 cartridges of 15 mg strength/day.

Lozenges: 1 lozenge every 1–2 h, those who smoke <20
cigarettes/day use lower-strength lozenges, those who smoke >20
cigarettes/day and who fail to stop smoking with low-strength
lozenges use the higher-strength lozenges, continue for 6–12 wk
before ↓dose, max 15 lozenges/day.

Oromucosal spray: 1–2 sprays, should not exceed 2 sprays/
episode (up to 4 sprays every hour), max 64 sprays/day.

Intranasal spray: 1 spray, up to twice every hour for 16 h/day,
continue for 8 wk before ↓dose, max 64 sprays/day.

Transdermal patches: those who smoke >10 cigarettes/day
apply high-strength patch/day for 6–8 wk, followed by medium-
strength patch for 2 wk, then low-strength patch for final 2 wk;
those who smoke <10 cigarettes/day start with medium-strength
patch for 6–8 wk, followed by low-strength patch for 2–4 wk;
slower titration schedule can be used in those who are not ready to
quit but want to ↓ consumption before a quit attempt; if abstinence
is not achieved/withdrawal symptoms, strength of patch should be
maintained/↑ until stabilised.

NIFEDIPINE

Ca^{2+} channel blocker (dihydropyridine): dilates smooth muscle,
esp arteries (inc coronaries). Reflex sympathetic drive ⇒ ↓HR
and ↑contractility ∴ ⇒ ↓HF cf other Ca^{2+} channel blockers (e.g.
verapamil, and to a lesser degree diltiazem), which ⇒ ↓HR +
↓contractility. Also diuretic fx.

Use: angina Px[1], HTN[2], Raynaud's[3].

CI: cardiogenic shock, clinically significant aortic stenosis, ACS (inc within 1 month of MI), acute/unstable angina, co-Rx with rifampicin ($\downarrow$fx of nifedipine*).

Caution: angina or LVF can worsen (consider stopping drug), $\downarrow$BP, DM, BPH, acute porphyria, L/H/P/B/E.

SE: flushing, headache, ankle oedema, dizziness, $\downarrow$BP, palpitations, poly-/nocturia, rash/pruritus, GI upset, weakness, myalgia, arthralgia, gum hyperplasia, rhinitis. Rarely PU, hepatotoxicity.

Interactions: metab by **P450 3A4**. $\uparrow$s fx of digoxin, theophylline and tacrolimus. $\downarrow$s fx of quinidine. Quinu-/dalfopristin, ritonavir and grapefruit juice $\uparrow$fx of nifedipine. Rifampicin*, phenytoin and carbamazepine $\downarrow$fx of nifedipine. Risk of $\downarrow\downarrow$BP with α-blockers, β-blockers or Mg^{2+} iv/im.

Dose: 5–20 mg tds po[3]; 10 mg bd or 20 mg od starting dose[1,2] titrating to max 90 mg od using long-acting preparations for HTN/angina, as normal-release preparations $\Rightarrow$ erratic BP control and reflex $\uparrow$HR, which can worsen IHD (e.g. Adalat LA or Retard and many others with differing fx and doses[SPC/BNF]). NB: $\downarrow$**dose if severe LF.**

NITRAZEPAM

Long-acting benzodiazepine: GABA$_A$ receptor positive allosteric modulator.

Use: insomnia (short-term use).

CI: respiratory depression, severe muscle weakness inc unstable MG, sleep apnoea, acute pulmonary insufficiency, chronic psychosis, depression (do not give nitrazepam alone).

Caution: respiratory disease, muscle weakness (inc MG), Hx of drug/alcohol abuse, personality disorder, porphyria, $\downarrow$albumin L/R/P/B/E.

Class SE: respiratory depression (rarely apnoea), drowsiness, dependence. Also ataxia, amnesia, headache, vertigo, GI upset, jaundice, $\downarrow$BP, $\downarrow$HR, visual/libido/urinary disturbances, blood disorders, paradoxical disinhibition in Ψ disorder.

Specific SE: movement disorders.
Warn: ↑fx of alcohol; occasional paradoxical agitation.
Interactions: ↑sedation with alcohol; ↑clearance with rifampicin.
Dose: 5–10 mg po od at bedtime.

☠ Overdose ⇒ **respiratory depression**, sedation and ataxia.

NITROFURANTOIN

Antibiotic: only active in urine (no systemic antibacterial fx).
Use: UTIs (but not pyelonephritis).
CI: G6PD deficiency, acute porphyria, **R** (if eGFR <45 mL/min; also ⇒ ↓activity of drug, as needs concentrating in urine), infants <3 years old, **P/B**.
Caution: DM, lung disease, ↓Hb, ↓vit B, ↓folate, electrolyte imbalance, susceptibility to peripheral neuropathy, **L/E**.
SE: GI upset, pulmonary reactions (inc effusions, fibrosis), peripheral neuropathy, hypersensitivity. Rarely, hepatotoxicity, cholestasis, pancreatitis, arthralgia, alopecia (transient), skin reactions (esp exfoliative dermatitis), blood disorders, BIH.
Dose: 50 mg qds po (↑ to 100 mg if severe chronic recurrent infection) or 100 mg bd (MR preparation); 50–100 mg od nocte if for Px. *Take with food.* Not available iv or im.

NB: can ⇒ false-positive urine dipstick for glucose and discolour urine.

NORETHISTERONE

Progestogen (testosterone analogue).
Use: endometriosis[1], dysfunctional uterine bleeding and menorrhagia[2], dysmenorrhoea[3], postponement of menstruation[4], breast Ca[5], contraception[6].
CI: liver/genital/breast cancers (unless progestogens being used for these conditions), atherosclerosis, undiagnosed vaginal bleeding, acute porphyria, Hx of idiopathic jaundice, severe pruritis, pemphigoid or severe pruritus during pregnancy.

Caution: risk of fluid retention, ↑susceptibility to TE disease, DM, epilepsy, migraine, HTN, depression, acute impairment of vision, L/H/R.

SE: menstrual cycle irregularities, ↑Wt, nausea, headache, dizziness, insomnia, drowsiness, breast tenderness, acne, depression, Δ libido, skin reactions, hirsutism and alopecia.

Interactions: metab by P450. fx ↓ by phenobarbital, phenytoin, carbamazepine, rifampicin, rifabutin, nevirapine, efavirenz, tetracyclines, ampicillin, oxacillin and cotrimoxazole. ↑s levels of ciclosporin.

Dose: 5 mg bd–tds po for ≥4–6 months, commencing on day 5 of cycle (can ↑ to max 25 mg/day if spotting occurs, ↓ing when stops)[1]; 5 mg tds po for 10 days for Rx (for Px: 5 mg bd po from day 19–26 of cycle)[2]; 5 mg tds po from day 5–24 for three to four cycles[3]; 5 mg tds po starting 3 days prior to expected menstruation onset (bleeding will commence 2–3 days after stopping)[4]; 40 mg od po[5]; 200 mg deep im injection within first 5 days of cycle or immediately after parturition *or* 350 micrograms po od at same time each day from day 1 of cycle[6].

NORTRIPTYLINE

TCA: blocks reuptake of NA (and 5-HT) through binding to noradrenaline transporter (NAT) and serotonin transport (SERT).

Use: depression[1], neuropathic pain (unlicensed)[2].

CI: recent MI (within 3 months), arrhythmias (esp HB), mania, L (if severe).

Caution: cardiac/thyroid disease, epilepsy, glaucoma (angle-closure)/↑IOP, ↑prostate, phaeo, porphyria. Also Hx of mania, psychosis or urinary retention, H/P/E.

SE: antimuscarinic fx (see p. 346, refer 'Cholinoceptors' section in 'Basic Psychopharmacology' chapter), **cardiac fx** (arrhythmias, HB, ↑HR, postural ↓BP, dizziness, syncope: **dangerous in OD**), ↑Wt, **sedation** (often ⇒ 'hangover'), seizures, GI upset, sexual dysfunction. Rarely hypomania, psychosis, fever, blood disorders, hypersensitivity, Δ LFTs, ↓Na⁺ (esp in elderly), agitation,

confusion, tinnitus, NMS, alopecia, gynaecomastia, ↑/↓BP,
paralytic ileus, fracture, infection, movement disorders, oedema
(inc testicular swelling), peripheral neuropathy, paraesthesia,
Δ sleep, stroke, tremor.

Warn: withdrawal fx, worse after regular administration for
8 wk+. ↓dose gradually over 4 wk+; ↑fx of alcohol.

Monitor: plasma nortriptyline concentration if dose >100 mg od.

Interactions: metab by P450 (CYP2D6); ☠ ↑risk of severe
toxic reaction with MAOIs (avoid with/for 14 days after stopping
MAOI); ☠ ↑risk of neurotoxicity with lithium; ↑fx of adrenaline,
noradrenaline, phenylephrine; ↑levels with bupropion, cinacalcet,
dronedarone, fluoxetine, paroxetine, terbinafine; ↓fx of ephedrine.

Dose: initiated at low dose, ↑ to 75–100 mg po od/in divided
doses, max 150 mg od[1]; initially 10 mg po od taken at night,
↑ gradually to 75 mg od[2].

☠ TCA overdose ⇒ dilated pupils, arrhythmias, ↓BP, hypothermia,
hyperreflexia, extensor plantar responses, seizures, respiratory
depression and coma.

NUROFEN see Ibuprofen; *NB:* 'over-the-counter' use can ⇒ poor
response to HTN and HF Rx.

NYSTATIN

Polyene antifungal.

Use: *Candida* infections: topically for skin/mucous membranes
(esp mouth/vagina); po for GI infections (not absorbed).

SE: GI upset (at ↑doses), skin reactions.

Dose: po suspension: 100,000 units qds, usually for 1 wk, for Rx
(can ↑ to 500,000 units qds). *Give after food.*

OLANZAPINE/ZYPREXA

'Atypical' (second generation) antipsychotic: D_1, D_2, D_4 and 5-HT_2,
H_1 (+ mild muscarinic) antagonist.

Use: schizophrenia^{NICE}, mania, bipolar Px, acute sedation, anorexia nervosa (rarely, for inpatients).

CI: known risk of narrow-angle glaucoma. If giving im, acute MI/ACS, ↓↓BP/HR, SSS or recent heart surgery.

Caution: as for other antipsychotics, plus BM suppression, ↓ leukocyte/neutrophil count, paralytic ileus, myeloproliferative disease, **H** (esp if Hx of cardiovascular disease/ ↑risk of CVA/TIA) **B**.

Class SE: EPSE, ↑prolactin and assoc Sx, sedation, ↑Wt, ↑QTc, VTE, blood dyscrasias, ↓seizure threshold, NMS.

Specific SE: high propensity for ↑Wt, lipids, BG*. Anticholinergic fx. Rarely ↓NØ.

Monitor: BG* (± HbA_{1C}) after 1 month then 4–6 monthly. LFTs, U&Es, FBC, prolactin (and CK if NMS suspected). Wt and lipids every 3 months for 1 year, then at least annually. If giving im, closely monitor cardiorespiratory function for ≥4 h post-dose, esp if given other antipsychotic or benzodiazepine.

Interactions: metab by **P450 (1A2)** ∴ many, but most importantly, levels ↓d by carbamazepine and smoking. ↑risk of ↓NØ with valproate. Levels may be ↑d by ciprofloxacin, fluvoxamine. ↑risk of arrhythmias with drugs that ↑QTc. ↑risk of ↓BP with general anaesthetics. ↓s fx of anticonvulsants.

Dose: 5–20 mg po nocte (consider 2.5 mg in the elderly). Available in 'melt' form if ↓compliance/swallowing (orodispersible). Available in quick-acting im form for acute sedation; give 5–10 mg (2.5–5 mg in elderly) repeating 2 h later if necessary to max total daily dose, inc po doses, of 20 mg (max 3 injections/day for 3 days).

NB: im doses not recommended with im/iv benzodiazepines (↑risk of respiratory depression) which should be given ≥1 h later; if benzodiazepines already given, use with caution and closely monitor cardiorespiratory function.

NB: a depot formulation exists (olanzapine Embonate) which is administered 2–4 wkly. ≥3 h post-dose monitoring by a HCP under medical supervision is required due to risk of rapid absorption: many organisations cannot facilitate this.

L/R/H = Liver, Renal and Heart failure. E = elderly. P = pregnancy. B = breastfeeding.

OLMESARTAN/OLMETEC

Angiotensin II antagonist: see Losartan.
Use: HTN.
CI: biliary obstruction, P/B.
Caution/SE/Interactions: see Losartan.
Dose: initially 10 mg od, ↑ing to max 40 mg (20 mg in LF, RF or elderly).

OMEGA-3-ACID ETHYL ESTERS 90

Essential fatty acid combination: 1 g capsule = eicosapentaenoic acid 460 mg and docosahexaenoic acid 380 mg.
Use: adjunct to diet in type IIb and III ↑TG[1] (with statin) or type IV. Added for 2° prevention within 3 months of acute MI[2].
CI: B.
Caution: bleeding disorders, anticoagulants (↑bleeding time), L/P.
SE: GI upset; rarer: taste disorder, dry nose, dizziness, hypersensitivity, hepatotoxicity, headache, rash, ↓BP, ↑BG.
Monitor: LFTs, INR.
Dose: Capsules: 2–4 g od[1]; 1 g od[2]. Take with food.

OMEPRAZOLE

PPI: inhibits H^+/K^+-ATPase of parietal cells ⇒ ↓acid secretion.
Use: PU Rx/Px (esp if on NSAIDs), GORD (if symptoms severe or complicated by haemorrhage/ulcers/stricture).NICE Also used for H. pylori eradication and ZE syndrome.
CI: avoid use with nelfinavir.
Caution: can mask symptoms of gastric Ca, B_{12} deficiency (may ↓absorption), severe ↓Mg^{2+} if Rx for >3 months, ↑risk of hip/wrist/spine fractures with ↑doses and long durations (>1 year), particularly in elderly or presence of other risk factors, development of SCLE, L/P/B.
SE: GI upset, headache, dizziness, arthralgia, weakness, skin reactions. Rarely, hepatotoxicity, blood disorders, hypersensitivity.
Interactions: ↓ (and ↑) P450 ∴ many, most importantly ↑s phenytoin, cilostazol, diazepam, raltegravir and digoxin levels.

↓s fx clopidogrel with high doses (80 mg/day), ↓s fx of ataza-/nelfi-/tipranavir, mild **W+**.

Dose: 20 mg od po, ↑ing to 40 mg in severe/resistant cases and ↓ing to 10 mg od for maintenance if symptoms stable; 20 mg bd for *H. pylori* eradication regimens. If unable to take po (e.g. perioperatively, ↓GCS, on ITU), give 40 mg iv od either over 5 min or as ivi over 20–30 min. In ZE syndrome: 60 mg od starting, maintenance dose of 20 mg od up to 120 mg/day in divided doses. *NB*: max dose 20 mg if LF.

NB: also specialist use iv for acute bleeds. Usually 80 mg stat then 8 mg/h ivi for 72 h if endoscopic evidence of PU (prescribed as divided infusions, as drug is unstable). Contact pharmacy ± GI team for advice on indications and exact dosing regimens.

ONDANSETRON

Antiemetic: 5-HT$_3$ antagonist: acts on central and GI receptors.

Use: N&V, esp if resistant to other Rx, post-operative or chemotherapy induced.

Caution: GI obstruction (inc subacute), ↑QTc*, avoid if hereditary galactose intolerance (Lapp lactase deficiency or glucose-galactose malabsorption), **L** (unless mild), **P/B**.

SE: constipation (or diarrhoea), headache, sedation, fatigue, dizziness. Rarely seizures, chest pain, ↓BP, Δ LFTs, rash, hypersensitivity.

Interactions: metab by **P450**. Levels ↓ by rifampicin, carbamazepine and phenytoin. ↓s fx of tramadol. Avoid with drugs that ↑QTc*.

Dose: 8 mg bd po; 16 mg od pr; 4–8 mg 2–8 hrly iv/im. Max 24 mg/day usually (8 mg/day if LF). Can also give as ivi at 1 mg/h for max of 24 h. Exact dose and route depend on indication.[SPC/BNF]

ORAMORPH

Oral morphine solution for severe pain, esp useful for prn or breakthrough pain.

Dose: multiply sc/im morphine dose by 2 to obtain approximately equivalent **Oramorph** dose. *NB:* ↓**dose if LF or RF.**

Solution most commonly used is 10 mg/5 mL, but can be 100 mg/5 mL ∴ *specify strength if prescribing in mL (rather than mg).*

ORPHENADRINE HYDROCHLORIDE

(No longer available in the UK; availability may vary in other countries.) Antimuscarinic; treats antipsychotic-induced parkinsonism by ↓ing downstream cholinergic fx.

Use: parkinsonism, drug-induced extrapyramidal symptoms (but not tardive dyskinesia).

CI: GI obstruction, MG, porphyria, urinary retention, tardive dyskinesia.

Caution: Glaucoma (angle-closure), substance misuse risk, psychosis, fever HTN, ↑prostate, H/E.

SE: dizziness, accommodation problems, anxiety, GI upset (C), sedation.

Warn: ↓dose gradually if long-term Rx.

Interactions: ↓absorption of levodopa.

Dose: initially 150 mg po od in divided doses, ↑ in steps of 50 mg every 2–3 days, usual dose 150–300 mg od in divided doses, max 400 mg od.

OXAZEPAM

Medium-acting benzodiazepine: GABA$_A$-receptor positive allosteric modulator.

Use: anxiety (short-term use)[1], insomnia with anxiety[2].

CI: respiratory depression, severe muscle weakness inc unstable MG, sleep apnoea, acute pulmonary insufficiency,v chronic psychosis, movement disorder, OCD, phobia, L (if severe).

Caution: respiratory disease, muscle weakness (inc MG), Hx of drug/alcohol abuse, personality disorder, porphyria, organic brain disease; liable to abuse, L/R/P/B/E.

SE: respiratory depression (rarely apnoea), drowsiness, dependence. Also ataxia, amnesia, headache, vertigo, GI upset, jaundice, cardiac fx (↓BP, ↓HR, syncope), visual/libido/urinary disturbances, blood dyscrasias, fever, oedema, paradoxical disinhibition in Ψ disorder.

Warn: ↑fx of alcohol; occasional paradoxical agitation.

Interactions: ↑sedation with alcohol.

Dose: 15–30 mg po tds/qds[1]; 15–25 mg od at bedtime, max 50 mg od[2].

OXYBUTYNIN

Anticholinergic (selective M3 antagonist); antispasmodic (↓s bladder muscle contractions).

Use: detrusor instability (also neurogenic bladder instability, nocturnal enuresis in paeds).

CI: bladder outflow or GI obstruction, urinary retention, severe UC/toxic megacolon, glaucoma (narrow angle), MG, **B**.

Caution: ↑prostate, Parkinson's, autonomic neuropathy, hiatus hernia (if reflux), ↑T4, IHD, arrhythmias, porphyria, cognitive disorders, L/R/H/P/E.

SE: antimuscarinic fx (see p. 346, refer 'Cholinoceptors' section in 'Basic Psychopharmacology' chapter), GI upset, palpitations/↑HR, skin reactions – mostly dose-related and reportedly less severe in MR preparations*.

Interactions: ↑anticholinergic SEs when co-Rx'd with other anticholinergic drugs, e.g. amantadine and other antiparkinsonian drugs, antihistamines, antipsychotics, TCAs, quinidine, digitalis, atropine.

Dose: initially 5 mg bd/tds po (2.5–3 mg bd if elderly), ↑ing if required to max of 5 mg qds (bd if elderly). Available as MR tablet (**Lyrinel XL*** 5–20 mg od) and transdermal patch (**Kentera** 36 mg; releases 3.9 mg/day and lasts 3–4 days).

OXYCODONE (HYDROCHLORIDE)

Opioid for moderate-to-severe pain (esp in palliative care).

CI: acute respiratory depression, coma, head injury, ↑ ICP, acute abdo, delayed gastric emptying, chronic constipation, cor pulmonale, **L** (if moderate/severe)/**R** (if severe).

Caution: ↓BP, respiratory diseases, IBD, MG, obstructive bowel disorders, ↑prostate, shock, urethral stenosis, P/B.
SE/Interactions: as morphine, but does not interact with baclofen, gabapentin and ritonavir.
Dose: 4–6 hrly po/sc/iv or as sc infusion. *NB:* 1 mg iv/sc = approximately 2 mg po. Available in immediate release (e.g. OxyNorm 4–6 hrly) or MR form as OxyContin (12 hrly). Available with naloxone (works locally to ↓GI SEs) as Targinact (12 hrly). *NB:* ↓dose if LF, RF or elderly.

OXYTETRACYCLINE
Tetracycline antibiotic: inhibits ribosomal protein synthesis.
Use: acne vulgaris (and rosacea).
CI/Caution/SE/Interactions: as tetracycline, plus caution in porphyria.
Dose: 500 mg bd po (1 h before food or on empty stomach) for ≥16 wk.

PABRINEX
Parenteral (iv or im) vitamins that come as a pair of vials. Vial 1 contains B_1 (thiamine*), B_2 (riboflavin) and B_6 (pyridoxine). Vial 2 contains C (ascorbic acid), nicotinamide and glucose.
Use: acute vitamin deficiencies (esp thiamine*), risk of Wernicke's encephalopathy (e.g. malnourished or unwell)[1], severe depletion at risk of Wernicke's encephalopathy[2], psychosis following narcosis or electroconvulsive therapy[3], toxicity from acute infections[4], haemodialysis[5].
Caution: rarely ⇒ anaphylaxis (esp if given iv too quickly; should be given over ≥30 min). *Ensure access to resuscitation facilities.*
Dose: 1 pair od for 3–5 days[1,BAP], 2–3 pairs tds[2], 1 pair bd up to 7 days[3,4], 1 pair every 2 wk[5].

*See p. 298, refer 'Wernicke's Encephalopathy' heading in 'Substance Misuse' part of 'Disorders' chapter for Wernicke's encephalopathy Px/Rx in alcohol withdrawal.

PALIPERIDONE

This is the po formulation. For depot, see later. Active metabolite of risperidone, 9-hydroxyrisperidone; dopamine D_2 and $5-HT_{2A}$ antagonist with weak H_1 and α_1/α_2 antagonism.

Use: schizophrenia, psychotic or manic symptoms of schizoaffective disorder.

CI: R (if creatinine clearance <10 mL/min).

Caution: cataract surgery (risk of intraoperative floppy iris syndrome), GI obstruction risk, prolactin-dependent tumours, Parkinson's/Lewy body dementia, jaundice, ↑prostate, severe respiratory disease, glaucoma (angle-closure), **R/H/E** (with dementia or risk factors for stroke).

SE: EPSE, ↑prolactin, sedation, ↑Wt, ↑QTc, VTE, blood dyscrasias, ↓seizure threshold, NMS, insomnia.

Monitor: prolactin (see p. 198, refer '↑prolactin' heading in 'Psychosis' section of 'Disorders' chapter), physical health monitoring (cardiovascular disease risk including Wt, BG, lipids) at least once/year.

Interactions: ↑risk of QT prolongation with class 1A and III antiarrhythmics (e.g. quinidine, disopyramide, amiodarone, sotalol), antihistamines, antibiotics (e.g. fluoroquinolones), antimalarials (e.g. mefloquine).

Dose: 6 mg po od in the morning, adjusted in steps of 3 mg over at least 5 days, usual dose 3–12 mg od.

PALIPERIDONE PALMITATE/XEPLION, TREVICTA

See Paliperidone.

Use: maintenance of schizophrenia.

CI: R (if creatinine clearance <50 mL/min).

Caution/SE/Monitor/Interactions: see Paliperidone.

Warn: Trevicta detected in plasma up to 18 months after single dose.

Dose: *1-monthly Xeplion pre-filled syringes (for those previously responsive to paliperidone/risperidone):* 150 mg im for 1 dose on day 1, then 100 mg for 1 dose on day 8, administered into deltoid muscle. Maintenance dose 1 month after second loading dose. Dose adjusted at monthly intervals, maintenance normally 75 mg

once a month. Following second dose, monthly maintenance doses administered into either deltoid/gluteal muscle.
3-monthly Trevicta pre-filled syringes (for those who are clinically stable on once-monthly im injection): initially 175–525 mg im every 3 months, administered into deltoid/gluteal, dose should be initiated in place of the next scheduled dose of monthly depot.

Approximate Equivalent Dosing[MPG]

PO risperidone	PO paliperidone	IM fortnightly risperidone depot	IM monthly paliperidone palmitate depot	IM 3/12ly paliperidone palmitate depot
1 mg	Unclear	No equivalent product	25 mg (unavailable in United Kingdom)	No equivalent product
2 mg	Unclear	25 mg	50 mg	175 mg
3 mg	6 mg	37.5 mg	75 mg	263 mg
4 mg	9 mg	50 mg	100 mg	350 mg
5 mg	Unclear	Not licensed	No equivalent product	No equivalent product
6 mg	12 mg	Not licensed	150 mg	525 mg

(DISODIUM) PAMIDRONATE

Bisphosphonate: ↓s osteoclastic bone resorption.
Use: ↑Ca^{2+} (esp metastatic: also ↓s pain)[1], Paget's disease, myeloma.
CI: P/B.
Caution: Hx of thyroid surgery, cardiac disease, L/R/H.
SE: flu-like symptoms (inc fever, transient pyrexia), **GI upset** (inc haemorrhage), **dizziness/somnolence** (common post-dose*), ↑ (or ↓) BP, seizures, musculoskeletal pain, osteonecrosis of jaw (esp in cancer patients; consider dental examination or preventative

Rx – MHRA advice), e'lyte Δs ($\downarrow PO_4$, $\downarrow$ or $\uparrow K^+$, $\uparrow Na^+$, $\downarrow Mg^{2+}$), RF, blood disorders.

Warn: not to drive/operate machinery immediately after Rx*.

Monitor: e'lytes (inc U&E before each dose), Ca^{2+}, PO_4, before starting biphosphonate consider dental check, as risk of osteonecrosis of the jaw.

Dose: 15–90 mg ivi according to indication ($\pm Ca^{2+}$ levels[1]). *NB: if RF, max rate of ivi 20 mg/h (unless for life-threatening $\uparrow Ca^{2+}$). Never given regularly for sustained periods.*

PANTOPRAZOLE

PPI; as omeprazole, but $\downarrow$interactions and can $\Rightarrow \uparrow$TGs.

Dose: 20–80 mg mane po 1 h before food ($\downarrow$ing to 20 mg maintenance if symptoms allow). If unable to take po (e.g. perioperatively, $\downarrow$GCS, on ITU), can give 40 mg iv over ≥ 2 min (or as ivi) od. $\uparrow$doses if ZE syndrome.[SPC/BNF] *NB:* $\downarrow$**dose if RF or LF.**

PARACETAMOL

Antipyretic and mild analgesic. Unlike NSAIDs, *has no anti-inflammatory fx.*

Use: mild pain (or moderate/severe in combination with other Rx), pyrexia.

Caution: alcohol dependence, L (CI if severe liver disease), R.

SE: *all rare:* rash, blood disorders, hepatic (rarely renal) failure – esp if over-Rx/OD (for Mx, see p. 383, refer 'Paracetamol Overdose' in 'Emergencies' chapter).

Interactions: may W+ if prolonged regular use.

Dose: 500 mg–1 g po/pr; 1 g (or 15 mg/kg if <50 kg) ivi. All doses 4–6 hrly, max 4 g/day (except max 3 g/day ivi in LF, dehydration, chronic alcoholism/malnutrition). Minimum iv dosing interval in RF (eGFR <30 mL/min) is 6 hrly. (For children, see Calpol.)

PAROXETINE/SEROXAT

SSRI antidepressant; as fluoxetine, but $\downarrow\downarrow t_{1/2}$*.

Use: depression[1], social/generalised anxiety disorder[1], PTSD[1], panic disorder[2], OCD[3].

CI/Caution/SE: as fluoxetine, but ↓frequency of agitation/insomnia, although ↑frequency of **antimuscarinic fx**, **extrapyramidal fx** and **withdrawal fx**. Avoid if <18 years old, as may ↑suicide risk and hostility. Stop if patient enters manic phase. P.

Interactions: risk of serotonin syndrome with other serotonergic drugs; ↓**P450** ∴ ↑levels of drugs primarily metabolised by CYP2D6 (e.g. pimozide, some TCAs, phenothiazine antipsychotics, risperidone, atomoxetine, propafenone, flecainide, metoprolol, **W+**). ↓**fx of tamoxifen.** ☠ ↑**risk of bleeding** with anticoagulants, antiplatelets, fibrinolytics. ↓fx of procyclidine. ☠ P450 inhibitors may ⇒ ↑paroxetine levels, so ↓paroxetine dose. **Never give with, or ≤2 wk after, MAOIs;** do not give MAOIs within 1 wk of stopping paroxetine.

Dose: initially 20 mg[1,3] (10 mg[2]) mane, ↑ing if required to max 50 mg[1] or 60 mg[2,3]. Max 40 mg in elderly for all indications. *NB:* ↓**dose if RF, LF.**

Taper down very slowly, as short $t_{1/2}$ ⇒ ↑risk of withdrawal syndrome.

PARVOLEX see Acetylcysteine; antidote for paracetamol poisoning.

PENICILLIN G see Benzylpenicillin.

PENICILLIN V see Phenoxymethylpenicillin.

PEPPERMINT OIL

Antispasmodic: direct relaxant of GI smooth muscle.
Use: GI muscle spasm, distension (esp IBS).
SE: perianal irritation, indigestion. Rarely rash or other allergy.
Dose: 1–2 capsules tds, before meals and with water.

PEPTAC

Alginate raft-forming oral suspension for acid reflux.
Dose: 10–20 mL after meals and at bedtime (*NB:* 3 mmol
Na+/5 mL).

PERINDOPRIL ERBUMINE

ACE-i; see Captopril.
Use: HTN, HF, Px of IHD.
CI/Caution/SE/Monitor/Interactions: as captopril, plus can ⇒
mood/sleep Δs.
Dose: 2–10 mg od$^{SPC/BNF}$, starting at 2–4 mg od. *NB:* **consider**
↓dose if RF, elderly, taking a diuretic, cardiac decompensation or
volume depletion.

PETHIDINE

Opioid; less potent than morphine but quicker action ⇒ ↑euphoria +
↑abuse/dependence potential ∴ not for chronic use, e.g. in palliative
care.
Use: moderate/severe pain, obstetric and peri-op analgesia.
CI: acute respiratory depression, risk of ileus, ↑ICP/head injury/
coma, phaeo.
Caution: any other condition where morphine CI/cautioned.
SE: as morphine, but ↓constipation.
Interactions: as morphine but ☠ ↑risk of hyperpyrexia/
CNS toxicity with **MAOIs** ☠. Ritonavir ⇒ ↓levels and ↑s toxic
metabolites. May ↑serotonergic effects of duloxetine. No known
interaction with gabapentin or baclofen.
Dose: 25–100 mg up to 4 hrly im/sc (can give 2 hrly post-op or
1–3 hrly in labour with max 400 mg/24 h); 25–50 mg up to 4 hrly

slow iv. Rarely used po: 50–150 mg up to 4 hrly. *NB:* ↓**dose if LF, RF or elderly.**

P

PHENELZINE

MAOI; non-selective and irreversible inhibitor of monoamine oxidase, ↑5-HT, NA and DA in CNS.

Use: depression.

CI: mania, cerebrovascular disease, Δ LFTs, phaeo, **L/H** ☠ interacting medication ☠.

Caution: agitation, blood dyscrasias, current ECT, DM, epilepsy, severe HTN due to drugs/foods, porphyria, surgery, **P/B/E**.

SE: dizziness, somnolence, fatigue, oedema, GI upset (N&V&C), antimuscarinic fx, postural ↓BP, twitching, ↑reflexes, ↑LFTs, sexual dysfunction, ☠ **hypertensive crisis** ☠, mania.

Warn: avoid tyramine- or dopa-rich food/drinks with/for 2–3 wks after stopping MAOI, withdrawal fx may occur within 1–3 days of stopping treatment, ↓dose gradually over 4 wk+.

Monitor: BP (risk of postural ↓BP and HTN).

Interactions: ☠ ↑risk of severe toxic reaction with serotonergics, dopaminergics and noradrenergics: SSRIs, SNRIs, NARIs, TCAs (and related drugs), other MAOIs (inc for Parkinson's disease), carbamazepine, linezolid, triptans, pethidine, tramadol. ☠

- Do not start phenelzine until these drugs have been stopped and they have cleared: 5 wk for fluoxetine, 3 wk for clomipramine/ imipramine, at least 7–14 days for other drugs.
- Wait 2 wk after stopping phenelzine before starting any of these medicines.

↑**risk of hypertensive crisis** with sympathomimetics, dopamine agonists, CNS stimulants, buspirone. ↑fx of CNS depressants, antimuscarinics, antidiabetics, antihypertensives.

Dose: initially 15 mg po tds, respond usually within first wk, ↑ after 2 wk to 15 mg qds (up to 30 mg tds may be used in inpatient); once satisfactory response achieved, ↓dose to lowest maintenance dose.

PHENOBARBITAL (= PHENOBARBITONE)

Barbiturate antiepileptic: potentiates GABA (inhibitory neurotransmitter), antagonises fx of glutamate (excitatory neurotransmitter).

Use: status epilepticus (SEs and interactions limit other uses).

Caution: respiratory depression, porphyria.

SE: hepatitis, cholestasis, respiratory depression, sedation, ↓BP, ↓HR, ataxia, skin reactions. Rarely paradoxical excitement (esp in elderly), blood disorders.

Interactions: ↑P450 ∴ many, most importantly ↓s levels/ fx of aripiprazole, antivirals, carbamazepine, Ca^{2+} antagonists, chloramphenicol, corticosteroids, ciclosporin, eplerenone, mianserin, tacrolimus, telithromycin, posa-/voriconazole and OCP. Anticonvulsant fx ↓d by antipsychotics, TCAs and SSRIs. Avoid with St John's wort. ↑s fx of sodium oxybate. Caution with other sedative drugs (esp benzodiazepines), W−.

Dose: total of 10 mg/kg as ivi at 100 mg/min (max total 1 g).

PHENOXYMETHYLPENICILLIN (= PENICILLIN V)

As benzylpenicillin (penicillin G) but active orally: used for ENT/skin infections (esp erysipelas), Px of rheumatic fever/S. *pneumoniae* infections (esp post-splenectomy).

Dose: 500 mg–1 g qds po (take on empty stomach; ≥1 h before food or ≥2 h after food).

PHENYTOIN

Antiepileptic: blocks Na^+ channels (stabilises neuronal membranes).

Use: all forms of epilepsy[1] (except absence seizures) inc status epilepticus[2].

CI: *if giving iv* (do not apply if po), sinus, ↓HR, Stokes-Adams syndrome, SAN block, second-/third-degree HB, acute porphyria.

Caution: DM, porphyria ↓BP, L/H/P (⇒ cleft lip/palate, congenital heart disease), B.

SE (acute): *dose dependent*: **drowsiness** (also confusion/dizziness), **cerebellar fx**, **rash** (common cause of intolerance and rarely ⇒ SJS/ TEN), N&V, diplopia, dyskinesia (esp orofacial). *If iv, risk of ↓BP,* arrhythmias* (esp ↑QTc), 'purple glove syndrome' (hand damage distal to injection site), CNS/respiratory depression.

SE (chronic): gum hypertrophy, coarse facies, hirsutism, acne, ↓folate (⇒ megaloblastic ↓Hb), Dupuytren's, peripheral neuropathy, osteomalacia. Rarely blood disorders, hepatotoxicity.

Warn: report immediately any rash, mouth ulcers, sore throat, fever, bruising, bleeding.

Monitor: FBC**, keep serum levels at 10–20 mg/L (narrow therapeutic index). 💀 If iv, closely monitor BP and ECG* (esp QTc) 💀.

Interactions: metab by and ↑s P450 ∴ many; most importantly ↓s fx of OCP, doxycycline, Ca^{2+} antagonists (esp nifedipine), imatinib, lapatinib, ciclosporin, keto-/itra-/posaconazole, indinavir, quinidine, theophyllines, eplerenone, telithromycin, aripiprazole, mianserin, mirtazapine, paroxetine, TCAs and corticosteroids. fx ↓d by rifampicin, rifabutin, theophyllines, mefloquine, pyrimethamine, sucralfate, antipsychotics, TCAs and St John's wort. Levels ↑d by NSAIDs (esp azapropazone), fluoxetine, mi-/flu-/voriconazole, diltiazem, disulfiram, trimethoprim, cimetidine, esomeprazole, amiodarone, metronidazole, chloramphenicol, isoniazid, sulphonamides, sulfinpyrazone, topiramate (levels of which are also ↓d by phenytoin) and ethosuximide. Complex interactions with other antiepileptics.[SPC/BNF] W− (or rarely W+).

Dose: po[1]: 150–500 mg/day in one to two divided doses.[SPC/BNF] iv[2]: load with 18 mg/kg ivi at max rate of 25–50 mg/min, then maintenance iv doses of approximately 100 mg tds/qds, adjusting to Wt, serum levels and clinical response. If available give iv as *fosphenytoin* (NB: doses differ). NB: ↓**dose if LF.**

💀 Stop drug if ↓WCC** is severe, worsening or symptomatic 💀

PHOSPHATE ENEMA

Laxative enemas; ⇒ osmotic H_2O retention ⇒ ↑evacuation.
Use: severe constipation (unresponsive to other Rx).

CI: acute GI disorders.
Caution: if debilitated or neurological disorder, R/E.
SE: local irritation.
Dose: 1 prn usually no more than once a day.

PHYTOMENADIONE

Iv vit K_1 for warfarin overdose/poisoning. Caution: give iv injections slowly. *NB:* not compatible with NaCl, P.

PIMOZIDE

DA antagonist; antagonises D_2 receptor in CNS.
Use: schizophrenia[1]; monosymptomatic hypochondriacal/paranoid psychosis[2].
CI: arrhythmia, personal Hx/FHx of congenital ↑QTc, drugs that ↑QTc, phaeo, CNS depression.
Caution: Parkinson's, epilepsy, MG, phaeo, glaucoma (angle-closure), ↑prostate, severe respiratory disease, jaundice, blood disorders, predisposition to postural ↓BP, photosensitivity, H.
SE: EPSE, ↑prolactin, **sedation,** ↑Wt, ↑QTc*, **photosensitisation,** VTE, blood dyscrasias, ↓seizure threshold, NMS, ↓appetite, depression, headache, hyperhidrosis, hypersalivation, sebaceous gland overactivity, urinary disorders, blurred vision.
Monitor: ECG before treatment and annually (review if QT prolonged)*.
Interactions: metab by P450 (CYP2D6, CYP3A4); ↑risk of QT prolongation* with drugs that ↑QTc (see p. 196, refer 'Prolonged QTc' heading in 'Psychosis' section of 'Disorders' chapter); ↑CNS depression with alcohol, hypnotics, sedatives, strong analgesics; ↓fx of levodopa.
Dose: initially 2 mg po od, ↑ in steps of 2–4 mg at intervals of not <1 wk, usual dose 2–20 mg od[1]; initially 4 mg po od, ↑ in steps of 2–4 mg at intervals of not <1 wk, max 16 mg od[2].

PIOGLITAZONE/ACTOS

Thiazolidinedione (glitazone) antidiabetic; ↓s peripheral insulin resistance (and, to lesser extent, hepatic gluconeogenesis).

Use: type 2 DM (second or third line) either as monotherapy, dual oral therapy (with a sulphonylurea [if metformin not tolerated] *or* metformin [if risk of ↓glucose with sulphonylurea unacceptable]) *or* triple oral therapy with a sulphonylurea + metformin (if obese, metabolic syndrome or human insulin unacceptable dt lifestyle/personal issues).[NICE] Can also be used in combination with insulin.
CI: ACS (inc Hx of), previous or active bladder cancer, uninvestigated macroscopic haematuria, H (inc Hx of), L/P/B.
Caution: peri-operatively cardiovascular disease. Omit pioglitazone peri-operatively as insulin needed. R.
SE: oedema (esp if HTN/CCF), ↓Hb, ↑Wt, GI upset (esp diarrhoea), headache, hypoglycaemia (if also taking sulphonylureas), ↑risk of distal fractures, rarely **hepatotoxicity**.
Monitor: LFTs. ☠ *Discontinue if jaundice develops.* ☠ Signs of HF.
Interactions: levels ↓ by rifampicin and ↑ by gemfibrozil. NSAIDs and selective COX-2 inhibitors can ↑ oedema.
Dose: initially 15–30 mg od (max 45 mg od).

PIPOTIAZINE PALMITATE/PIPORTIL
(Not readily available in the United Kingdom – requires importing.)
Phenothiazine antipsychotic; dopamine ($D_1/D_2/D_3/D_4$), serotonin ($5\text{-}HT_1/5\text{-}HT_2$), histamine ($H_1$), adrenergic ($\alpha_1/\alpha_2$) and muscarinic ($M_1/M_2$) receptor antagonist.
Use: maintenance treatment of schizophrenia or paranoid psychosis.
CI: CNS depression, phaeo, severe cerebral atherosclerosis, L/R/H.
Caution: Parkinson's, epilepsy, MG, phaeo, glaucoma (angle-closure), ↑prostate, severe respiratory disease, jaundice, blood disorders, predisposition to postural ↓BP, photosensitivity, alcohol withdrawal, brain damage, severe antipsychotic-induced EPSEs, ↓/↑thyroid.
Class SE: EPSE, ↑prolactin and assoc Sx, sedation, ↑Wt, QT prolongation, VTE, blood dyscrasias, ↓seizure threshold, NMS.

SE: postural ↓BP, insomnia, abnormal LFTs, contact skin sensitisation, visual changes, ↑blood glucose.

Monitor: glucose and ECG monitoring during treatment.

Interactions: ↑risk of arrhythmias with concomitant QT prolonging drugs; ↑fx of alcohol, barbiturates, sedatives; ↑EPSE with tetrabenazine, lithium; ↑CNS toxicity with lithium, ritonavir may ↑levels.

Dose: initially 25 mg im, ↑ by 25–50 mg, administered into gluteal muscle, usual maintenance dose 50–100 mg every 4 wk, max 200 mg every 4 wk.

PIRITON see Chlorphenamine; antihistamine for allergies.

PLAVIX see Clopidogrel; anti-Pt agent for Px of IHD (and CVA).

POTASSIUM TABLETS see **Kay-cee-L** (syrup 1 mmol/mL), **Sando-K** (effervescent 12 mmol/tablet) and **Slow-K** (MR non-effervescent 8 mmol/tablet, reserved for when syrup/effervescent preparations are inappropriate; avoid if ↓swallow). Swallow whole with fluid during meals while sitting or standing.

PRAMIPEXOLE/MIRAPEXIN

Dopamine agonist (non-ergot derived); use in early Parkinson's ⇒ ↓motor complications (e.g. dyskinesias) but ↓motor performance cf L-dopa.

Use: Parkinson's[1], moderate-to-severe restless legs syndrome (RLS)[2].

CI: B

Caution: psychotic disorders, severe cardiovascular disease, R/H/P.

SE: GI upset, sleepiness (inc sudden onset sleep), ↓BP (inc postural, esp initially), Ψ disorders (esp psychosis and impulse control disorders, e.g. gambling and ↑sexuality), amnesia, headache, oedema.

Warn: sleepiness and ↓BP may impair skilled tasks (inc driving). Avoid abrupt withdrawal.

Monitor: ophthalmological testing if visual Δs occur.
Interactions: antipsychotics can ↓fx.
Dose: initially 88 micrograms tds[1] (or 88 micrograms nocte for RLS[2]), ↑ing if tolerated/required to max 1.1 mg tds[1] (or 540 micrograms nocte[2]). *NB:* **doses given for BASE (not SALT) and ↓dose if RF.**

PRAVASTATIN/LIPOSTAT
HMG-CoA reductase inhibitor: 'statin'; ↓s cholesterol/LDL (and TG).
Use/CI/Caution/SE/Monitor: see Simvastatin.
Interactions: ↑risk of myositis (± ↑levels) with 🐝 fibrates 🐝, nicotinic acid, daptomycin, ciclosporin and ery-/clarithromycin.
Dose: 10–40 mg nocte. *NB:* ↓dose if RF (10 mg if moderate-to-severe RF).

PREDNISOLONE
Glucocorticoid (and mild mineralocorticoid activity).
Use: anti-inflammatory (e.g. rheumatoid arthritis, IBD, asthma, eczema), immunosuppression (e.g. transplant rejection Px, acute leukaemias), glucocorticoid replacement (e.g. Addison's disease, hypopituitarism).
CI: systemic infections (without antibiotic cover).
Caution: DM, epilepsy, HTN, glaucoma, osteoporosis, PU, TB, severe mood disorders, L/R.
SE: ↑infections, metabolic (fluid retention, ↑lipids, ↑Wt, DM, ↑Na+, ↓K+), adrenal suppression, bruising, cardiac (HTN, CCF, myocardial rupture post-MI, TE), musculoskeletal (proximal myopathy, osteoporosis), worsening of seizures, Ψ fx (anxiety, depression, psychosis), ocular (cataract, glaucoma, corneal/scleral thinning), GI (peptic/duodenal ulcer – give PPI if on ↑doses, pancreatitis).
Warn: avoid contact with chickenpox if not infected previously. Carry steroid card. 🐝 Risk of Addisonian crisis if abrupt withdrawal – must ↓ slowly if >3 wk Rx 🐝.

Interactions: fx can be ↓d by rifampicin, carbamazepine, phenytoin and phenobarbital. fx (and risk of adrenal suppression) can be ↑d by erythromycin, ritonavir, ketoconazole, itraconazole and ciclosporin (whose own fx are ↑d by methylprednisolone). ↑risk of ↓K⁺ with amphotericin and digoxin. Risk of ↑ or ↓anticoagulant effect of coumarins.

Dose: usually 2.5–15 mg od po for maintenance. In acute/initial stages, 20–60 mg od often needed (depends on cause and often physician preference), e.g. acute asthma (40 mg od), acute COPD (30 mg od), temporal arteritis (40–60 mg daily). Take with food (↓Na⁺, ↑K⁺ diet recommended if on long-term Rx). For other causes, consult^SPC/BNF, pharmacy or local specialist relevant to the disease. Also available as once- or twice-wkly im injection.

> 💀 Warn patient not to stop tablets suddenly (*can ⇒ Addisonian crisis*). Requirements may ↑ if intercurrent illness/surgery. Consider Ca/vit D supplements/bisphosphonate to ↓risk of osteoporosis and PPI to ↓risk of GI ulcer 💀.

PREGABALIN/LYRICA
Antiepileptic; GABA analogue.

Use: epilepsy (partial seizures with or without 2° generalisation), neuropathic pain, generalised anxiety disorder.

CI: B.

Caution: avoid abrupt withdrawal, H (if severe)/ R/P/E.

SE: neuro-Ψ disturbance; esp somnolence/dizziness (↑falls in elderly), confusion, visual Δ (esp blurred vision), mood ↑ or ↓ (and possibly suicidal ideation/behaviour†), ↓libido, sexual dysfunction and vertigo. Also GI upset, ↑appetite/Wt, oedema and dry mouth. Rarely HF (esp if elderly and/or CVS disease).

Warn: seek medical advice if ↑suicidality or mood ↓. Do not stop abruptly as can ⇒ withdrawal fx (insomnia, headache, N&D, flu-like symptoms, pain, sweating, dizziness).

Dose: 50–600 mg/day po in two to three divided doses.
NB: stop over ≥1 wk* and ↓dose if RF.

PROCHLORPERAZINE/STEMETIL

Antiemetic: DA antagonist (phenothiazine ∴ also antipsychotic, but now rarely used for this).

Use: N&V (inc labyrinthine disorders).

CI/Caution/SE/Warn/Monitor/Interactions: as chlorpromazine, but CI are relative and ⇒ ↓sedation. *NB:* can ⇒ extrapyramidal fx (esp if elderly/debilitated); see p. 348, refer 'Extrapyramidal Effects' in 'Basic Psychopharmacology' chapter

Dose: *po:* acutely 20 mg, then 10 mg 2 h later (5–10 mg bd/tds for Px and labyrinthine disorders); *im:* 12.5 mg, then po doses 6 h later. Available as quick-dissolving 3 mg tablets to be placed under lip (Buccastem); give 1–2 bd. *NB:* ↓dose if RF.

PROCYCLIDINE

Antimuscarinic: ↓s cholinergic to dopaminergic ratio in extrapyramidal syndromes ⇒ ↓tremor/rigidity. No fx on bradykinesia (or tardive dyskinesia; may even worsen).

Use: extrapyramidal symptoms (e.g. parkinsonism), esp if drug induced[1] (e.g. antipsychotics).

CI: urinary retention (if untreated), glaucoma* (angle-closure), GI obstruction, MG.

Caution: ↑prostate, tardive dyskinesia, H/E.

SE: antimuscarinic fx, Ψ disturbances, euphoria (can be drug of abuse), glaucoma*.

Dose: 2.5 mg tds po prn[1] (↑ if necessary to max of 10 mg tds); 5–10 mg im/iv if acute dystonia or oculogyric crisis.

NB: do not stop suddenly: can ⇒ rebound antimuscarinic fx.

PROMETHAZINE HYDROCHLORIDE

Sedating antihistamine. Anticholinergic fx.

Use: insomnia[1]. Also used iv/im for anaphylaxis and po for symptom relief in chronic allergies. Used in rapid tranquilisation.

CI: CNS depression/coma, MAOI within 14 days.

Caution: urinary retention, ↑prostate, glaucoma, epilepsy, IHD, asthma, porphyria, pyloroduodenal obstruction, R (↓dose), L (avoid if severe)/P/B/E (anticholinergic: caution in dementia).

SE: antimuscarinic fx, hangover sedation, headache.
Interactions: ↑s fx of anticholinergics, TCAs and sedatives/hypnotics.
Dose: 25 mg nocte[1] (can ↑dose to 50 mg).

PROPRANOLOL

β-blocker (non-selective): β1 ⇒ ↓HR and ↓contractility, $β_2$ ⇒ vasoconstriction (and bronchoconstriction). Also blocks fx of catecholamines, ↓s renin production, slows SAN/AVN conduction.

Use: HTN[1], IHD (angina Rx[2], MI Px[3]), portal HTN[4] (Px of variceal bleed; *NB: may worsen liver function*), essential tremor[5], Px of migraine[6], anxiety[7], ↑T_4 (symptom relief[8], thyroid storm[9]), arrhythmias[8] (inc severe[9]).

CI: asthma/Hx of bronchospasm, peripheral arterial disease (if severe), Prinzmetal's angina, severe ↓HR or ↓BP, SSS, second-/third-degree HB, cardiogenic shock, metabolic acidosis, phaeo (unless used specifically with α-blockers), **H** (if uncontrolled).

Caution: COPD, first-degree HB, DM*, MG, Hx of hypersensitivity (may ↑ to *all* allergens), **L/R/P/B**.

SE: ↓HR, ↓BP, HF, peripheral vasoconstriction (⇒ cold extremities, worsening of claudication/Raynaud's), fatigue, depression, sleep disturbance (inc nightmares), hyperglycaemia (and ↓sympathetic response to hypoglycaemia*), GI upset. Rarely conduction/blood disorders.

Interactions: 💀 verapamil and diltiazem ⇒ risk of HB and ↓HR 💀. Risk of ↓BP and HF with nifedipine. Risk of ↓BP with α-blockers. ↑s risk of bupiva-/lidocaine toxicity. ↑s risk of AV block, myocardial depression and ↓HR with amiodarone, flecainide. Levels of both drugs can ↑ with chlorpromazine. Risk of ↓BP with moxisylyte. Risk of ↑BP (and ↓HR) with dobutamine, adrenaline and noradrenaline. Risk of withdrawal ↑BP with clonidine (stop β-blocker before slowly ↓ing clonidine).

Dose: 80–160 mg bd po[1]; 40–120 mg bd po[2]; 40 mg qds for 2–3 days, then 80 mg bd po[3] (start 5–21 days post-MI); 40 mg bd po[4] (↑dose if necessary); 40 mg bd/tds po[5,6]; 40 mg od po[7] (↑dose to

tds if necessary); 10–40 mg tds/qds[8]; 1 mg iv over 1 min[9] repeating
every 2 min if required, to max total 10 mg (or 5 mg in anaesthesia).

NB: ↓po dose in LF and ↓initial dose in RF. Withdraw slowly (esp in
angina); if not can ⇒ rebound ↑ of symptoms.

PROSCAR see Finasteride; antiandrogen for BPH (and baldness).

PROTAMINE (SULPHATE)

Protein (basic) that binds heparin (acidic).
Use: reversal of heparin (or LMWH) following over-Rx/OD or
after temporary anticoagulation for extracorporeal circuits (e.g.
cardiopulmonary bypass, haemodialysis).
Caution: ↑risk of hypersensitivity reaction in patients who have
been previously exposed to protamine or may have antibodies to
this including: (1) past coronary angioplasty or cardiopulmonary
bypass, (2) DM treated with protamine insulin, (3) fish allergy,
(4) vasectomy or infertility.
SE: ↓BP, ↓HR, N&V, flushing, dyspnoea. Rarely pulmonary
oedema, HTN, hypersensitivity reactions.
Dose: 1 mg per 80–100 units of heparin to be reversed (max
50 mg) iv/ivi at rate ≤5 mg/min; exact regimen depends on whether
reversing heparin or LMWH and whether given iv or sc.[BNF/SPC]
NB: $t_{1/2}$ of iv heparin is short; ↓doses of protamine if giving to
reverse iv heparin >15 min after last dose – see SPC.

Max total dose 50 mg: ☠ *high doses can ⇒ anticoagulant fx!* ☠

PYRIDOSTIGMINE

Anticholinesterase: inhibits cholinesterase at neuromuscular
junction ⇒ ↑ACh ⇒ ↑neuromuscular transmission.
Use: myasthenia gravis.
CI: GI/urinary obstruction.
Caution: asthma or COPD, recent MI, ↓HR/BP, arrhythmias,
vagotonia, ↑T_4, PU, epilepsy, parkinsonism, R/P/B/E.
SE: cholinergic fx (see p. 346, refer 'Cholinoceptors' in 'Basic
Psychopharmacology' chapter) – esp if xs Rx/OD, where ↓BP,

bronchoconstriction and (confusingly) weakness can also occur (= cholinergic crisis*); ↑secretions (sweat/saliva/tears) and miosis are good clues** of xs ACh.

Interactions: fx ↓d by aminoglycosides (e.g. gentamicin), polymixins, clindamycin, lithium, quinidine, chloroquine, propranolol and procainamide. ↑s fx of suxamethonium. Atropine and hyoscine antagonise the muscarinic fx.

Dose: 30–120 mg po up to qds (can ↑ to max total 1.2 g/24 h; if possible give <450 mg/24 h to avoid receptor downregulation). *NB:* ↓**dose if RF.**

> ☠ ↑ing weakness can be due to *cholinergic crisis** as well as MG exacerbation; if unsure which is responsible**, get senior help (esp if ↓respiratory function) before giving Rx, as the wrong choice can be fatal! ☠

QUETIAPINE/SEROQUEL

Atypical (second generation) antipsychotic. $5-HT_2$ antagonist, α_1 and histamine antagonism. Weak DA antagonism. Some anticholinergic activity.

Use: schizophrenia[1], mania[2], depression in bipolar disorder[3]. Off-licence use for psychosis/behavioural disorders (esp in dementias, but use of antipsychotics in dementia generally not recommended).

CI: B. CYP3A4 inhibitors (e.g clarithromycin, erythromycin).

Caution: Hx of epilepsy, drugs that ↑QTc, **H**.

SE: Sedation (esp initially*), ↑Wt, ↑QTc EPSE, ↑prolactin, VTE, blood dyscrasias, ↓seizure threshold, NMS, ↓BP.

Warn/Monitor/Interactions: as olanzapine, but also levels ↑ by ery-/clarithromycin.

Dose: *needs titration** (*see SPC/BNF*): initially 25 mg bd ↑ing daily to max 750 mg od[1]; initially 50 mg bd ↑ing daily to max 800 mg od[2]; initially 50 mg od ↑ing daily to max 600 mg od[3]. If RF, LF or elderly start at 25 mg od ↑ing less frequently. Available in MR form; initially, 300 mg od then 600 mg od the next day[2], then adjust to response (if giving for depression[3] or if RF, LF or elderly start at 50 mg od then ↑cautiously[SPC/BNF]).

R

QUININE

Antimalarial: kills bloodborne schizonts.

Use: malaria Rx[1] (esp falciparum), nocturnal leg cramps[2].

CI: optic neuritis, tinnitus, haemoglobinuria, MG.

Caution: cardiac disease (inc conduction dfx, AF, HB), G6PD deficiency, H/P/E.

SE: visual Δs (inc temporary blindness, esp in OD), tinnitus (and vertigo/deafness), GI upset, headache, rash/flushing, hypersensitivity, confusion, hypoglycaemia*. Rarely blood disorders, AKI, cardiovascular fx (can $\Rightarrow$ severe $\downarrow$BP in OD). Dose-dependent $\uparrow$QTc.

Monitor: blood glucose*, ECG (if elderly) and e'lytes (if given iv).

Interactions: $\uparrow$s levels of flecainide and digoxin. $\uparrow$s risk of arrhythmias with pimozide, moxifloxacin and amiodarone. $\uparrow$risk of seizures with mefloquine. Avoid artemether/lumefantrine.

Dose: 200–300 mg nocte po as quinine *sulphate*[2]. (*NB:* $\downarrow$iv maintenance dose if RF).

RAMIPRIL/TRITACE

ACE-i; see Captopril.

Use: HTN[1], HF[2], Px post-MI[3]. Also Px of cardiovascular disease (if age >55 years and at risk)[4] and renal disease inc nephropathy.

CI/Caution/SE/Monitor/Interactions: as captopril.

Dose: initially 1.25 mg od ($\uparrow$ing slowly to max of 10 mg daily)[1,2]; initially 2.5 mg bd then $\uparrow$ to 5 mg bd after 3 days[3] (start $\geq$48 h post-MI), then maintenance 2.5–5 mg bd; initially 2.5 mg od ($\uparrow$ing to 10 mg)[4]. *NB:* $\downarrow$dose if RF.

RANITIDINE/ZANTAC

H_2 antagonist $\Rightarrow$ $\downarrow$parietal cell H^+ secretion.

Use: PU (Px if on long-term high-dose NSAIDs[1], chronic Rx[2], acute Rx[3]), reflux oesophagitis.

Caution: L/R/P/B. ☠*May mask symptoms of gastric cancer* ☠.

SE: *all rare:* GI upset (esp diarrhoea), dizziness, confusion, fatigue, blurred vision, headache, Δ LFTs (rarely hepatitis), rash.

Very rarely arrhythmias (esp if given iv), hypersensitivity, blood disorders.

Dose: initially 150 mg bd po (or 300 mg nocte)[1,2], ↑ing to 600 mg/day if necessary but try to ↓ to 150 mg nocte or bd for maintenance; 50 mg tds/qds iv[3] (or im/ivi[SPC/BNF]).

NB: ↓dose if RF.

REBOXETINE

NA reuptake inhibitor; binds to noradrenaline transporter (NAT) > serotonin transporter (SERT).

Use: depression.

Caution: epilepsy, ↑prostate/urinary retention, CVD, BPAD, glaucoma (angle-closure), H.

SE: ↓sleep, dizziness, dry mouth, GI upset (C&N&V), ↑sweating, ↓appetite, agitation, headache, paraesthesia, visual disorders, cardiac fx (↑HR, palpitations, ↑/↓BP), rash, urinary disturbance, sexual dysfunction, chills.

Warn: avoid sudden withdrawal.

Interactions: metab by P450 (CYP3A4); ☠ ↑risk of hypertensive crisis with MAOIs & linezolid. ☠

Dose: 4 mg po bd for 3–4 wk, ↑ to 10 mg od in divided doses, max 12 mg od.

RIFAMPICIN

Rifamycin antibiotic: 'cidal' ⇒ ↓RNA synthesis.

Use: TB Rx, *N. meningitidis* (meningococcal)/*H. influenzae* (type b) meningitis Px. Rarely for *Legionella/Brucella/Staphylococcus* infections.

CI: jaundice, concurrent saquinavir/ritonavir therapy, hypersensitivity to rifamycins or excipients.

Caution: acute porphyria, L/R/P.

SE: hepatotoxicity, GI upset (inc AAC), headache, fever, flu-like symptoms (esp if intermittent use), orange/red body secretions*, SOB, blood disorders, skin reactions, shock, AKI.

Warn: of symptoms/signs of liver disease; report jaundice/
persistent N&V/malaise immediately. Take 30–60 min before food.
Warn about secretions and can discolour soft contact lenses*.
Monitor: LFTs, FBC (and U&Es if dose >600 mg/day).
Interactions: ↑P450 ∴ many^SPC/BNF; most importantly ↓s fx
of OCP**, atovaquone, lamotrigine, phenytoin, sulphonylureas,
tolbutamide, canagliflozin, nateglinide, quinine, mefloquine,
gefi-/nilotinib, keto-/flu-/itra-/posa-/voriconazole, terbinafine,
antivirals, telithromycin, nevirapine, ciclosporin, siro-/tacrolimus,
mycophenolate, dronedarone, rivaroxaban, dabigatran, cytotoxics,
corticosteroids, abiraterone, ivacaftor, macitentan, ranolazine,
roflumilast, tadalafil, ticagrelor, haloperidol, aripiprazole,
disopyramide, bosentan, propafenone, eplerenone and Ca^{2+}
antagonists. ↑risk of hepatotoxicity with isoniazid, W–.
Dose: see SPC/BNF. (*NB:* well-absorbed po; give iv *only* if
↓swallow.) *NB:* ↓dose if LF or RF.

Other contraception** needed during Rx.

RISEDRONATE

Bisphosphonate: ↓s osteoclastic bone resorption.
Use: osteoporosis (Px[1]/Rx[2], esp if post-menopausal or steroid
induced), Paget's disease[3].
CI: ↓Ca^{2+}, R (if eGFR ≤ 30 mL/min), P/B.
Caution: delayed GI transit/emptying (esp oesophageal
abnormalities). Correct Ca^{2+} and other bone/mineral metabolism
Δ (e.g. vit D and PTH function) before Rx, dental procedures in
patients at risk of osteonecrosis of the jaw (e.g. chemotherapy).
SE: GI upset, bone/joint/muscle pain, headache, rash. Rarely iritis,
dry eyes/corneal lesions, oesophageal stricture/inflammation/
ulcer*, osteonecrosis of the jaw and atypical femoral fractures.
Warn: of symptoms of oesophageal irritation and if develop to
stop tablets/seek medical attention. Must swallow tablets whole
with full glass of water on an empty stomach ≥30 min before, and
stay upright until breakfast/other food/oral medications*. Need to
report thigh, hip or groin pain.

Interactions: Ca^{2+}-containing products (inc milk) and antacids ($\Rightarrow$ ↓absorption) ∴ separate doses as much as possible from risedronate. Also avoid iron and mineral supplements.

Dose: 5 mg od[1,2] (or 1 × 35 mg tablet/wk as **Actonel Once a Week**[2]); 30 mg daily for 2 months[3].

▼ RISPERIDONE/RISPERDAL

'Atypical' antipsychotic: similar to olanzapine ($\Rightarrow$ ↓extrapyramidal fx cf 'typical' antipsychotics, esp tardive dyskinesia; however, causes more EPSEs than most 'atypical' antipsychotics). DA, 5-HT_2 and α antagonism. Prodrug: active form paliperidone.

Use: psychosis/schizophrenia (acute and chronic)[NICE], mania and short-term Rx (<6 wk) of persistent aggression unresponsive to non-pharmacological Rx in Alzheimer's.

CI: phenylketonuria.

SE: ↑**prolactin, sedation,** ↑Wt, EPSE, ↓BP, QT prolongation, VTE, blood dyscrasias, ↓seizure threshold.

Caution: similar to olanzapine, but also caution if dementia with Lewy bodies, prolactin-dependent tumours, dehydration, cataract surgery, acute porphyria.

Interactions: levels may be ↓ by carbamazepine and ↑ by ritonavir, fluoxetine and paroxetine. ↑mortality rate in elderly if taking furosemide. ↑risk of arrhythmias with drugs that ↑QTc and atomoxetine. ↑risk of ↓BP with general anaesthetic. ↓s fx of anticonvulsants.

Dose: initially 2 mg od titrating up if necessary, generally to 4–6 mg od (if elderly, initially 500 micrograms bd titrating up if required to max 2 mg bd po). Also available as liquid or quick dissolving 1, 2, 3 or 4 mg tablets and as long-acting im 2-wkly injections ('**Consta**') for ↑compliance. *NB:* ↓**dose if LF or RF.**

▼ RIVAROXABAN/XARELTO

Oral anticoagulant; direct inhibitor of activated factor X (factor Xa).

Use: Px of VTE following knee[1] or hip[2] replacement surgery, initial Rx of DVT[3] or PE[3], continued Rx of DVT or PE[4], Px of recurrent DVT or PE[4], Px of stroke and systemic embolism in non-valvular AF and at ≥1 risk factor (e.g. CHF, HT, previous stroke or TIA, symptomatic HF, E ≥75 years of age, DM)[5], Px of atherothrombotic events after ACS with ↑cardiac biomarkers (in combination with aspirin alone or aspirin and clopidogrel)[6].

CI: active bleeding or significant risk of major bleeding[BNF], in ACS–previous stroke, in ACS–TIA, malignant neoplasms, oesophageal varices, recent brain surgery, recent GI ulcer, recent intracranial haemorrhage, ophthalmic surgery or spine surgery, vascular aneurysm, **L** (if coagulopathy present)/ **R**(if severe)/**P/B**.

Caution: ☠ anaesthesia with post-operative indwelling epidural catheter (risk of paralysis), see BNF; bronchiectasis, prosthetic heart valve (efficacy not established), risk of bleeding; ☠ do not use as alternative to unfractionated heparin in patients with PE and haemodynamic instability, or who may receive thrombolysis or pulmonary embolectomy; severe HTN, vascular retinopathy, mild-to-moderate liver impairment.

SE: anaemia, haemorrhage, menorrhagia, ↓BP/dizziness, GI upset, headache, fever, oedema, pain in extremity, renal impairment, skin reactions, wound complications. Less common: allergic oedema, angioedema, dry mouth, hepatic disorders, intracranial haemorrhage, syncope, ↑HR, ↓ or ↑Pt. Rarely vascular pseudoaneurysm.

Dose: To be taken with food[1,2], to be started 6–10 h after surgery – 10 mg bd po for 2 wk[1]; for 5 wk[2]. 15 mg bd po for 21 days, to be taken with food[3]. 20 mg od po (see SPC for duration of treatment and dose[4]), 20 mg od po[5]; 2.5 mg bd po (usual duration 12 months[6]). ↓dose in RF.[BNF] See SPC for how to change from, or to, other anticoagulants.

RIVASTIGMINE/EXELON

Acetylcholinesterase inhibitor that acts centrally (crosses blood-brain barrier): replenishes ACh, which is ↓d in certain dementias.
Use: Alzheimer's disease[NICE] and Parkinson's disease dementia.
CI: **L** (if severe, otherwise caution), **B**.
Caution: conduction defects (esp SSS), PU susceptibility, Hx of COPD/asthma/seizures, bladder outflow obstruction, **R/P**.
SE: cholinergic **fx**, ↓Wt, GI upset (esp nausea initially), headache, dizziness, behavioural/Ψ reactions. Rarely GI haemorrhage, ↓HR, AV block, angina, seizures, rash.
Monitor: Wt, pulse.
Dose: 1.5 mg bd po initially (↑ing slowly to 3–6 mg bd: specialist review needed for clinical response and tolerance). Give with morning and evening meals. Available as daily transdermal patch releasing 4.6 mg or 9.5 mg/24 h.

NB: If >3 days are missed for any formulation, retitration at the lowest dose is necessary.

RIZATRIPTAN/MAXALT

$5\text{-HT}_{1B/1D}$ agonist for acute migraine.
Use/CI/Caution/SE/Interactions: see Sumatriptan.
Dose: 10 mg po (can repeat after ≥2 h if responded then recurs). Max 20 mg/24 h. Absorption delayed by approximately 1 h if taken with food. *NB:* give 5 mg doses if **RF** or **LF** (and avoid if either severe).

ROPINIROLE/REQUIP[1] or ADARTREL[2]

Dopamine agonist (non-ergot derived); use in early Parkinson's ⇒ ↓motor complications (e.g. dyskinesias) but ↓motor performance cf

L-dopa. Also adjunctive use in Parkinson's with motor fluctuations.

Use: Parkinson's[1], moderate-to-severe restless legs syndrome (RLS)[2].

CI: P/B.

Caution: major psychotic disorders, severe cardiovascular disease, L/R.

SE: GI upset, sleepiness (inc sudden-onset sleep), ↓BP (inc postural, esp initially), Ψ disorders (esp psychosis and impulse control disorders, e.g. gambling and ↑sexuality), confusion, hallucinations, leg oedema, paradoxical worsening of restless legs syndrome symptoms or early morning rebound (may need to withdraw or reduce dose).

Warn: sleepiness and ↓BP may impair skilled tasks (inc driving). Avoid abrupt withdrawal. Take with food.

Dose: initially 250 micrograms tds[1] (or 250 micrograms nocte for RLS[2]) ↑ing if tolerated/required to max 8 mg tds[1] (or 4 mg nocte for RLS[2]). Available in MR preparation 2–24 mg od[1].

ROSUVASTATIN/CRESTOR

HMG-Co A reductase inhibitor; 'statin' to ↓cholesterol (and TG).

Use/CI/Caution/SE: as simvastatin, but can ⇒ DM and proteinuria (and rarely haematuria). Avoid if severe RF.

Interactions: ↑risk of myositis with ☠ fibrates and ciclosporin ☠, daptomycin, protease inhibitors, fusidic and nicotinic acid. Levels ↓ by antacids, erythromycin. Mild **W+**.

Dose: initially 5–10 mg od. If necessary ↑ to 20 mg after ≥4 wk (if not of Asian origin or risk factors for myopathy/rhabdomyolysis, can ↑ to 40 mg after further 4 wk). *NB:* ↓dose if RF, Asian origin or other ↑risk factor for myopathy.

SALBUTAMOL

β_2 agonist, short acting: dilates bronchial smooth muscle (and endometrium). Also inhibits mast-cell mediator release.

Use: chronic[1] and acute[2] asthma. Rarely ↑K+(give nebs prn), premature labour (iv).

Caution: cardiovascular disease (esp arrhythmias*, susceptibility to ↑QTc, HTN), DM (can ⇒ DKA, esp if iv ∴ monitor CBGs), ↑T$_4$, P/B.

SE: *neurological:* fine tremor, headache, nervousness, behavioural/sleep Δs (esp in children); CVS: ↑**HR**, palpitations/ arrhythmias (esp if iv), ↑QTc*; *other:* ↓K+, muscle cramps. Rarely hypersensitivity, paradoxical bronchospasm. Lactic acidosis with high doses.

Monitor: K+ and glucose (esp if ↑ or iv doses).

Interactions: iv salbutamol ⇒ ↑risk of ↓↓BP with methyldopa.

Dose: 100–200 micrograms (aerosol) or 200–400 micrograms (powder) inh prn up to qds[1]; 2.5–5 mg qds 4-hrly neb[2]. If life-threatening (see p. 408, refer 'Acute Asthma' section in 'Emergencies' chapter), can ↑nebs to every 15 min or give as ivi (initially 5 micrograms/min, then up to 20 micrograms/min according to response).

SALMETEROL/SEREVENT

Bronchodilator: long-acting β_2 agonist (LABA).

Use: first choice add-on for asthma Rx[1] (on top of short-acting β_2 agonist and inh steroids). Also COPD[2].

Not for acute Rx.

Caution/SE/Monitor: as salbutamol.

Dose: 50–100 micrograms bd inh[1]; 50 micrograms bd inh[2].

SANDOCAL

Calcium supplement; available as '1000' (1 g calcium = 25 mmol Ca^{2+}) effervescent tablets.

SANDO-K

Effervescent oral KCl (12 mmol K+/tablet).

Use: ↓K⁺.
CI: K⁺ >5 mmol/L, **R** (if severe, otherwise caution).
Caution: GI ulcer/stricture, hiatus hernia, taking other drugs that ↑K⁺ and cardiac disease.
SE: N&V, GI ulceration, flatulence.
Dose: according to serum K+: start with 2–4 tablets/day if diet normal. Take with food. *NB:* **↓dose in RF/elderly** (↑ if established ↓K⁺).

SAXAGLIPTIN/ONGLYZA

Oral antidiabetic (dipeptidylpeptidase-4 inhibitor): ⇒ ↑insulin secretion and ↓glucagon secretion. Does not appear associated with ↑Wt. ↓incidence of hypoglycaemia than with sulfonylureas.
Use: type 2 DM as monotherapy (if metformin inappropriate), or combined with other antidiabetic drugs (including insulin) if existing Rx fails to achieve glycaemic control.
CI: history of serious hypersensitivity to dipeptidylpeptidase-4 inhibitors. **L** (if severe)/**P**/**B**.
Caution: history of pancreatitis **L**/**R**/**E**.
SE: abdominal pain, constipation, vomiting, dizziness, tiredness, headache, ↑risk of infection, skin reactions. Uncommon: pancreatitis. Rarely angioedema.
Dose: 5 mg od po. Dose of concomitant sulphonylurea or insulin may need to be ↓d. ↓dose in RF.

▼ SEMISODIUM VALPROATE/DEPAKOTE

See (Sodium) valproate: semisodium valproate = equimolar amounts of sodium valproate and valproic acid.
Use: treatment of mania[1]; migraine prophylaxis (unlicensed)[2].
CI/Caution/SE/Warn/Monitor/Interactions: see (Sodium) valproate.
Dose: initially 750 mg po od in two to three divided doses, ↑ to 1–2 g od, doses >45 mg/kg od require careful monitoring[1]; initially 250 mg bd, ↑ to 1 g od in divided doses[2].

NB: semisodium valproate and sodium valproate have the same adverse effects but the severity/frequency may differ slightly due to different times to convert to free valproate.

Women of childbearing age must not be prescribed valproate without being enrolled on a Pregnancy Prevention Programme (MHRA April 2018 alert)*. Patients must sign a risk acknowledgement form.

SENNA/SENOKOT

Stimulant laxative; takes 8–12 h to work.
Use: constipation.
CI: GI obstruction.
Caution: P (try bulk-forming or osmotic laxative first).
SE: GI cramps. If chronic use atonic non-functioning colon, $\downarrow K^+$.
Dose: 2 tablets nocte (can ↑ to 4 tablets nocte). Available as syrup.

SEPTRIN see Co-trimoxazole (sulphamethoxazole + trimethoprim).

SERETIDE: combination asthma or COPD inhaler with possible synergistic action: long-acting β_2 agonist (LABA) salmeterol 50 micrograms (Accuhaler) or 25 micrograms (**Evohaler**) + fluticasone (steroid) in varying quantities (50, 100, 125, 250 or 500 micrograms/puff). Note different devices have different licensed indications.

SEROXAT see Paroxetine; SSRI antidepressant.

SERTRALINE/LUSTRAL

SSRI antidepressant; also increases dopamine levels; see Fluoxetine.
Use: depression[1] (also PTSD, OCD, social anxiety disorder and panic disorder). Relatively good safety record in pregnancy and breastfeeding (can use if benefits > risks).
CI/Caution/SE/Warn/Interactions: as fluoxetine, but ↑agitation/insomnia, does not ↑carbamazepine/phenytoin levels, but does ↑pimozide levels (CI with pimozide).

Dose: initially 50 mg od (25 mg for PTSD and anxiety disorders), ↑ing in 50 mg increments over several weeks to max daily dose 200 mg. *NB:* ↓**dose or frequency if LF.**

SEVELAMER HYDROCHLORIDE

PO_4 binding agent; contains no Al/Ca^{2+} ∴ no risk of ↑ing Al/Ca^{2+} (which can occur with other drugs, esp if on dialysis). Also ↓s cholesterol.

Use: ↑PO_4 (if on dialysis). Also chronic kidney disease not on dialysis with PO_4 ≥1.78 mmol/L.

CI: GI obstruction, ↓PO_4.

Caution: GI disorders, P/B.

SE: GI upset.

Interactions: can ↓plasma levels of ciprofloxacin, levothyroxine, ciclosporin and immunosuppressants used in renal transplant patients.

Dose: initially 800–1600 mg tds po with meals, then adjust to response.[SPC/BNF]

SILDENAFIL/VIAGRA OR REVATIO

Phosphodiesterase type-5 inhibitor: ↑s local fx of NO (⇒ ↑smooth-muscle relaxation ∴ ↑blood flow into corpus cavernosum).

Use: erectile dysfunction[1], pulmonary artery hypertension[2] (and digital ulceration under specialist supervision).

CI: recent CVA/MI/ACS, ↓BP (systolic <90 mm Hg), hereditary degenerative retinal disorders, Hx of non-arteritic anterior ischaemic optic neuropathy and conditions where vasodilation/sexual activity is inadvisable, L/H (if either severe).

Caution: cardiovascular disease, LV outflow obstruction, bleeding disorders (inc active PU), anatomical deformation of penis, predisposition to prolonged erection (e.g. multiple myeloma/leukaemias/sickle cell disease), R/P/B.

SE: headache, flushing, GI upset, dizziness, visual disturbances, nasal congestion, hypersensitivity reactions. Rarely serious cardiovascular events, priapism and painful red eyes.

Interactions: ☠ *Nitrates (e.g. GTN/ISMN/ISDN) and nicorandil can ↓↓BP ∴ never give together.* ☠ Antivirals (esp rito-/ataza-/indinavir) ↑ its levels. ↑s hypotensive fx of α-blockers; avoid concomitant use. Levels ↑d by keto-/itraconazole and grapefruit juice.
Dose: initially 50 mg po approximately 1 h before sexual activity[1], adjusting to response (1 dose per 24 h, max 100 mg per dose); 20 mg po or 10 mg iv tds[2]. *NB:* ↓**dose if RF or LF.**

SIMVASTATIN/ZOCOR

HMG-CoA reductase inhibitor ('statin'): ⇒ ↓cholesterol (↓s synthesis), ↓LDL (↑s uptake), mildly ↓s TG.
Use: ↑cholesterol, Px of atherosclerotic disease: IHD (inc 1° prevention), CVA, PVD.
CI: **L** (inc active liver disease or Δ LFTs), **P** (contraception required during, and for 1 month after, Rx), **B**.
Caution: ↓T_4, alcohol abuse, Hx of liver disease, **R** (if severe).
SE: hepatitis and myositis* (both rare but important), headache, GI upset, rash. Rarely pancreatitis, hypersensitivity, anaemia, tendinopathy.
Monitor: LFTs (and CK if symptoms develop*).
Interactions: ↑risk of myositis (±↑levels) with ☠ fibrates ☠, clari-/ery-/telithromycin, itra-/keto-/mi-/posaconazole, ciclosporin, protease inhibitors, nicotinic acid, fusidic acid, colchicine, danazol, amiodarone, dronedarone, verapamil, diltiazem, amlodipine, ranolazine and grapefruit juice, mild **W+**.
Dose: 10–80 mg nocte (usually start at 10–20 mg[SPC/BNF]), ↑ing at intervals ≥4 wk. ↓max dose if significant drug interactions.[SPC/BNF] *NB:* ↓**dose if RF** or other ↑risk factor for myositis*.

☠ Myositis* can rarely ⇒ rhabdomyolysis; ↑risk if ↓T_4, RF or taking drugs that ↑levels/risk of myositis (see previous discussion) ☠.

SINEMET see Co-careldopa; L-dopa for Parkinson's.

SLOW-K

Slow-release (non-effervescent) oral KCl (8 mmol K^+/tablet).

Use: ↓K⁺ where liquid/effervescent tablets inappropriate.
CI/Caution/SE: as Sando-K, plus caution if ↓swallow.
Dose: according to serum K⁺: average 3–6 tablets/day. *NB:* ↓**dose if RF** (and caution if taking other drugs that ↑K⁺) and should be taken whole with plenty of water, during meals while sitting upright.

▼ (SODIUM) VALPROATE

Antiepileptic and mood stabiliser: potentiates and ↑s GABA levels.
Use: epilepsy[1], mania[2] (and off-licence for other Ψ disorders).
CI: acute porphyria, personal or family Hx of severe liver dysfunction, **L** (inc active liver disease); women and girls of childbearing potential unless conditions met of Pregnancy Prevention Programme.[MHRA]
Caution: SLE, ↑bleeding risk*, women of childbearing age **R**, **P** (⇒ neural-tube/craniofacial and other developmental defects**; therefore, give Px folate), **B**.
SE: sedation, **cerebellar fx** (see p. 348, refer 'Cerebellar Effects' in 'Side Effect Profiles' in 'Basic Psychopharmacology' chapter; esp tremor, ataxia), **headache, GI upset,** ↑Wt, SOA, alopecia, skin reactions, ↓cognitive/motor function, Ψ disorders, encephalopathy (2° to ↑ammonia). Rarely but seriously **hepatotoxicity, blood disorders** (esp ↓Pt*), **pancreatitis** (mostly in first 6 months of Rx).
Warn: of clinical features of pancreatitis and liver/blood disorders. Inform women of childbearing age of teratogenicity/need for contraception**.
Monitor: LFTs, FBC ± serum levels *pre-dose* (therapeutic range 50–100 mg/L; useful for checking compliance but ↓use for efficacy).
Interactions: fx ↓d by antimalarials (esp mefloquine), orlistat, carbapenems, antidepressants (inc St John's wort), antipsychotics and some antiepileptics.[SPC/BNF] Levels ↑ by cimetidine. ↑s fx of aspirin and primidone. ↑risk of ↓NØ with olanzapine. Mild **W+**.
Dose: initially 300 mg bd, ↑ing to max of 2.5 g/day[1]; initially 750 mg in 1–2 divided doses, ↑ing to usual dose of 1–2 g in 1–2 divided doses[2]. *NB:* ↓**dose if RF**.

Can give false-positive urine dipstick for ketones.

SPIRIVA see Tiotropium; new inhaled muscarinic antagonist.

SPIRONOLACTONE

K⁺-sparing diuretic: aldosterone antagonist at distal tubule (also potentiates loop and thiazide diuretics).
Use: ascites (esp 2° to cirrhosis or malignancy), oedema, HF (adjunct to ACE-i and/or another diuretic), nephrotic syndrome, 1° aldosteronism.
CI: ↑K⁺, ↓Na⁺, Addison's, **P/B**.
Caution: porphyria, **L/R/E**.
SE: ↑K⁺, gynaecomastia, GI upset (inc N&V), impotence, ↓BP, ↓Na⁺, rash, confusion, headache, hepatotoxicity, blood disorders.
Monitor: U&E.
Interactions: ↑s digoxin and lithium levels. ↑s risk of RF with NSAIDs (which also antagonise its diuretic fx).
Dose: 100–400 mg/day po (25 mg od if for HF).

> 🕮 Beware if on other drugs that ↑K⁺, e.g. amiloride, triamterene, ACE-i, angiotensin II antagonists and ciclosporin. Do not give with oral K⁺ supplements inc dietary salt substitutes 🕮.

STEMETIL see Prochlorperazine; DA antagonist antiemetic.

ST JOHN'S WORT

Herbal medicinal product – unlicensed.
Use: mild low mood and anxiety. Not recommended.ᴺᴵᶜᴱ
CI: photosensitivity, phototherapy, concomitant use of interacting medications (see Interactions).
SE: GI upset (N&D), abdominal pain, photosensitivity, ↓appetite, dizziness, confusion, fatigue, sedation, restlessness, headache.
Interactions: ↑P450 (**CYP3A4, CYP1A2**); fx vary between preparations; ↓levels of antiretrovirals, benzodiazepines (e.g. alprazolam, midazolam), COCP, immunosuppressants

S

(e.g. cyclosporine, tacrolimus), antiarrhythmics (e.g. amiodarone, flecainide, mexiletine), β-blockers (e.g. metoprolol, carvedilol), calcium channel blockers (e.g. verapamil, diltiazem, amlodipine, pregabalin), statins (e.g. lovastatin, simvastatin, atorvastatin), digoxin, methadone, omeprazole, phenobarbital, theophylline, warfarin, levodopa, buprenorphine; ↑serotonergic fx with TCA (e.g. amitriptyline, clomipramine), MAOI (e.g. moclobemide), SSRI (e.g. citalopram, escitalopram, fluoxetine, fluvoxamine, paroxetine, sertraline), duloxetine, venlafaxine, anxiolytics (e.g. buspirone), 5-HT agonists (e.g. Sumatriptan).
Dose: preparations vary – see relevant SPC.

☠ Multiple drug interactions.

▼ STRONTIUM RANELATE/ARISTO
↑s bone formation and ↓s bone resorption.
Use: osteoporosis^NICE if at ↑risk and other treatments such as bisphosphonates CI/not tolerated.^SPC/BNF
CI: VTE (inc Hx of), temporary or prolonged immobilisation, IHD (inc PHx of), peripheral arterial/cerebrovascular disease, uncontrolled HTN, phenylketonuria (contains aspartame), **P/B.**
Caution: ↑risk of VTE (must assess risk if >80 years old), Δs urinary and plasma Ca^{2+} measurements, R (avoid if severe).
SE: severe allergic reactions*, GI upset.
Warn: to report any skin rash* and immediately stop drug.
Interactions: absorption ↓ by concomitant ingestion of Ca^{2+} (e.g. milk) and Mg^{2+}. ↓s absorption of quinolones and tetracycline.
Dose: 2 g (1 sachet in water) po od at bedtime.^SPC/BNF *Avoid food/milk 2 h before and after taking.* **NB** specialist use only.

☠ Rash* can be early DRESS syndrome: Drug Rash, Eosinophilia and Systemic Symptoms (e.g. fever); lymphadenopathy and ↑WCC also seen early. Can ⇒ LF, RF or respiratory failure ± death. ☠

SULPIRIDE

Benzamide, atypical antipsychotic; selective dopamine D_2 antagonist.

Use: schizophrenia, predominantly –ve symptoms[1]; schizophrenia, predominantly +ve symptoms[2].

CI: CNS depression, phaeo, prolactin-elevating tumour, **H**.

Caution: Parkinson's, epilepsy, MG, phaeo, glaucoma (angle-closure), ↑prostate, severe respiratory disease, jaundice, blood disorders, predisposition to postural ↓BP, photosensitivity, aggression/agitation (even low doses may ↑symptoms), Hx/FHx of Ca breast (due to ↑prolactin).

SE: ↑prolactin and assoc Sx, ↓sleep, sedation, **EPSEs**, constipation, ↑LFTs, rash, ↑Wt, **cardiac fx** (↑QTc, arrhythmia), **VTE**, blood dyscrasias, **NMS**, ↓seizure threshold.

Warn: EPSEs and withdrawal fx in neonate if used in third trimester, ↑fx of alcohol.

Monitor: ECG may be required, esp if (risk factors for) CVD or inpatient admission; prolactin at start of therapy, 6 months and then yearly; physical health monitoring (CVD risk) at least once/year.

Interactions: ↑risk of ↑QTc/torsade de pointes with β-blockers, calcium channel blockers, diuretics, stimulant laxatives, class 1A and III antiarrhythmics (e.g. quinidine, disopyramide, amiodarone, sotalol), ↑sedative fx of alcohol, ↓fx of levodopa, ropinirole.

Dose: 200–400 mg po bd, max 800 mg od[1]; 200–400 mg po bd, max 2.4 g od[2].

SUMATRIPTAN/IMIGRAN

$5\text{-HT}_{1B/1D}$ agonist.

Use: migraine (acute). Also cluster headache (sc route and intranasally).

CI: IHD, coronary vasospasm (inc Prinzmetal's), PVD, HTN (moderate, severe or uncontrolled). Hx of MI, CVA or TIA.

Caution: predisposition to IHD (e.g. cardiac disease), L/H/P/B/E.

SE: sensory Δs (tingling, heat, pressure/tightness), dizziness, flushing, fatigue, N&V, seizures, visual Δs and drowsiness.

Interactions: ↑risk of CNS toxicity with SSRIs, MAOIs, moclobemide and St John's wort. ↑risk of vasospasm with ergotamine and methysergide.

Dose: 50 mg po (can repeat after ≥2 h if responded then recurs and can ↑doses, if no **LF**, to 100 mg if required). Max 300 mg/24 h. Available sc or intranasally.[BNF/SPC]

NB: frequent use may ⇒ xmedication overuse headache.

SYMBICORT

Combination asthma/COPD inhaler: each puff contains x microgram budesonide (steroid) + y microgram formoterol (long-acting β_2 agonist) in the following 'x/y' strengths; '100/6', '200/6' and '400/12'. *NB: different strengths have different licenses.*

TADALAFIL/CIALIS/ADCIRCA

Phosphodiesterase type-5 inhibitor; see Sildenafil.

CI/Use/Caution/SE/Interactions: as sildenafil plus CI in moderate HF and uncontrolled HTN/arrhythmias.

Dose *(for erectile dysfunction)*: initially 10 mg ≥30 min before sexual activity, adjusting to response (1 dose per 24 h, max 20 mg per dose, unless RF or LF when max 10 mg).

TAMOXIFEN

Oestrogen receptor antagonist.

Use: oestrogen receptor-positive Ca breast[1] (as adjuvant Rx: ⇒ ↑survival, delays metastasis), anovulatory infertility[2].

CI: P** (exclude pregnancy before starting Rx), history of TE.

Caution: ↑risk of **TE*** (if taking cytotoxics), porphyria, B.

SE: hot flushes, GI upset, menstrual/endometrial Δs (🔬 inc Ca: if Δ vaginal bleeding/discharge or pelvic pain/pressure ⇒ urgent Ix 🔬. Also fluid retention, exac bony metastases pain. Many other gynaecological/blood/skin/metabolic Δs (esp lipids, LFTs).

Warn: of symptoms of endometrial cancer and TE* (and to report calf pain/sudden SOB). If appropriate, advise non-hormonal contraception**.

Interactions: W+, SSRIs.
Dose: 20 mg od po[1]; for anovulatory infertility[2], see SPC/BNF.

TAMSULOSIN/FLOMAXTRA XL

α-Blocker $\Rightarrow$ internal urethral sphincter relaxation ($\therefore \Rightarrow \uparrow$bladder outflow) and systemic vasodilation.
Use: BPH.
CI/Caution/SE/Interactions: as doxazosin plus **L** (if severe).
Dose: 400 micrograms mane (after food).

TEGRETOL see Carbamazepine; antiepileptic.

TELMISARTAN/MICARDIS

Angiotensin II antagonist; see Losartan.
Use: HTN[1]. Px of cardiovascular events if established atherosclerosis or type 2 DM with organ damage[2].
CI: biliary obstruction, **L** (if severe, otherwise caution), **P/B**.
Caution/SE/Interactions: as losartan, plus $\uparrow$s digoxin levels.
Dose: 20–80 mg od[1] (usually 40 mg od); 80 mg od[2]. *NB:* ↓**dose if LF or RF.**

TEMAZEPAM

Benzodiazepine, short-acting.
Use: insomnia (short-term management)
CI/Caution/SE/Interactions: see Diazepam.
Dose: 10 mg nocte (can ↑dose if tolerant to benzodiazepines, but beware respiratory depression) max dose 40 mg od.
NB: **Dependency common: max 4 wk Rx.** *NB:* ↓**dose if LF, severe RF or elderly.**

TERAZOSIN/HYTRIN

α-Blocker $\Rightarrow$ internal urethral sphincter relaxation ($\therefore \Rightarrow \uparrow$bladder outflow) and systemic vasodilation.
Use: BPH[1] (and rarely HTN[2]).
Caution: Hx of micturition syncope or postural ↓BP, **P/B/E**.
SE/Interactions: see Doxazosin. 'First-dose collapse' common.

T

Dose: initially 1 mg nocte, ↑ing as necessary to max 10 mg/day[1] (or 20 mg/day[2]).

TERBINAFINE/LAMISIL

Antifungal: oral[1,2] or topical cream[3].
Use: ringworm[1] (*Tinea* spp), dermatophyte nail infections[2], fungal skin infections[3]. *NB: Ineffective in yeast infections.*
Caution: psoriasis (may worsen), autoimmune disease (risk of lupus-like syndrome), L/R (neither apply if giving topically), P/B.
SE: headache, GI upset, mild rash, joint/muscle pains. Rarely neuro-Ψ disturbances, blood disorders, hepatic dysfunction, serious skin reactions (stop drug if progressive rash).
Dose: 250 mg od po for 2–6 wk[1] or 6 wk–3 months[2]; 1–2 topical applications/day for 1–2 wk[3].

TERBUTALINE/BRICANYL

Inhaled β_2 agonist similar to salbutamol.
Dose: 500 micrograms od-qds inh (powder or aerosol); 5–10 mg up to qds neb. Can also give po/sc/im/iv.[SPC/BNF]

TETRACYCLINE

Tetracycline broad-spectrum antibiotic: inhibits ribosomal (30S subunit) protein synthesis.
Use: acne vulgaris[1] (or rosacea), genital/tropical infections (*NB:* doxycycline often preferred).
CI: age <12 years (stains/deforms teeth), acute porphyria, R/P/B.
Caution: may worsen MG or SLE, L.
SE: GI upset (rarely AAC), oesophageal irritation, headache, dysphagia. Rarely hepatotoxicity, blood disorders, photosensitivity, hypersensitivity, visual Δs (rarely 2° to BIH; stop drug if suspected).
Interactions: ↓absorption with milk (do not drink 1 h before or 2 h after drug), antacids and Fe/Al/Ca/Mg/Zn salts. ↓s fx of OCP (small risk). ↑risk of BIH with retinoids. Mild W+.
Dose: 500 mg bd po[1], otherwise 250–500 mg tds/qds po. *NB:* max 1 g/24 h in LF.

NB: swallow tablets whole with plenty of fluid while sitting or standing and take ≥30 min before food.

THIAMINE (= VITAMIN B1)
Use: replacement for nutritional deficiencies (esp in alcoholism).
Dose: 100 mg bd/tds po in severe deficiency (25 mg od if mild/chronic).

For iv preparations, see Pabrinex and p. 298, refer 'Wernicke's Encephalopathy' heading in 'Substance Misuse' section of 'Disorders' chapter for Mx of acute alcohol withdrawal.

THYROXINE (= LEVOTHYROXINE)
Synthetic T_4 (*NB:* thyroxine often now called 'levothyroxine').
Use: $\downarrow T_4$ Rx (for maintenance). *NB:* acutely, e.g. myxoedema coma, liothyronine (T_3) often needed.
CI: $\uparrow T_4$, adrenal insufficiency.
Caution: panhypopituitarism/other predisposition to adrenal insufficiency (*corticosteroids needed first*), chronic $\downarrow T_4$, cardiovascular disorders (esp HTN/IHD; can worsen)*, DI, DM, P/B/E.
SE: features of $\uparrow T_4$ (should be minimal unless xs Rx): D&V, tremors, restlessness, headache, flushing, sweating, heat intolerance, angina, arrhythmias, palpitations, $\uparrow$HR, muscle cramps/weakness, $\downarrow$Wt. Also osteoporosis (esp if xs dose given; use min dose necessary).
Interactions: can Δ digoxin and antidiabetic** requirements, $\uparrow$fx of TCAs and $\downarrow$levels of propranolol. W+.
Monitor: baseline ECG to help distinguish Δs due to ischaemia or $\downarrow T_4$.
Dose: 25–200 micrograms mane (titrate up slowly, esp if >50 years old/$\downarrow\downarrow T_4$/HTN/IHD*).

NB: For T_3 see Liothyronine.

TICAGRELOR/BRILIQUE

Antiplatelet agent (purinergic [P2Y$_{12}$] receptor antagonist): prevents ADP-mediated P2Y$_{12}$-dependent Pt activation and aggregation.
Use: Px of atherothrombotic events in ACS[1] (in combination with aspirin)[NICE], Px of atherothrombotic events if previous AMI and ↑risk of atherothrombotic events[2] (in combination with aspirin).[NICE]
CI: active bleeding; history of intracranial haemorrhage, severe LF, P/B.
Caution: asthma, COPD; unless pacemaker fitted – bradycardia, second- or third-degree AV block or SSS; stop 5 days before elective surgery if antiplatelet effect not desirable, history of hyperuricaemia; ↑risk of bleeding[BNF] (unless pacemaker fitted), LF, monitor renal function for 1 month if Rx for ACS.
SE: haemorrhage, GI upset, dizziness/syncope, dyspepsia, dyspnoea; hyperuricaemia/gout/gouty arthritis, headache; skin reactions, angioedema; confusion.
Dose: initially 1 dose of 180 mg po, then 90 mg bd po (usually for ≤12 months)[1]; 60 mg bd po, extended Rx may be started without interruption after initial 12-month therapy for ACS[2]. Rx[2] may also be started <2 years from AMI, ≤1 year after stopping previous ADP receptor inhibitor Rx (limited data on continuing Rx[2] beyond 3 years[BNF]).

TIMOLOL EYE DROPS/TIMOPTOL

β-blocker eye drops; ↓aqueous humour production.
Use: glaucoma (second line), ocular HTN (first line); not useful if on systemic β-blocker.
CI: asthma, ↓HR, HB, H (if uncontrolled).
Caution/SE/Interactions: as propranolol* plus can ⇒ local irritation.
Dose: 1 drop bd (0.25% or 0.5%). Also available in long-acting od preparations **TIMOPTOL LA** (0.25% and 0.5%) and **NYOGEL/TIOPEX** (0.1%). Timolol 0.5% also available in

combination with other classes of glaucoma medications; carbonic anhydrase inhibitors (dorzolamide **Cosopt**, brinzolamide **Azarga**), PG analogues (latanoprost **Xalacom**, travoprost **DuoTrav**, bimatoprost **Ganfort**), α-agonists (brimonidine **Combigan**).

💀 Systemic absorption possible despite topical application 💀.

TIOTROPIUM/SPIRIVA

Long-acting inh muscarinic antagonist for COPD (and asthma as **Respimat** solution); similar to ipratropium, but only for chronic use and caution in RF. Also caution in arrhythmias, IHD or HF for Respimat.

SE: dry mouth, urinary retention, glaucoma.
Dose: 18 micrograms (**Spiriva**) or 10 micrograms (**Braltus**) dry powder inhaler od inh; 5 micrograms by solution inhaler (**Respimat**) od inh.

TOLBUTAMIDE

Oral antidiabetic (short-acting sulphonylurea).
Use/CI/Caution/SE/Interactions: as gliclazide. Can also ⇒ headache and tinnitus.
Dose: 500 mg–2 g daily in divided doses, with food. *NB:* ↓dose if LF.

TOLTERODINE/DETRUSITOL

Antimuscarinic, antispasmodic.
Use: detrusor instability; urinary incontinence/frequency/urgency.
CI/Caution/SE: as oxybutynin (SEs mostly antimuscarinic fx; see p. 346, refer 'Cholinoceptors' heading in 'Basic Psychopharmacology' chapter) plus caution if Hx of, or taking drugs that, ↑QTc, **P/B**.
Interactions: ↑risk of ventricular arrhythmias with amiodarone, disopyramide, flecainide and sotalol.
Dose: 1–2 mg bd po. *NB:* ↓**dose if RF or LF**. (MR preparation available as 4 mg od po; not suitable if RF or LF.)

TOPIRAMATE

Anticonvulsant; exact mechanism unknown – acts to stabilise cell membrane via Na^+ or Cl^- channels.

Use: monotherapy for generalised tonic-clonic or focal seizures[1], adjunctive treatment in epilepsy[2], migraine prophylaxis[3].

CI: women of childbearing potential if not on highly effective contraception, **P** (if for migraine).

Caution: risk of renal stones/metabolic acidosis, porphyria, cognitive impairment, ↑ammonia, **B/P**.

SE: nasopharyngitis, Ψ fx (depression, mood Δs, agitation, expressive dysphasia), paraesthesia, somnolence, dizziness, GI upset (V&C, abdo discomfort), fatigue, ↓Wt/appetite, blood dyscrasias, hypersensitivity (rash), impaired cognition, ataxia, visual problems, tinnitus, muscle/joint pain, twitching, renal stones, pyrexia.

Warn: risk of major congenital malformations/need for contraception if given to women of childbearing age. Ensure high fluid intake to avoid renal stones.

Monitor: prenatal monitoring (e.g. foetal growth).

Interactions: ↓fx of COCP, desogestrel, etonogestrel, levonorgestrel, norethisterone, ulipristal; ↑risk of toxicity with valproate (encephalopathy); ↑risk of renal calculi with zonisamide, ↓levels by carbamazepine, phenytoin and primidone.

Dose: initially 25 mg po od at night for 1 wk, ↑ in steps of 25–50 mg every 1–2 wk, usually dose 100–200 mg od in two divided doses, max 500 mg od[1]; initially 25–50 mg po od at night for 1 wk, ↑ in steps of 25–50 mg every 1–2 wk, usual dose 200–400 od in two divided doses, max 400 mg od[2]; initially 25 mg po od at night for 1 wk, ↑ in steps of 25 mg every wk, usual dose 50–100 mg od in two divided doses, max 200 mg od[3].

TRAMADOL

Opioid. Also ↓s pain by ↑ing 5-HT/noradrenergic transmission.

Use: moderate-to-severe pain (esp musculoskeletal).

CI/Caution: as codeine, but also CI in uncontrolled epilepsy, patients taking MAOIs, **P/B**. Not suitable as substitute in opioid-dependent patients.

SE: as morphine, but ↓respiratory depression, ↓constipation, ↓addiction. ↑confusion (esp in elderly) compared to codeine.

Interactions: as codeine; also ↑risk convulsions with SSRIs/TCAs/antipsychotics, ↑risk serotonin syndrome with SSRIs. Carbamazepine and ondansetron ↓ its fx, **W+**.

Dose: initially 100 mg, then 50–100 mg up to 4-hrly po/im/iv, max 400 mg/day. Post-op: initially 100 mg im/iv, then 50 mg every 10–20 min prn (max total dose of 250 mg in first hour), then 50–100 mg 4–6 hrly (max 400 mg/day). *NB:* ↓dose if RF, LF or elderly; see BNF for dosing differences between formulations.

TRANDOLAPRIL/GOPTEN

ACE-i for HTN, HF and LVF post-MI.

CI/Caution/SE/Monitor/Interactions: see Captopril.

Dose: initially 500 micrograms od, ↑ing at intervals of 2–4 wk if required to max 4 mg od (max 2 mg if RF). ↓doses if given with diuretic. If for LVF post-MI, start ≥3 days after MI.

TRANEXAMIC ACID

Antifibrinolytic: inhibits activation of plasminogen to plasmin.

Use: bleeding: acute bleeds[1] (esp 2° to anticoagulants, thrombolytic/anti-Pt agents, epistaxis, haemophilia), menorrhagia[2], hereditary angioedema[3].

CI: TE disease, Hx of convulsions, **R** (if severe, otherwise caution).

Caution: gross haematuria (can clot and obstruct ureters), DIC, **P**.

SE: GI upset, colour vision Δs (stop drug), TE.

Dose: 15–25 mg/kg bd/tds po (if severe, 500 mg–1 g tds iv)[1]; 1 g tds po for 4 days (max 4 g/day)[2]; 1–1.5 g bd/tds po[3]. *NB:* ↓dose if RF.

TRANYLCYPROMINE

MAOI; non-selective and irreversible inhibitor of monoamine oxidase, ↑5-HT, NA and DA in CNS.

Use: depression.

CI: mania, phaeo, cerebrovascular disease, ↑T$_4$, porphyria, concomitant amphetamine use, **L/H**.

Caution: agitation, concurrent ECT, Hx of dependence, suicidal ideation, blood dyscrasias, DM, epilepsy, surgery, severe hypertensive reactions, **P/B/E**.

SE: insomnia, chest pain, diarrhoea, drug dependence, extrasystole, flushing, hypomania, mydriasis, pain, pallor, photophobia, sleep Δs, headache, liver injury (rare), ☠ hypertensive crisis ☠.

Warn: avoid tyramine-rich or dopa-rich food/drinks with/for 2–3 wk after stopping MAOI; withdrawal fx may occur within 5 days of stopping treatment, worse after regular administration for 8 wk+; ↓dose gradually over 4 wk+ (longer if used long term).

Monitor: BP (risk of HTN and postural ↓BP), LFTs.

Interactions: ↓P450 (CYP2A6); ☠ ↑risk of severe toxic reaction with serotonergics, dopaminergics and noradrenergics: SSRIs, SNRIs, NARIs, TCAs (and related drugs), other MAOIs (inc for Parkinson's), carbamazepine, linezolid, triptans, pethidine, tramadol. ☠

- Do not start tranylcypromine until these drugs have been stopped and they have cleared: 5 wk for fluoxetine, 3 wk for clomipramine/imipramine, at least 7–14 days for other drugs.
- Wait 2 wk after stopping tranylcypromine before starting any of these medicines.

↑risk of hypertensive crisis with sympathomimetics, dopamine agonists, CNS stimulants, buspirone. ↑fx of CNS depressants, antimuscarinics, antidiabetics, antihypertensives.

Dose: initially 10 mg po bd taken no later than 3 p.m., ↑ after 1 wk to 10 mg in the morning and 20 mg in the afternoon, maintenance 10 mg od, closer supervision if doses >30 mg od.

☠ Hypertensive crisis may develop if taken with food high in tyramine or DOPA. See p. 236, refer 'MAOI tyramine effect' heading in 'Depression' section of 'Disorders' chapter ☠.

TRAVOPROST EYE DROPS/TRAVATAN

Topical PG analogue for glaucoma; see Latanoprost.
Use/CI/Caution/SE: see Latanoprost.
Dose: 1 drop od, preferably in the evening.

TRAZODONE HYDROCHLORIDE

Antidepressant and anxiolytic; binds at $5-HT_2$ receptors and ↓5-HT reuptake, with α-adrenergic and histaminergic blockade (sedative fx).
Use: depression[1], anxiety[2].
CI: arrhythmia (esp HB), mania, post-MI, **L** (if severe).
Caution: acute MI, phaeo, ↑T_4, sedative intoxication, chronic constipation, DM, epilepsy, Hx of bipolar disorder/psychosis, ↑intraocular pressure, suicide risk, urinary retention, ↑prostate, glaucoma (angle-closure), **L/R** (if severe).
SE: drowsiness, headache, ↑/↓appetite, cardiac fx (↑QTc, ↑BP, postural ↓BP, arrhythmia, syncope), blood dyscrasias, antimuscarinic fx (mild; see p. 346, refer 'Cholinoceptors' heading in 'Basic Psychopharmacolog' chapter), GI upset (C&D&N&V), SOB, ↓Na, sexual dysfunction, liver disorders, Ψ fx (agitation, confusion, psychosis, mania, suicidal ideation), amnesia, movement disorder, **paralytic ileus, serotonin syndrome, seizure**, rash, ↓Wt, sleep Δs, paraesthesia.
Warn: ↑fx of alcohol.
Interactions: metab by P450 (CYP3A4); ☠ ↑risk of serotonin syndrome with TCA ☠; ↑levels with CYP3A4 inhibitors (e.g. erythromycin, ritonavir), ↓levels with COCP, **phenytoin, carbamazepine,** barbiturates.
Dose: initially 150 mg po od at bedtime/taken after food in divided doses, ↑ to 300–600 mg od[1]; 75 mg po od, ↑ to 300 mg od[2].

TRIFLUOPERAZINE/STELAZINE

Phenothiazine, typical antipsychotic; blocks post-synaptic dopamine D_1/D_2 receptors.

Use: high dose: psychosis, short-term adjunctive management of agitated/aggressive behaviour[1]; **low dose:** adjunctive treatment of severe anxiety[2]; severe N&V[3].

CI: CNS depression, phaeo, L.

Caution: Parkinson's, drugs that ↑QTc, epilepsy, MG, phaeo, glaucoma (angle-closure), ↑prostate, severe respiratory disease, jaundice, blood disorders, H/P/B.

Class SE: EPSE, ↑prolactin and assoc Sx, sedation, ↑Wt, QT prolongation, VTE, blood dyscrasias, ↓seizure threshold, NMS.

SE: anxiety, ↓appetite, blood dyscrasia, jaundice, cataract, weakness, oedema, skin reactions, antimuscarinic fx (see p. 346, refer 'Cholinoceptors' heading in 'Basic Psychopharmacology' chapter).

Warn: if used in third trimester, monitor for EPSEs in neonate; avoid direct sunlight at higher doses (photosensitisation), ↑fx of alcohol. Gradual withdrawal advised if on high doses – risk of withdrawal Sx (N&V, insomnia, involuntary movements).

Monitor: ECG may be required, esp if (risk factors for) CVD or inpatient admission; prolactin concentration at start of therapy, 6 months, then yearly.

Interactions: ☠ ↑risk of neuroleptic malignant syndrome with MAOIs ☠; ↑risk of neurotoxicity with lithium and reduced levels by lithium; ↓fx of levodopa.

Dose: initially 5 mg po bd, ↑ by 5 mg after 1 wk, then further ↑ in steps of 5 mg at intervals of 3 days (when satisfactory control achieved, ↓ gradually until effective maintenance level established), max dose in practice 30 mg/day[1]; 2–4 mg po od in divided doses, max 6 mg od.[2,3]

TRI-IODOTHYRONINE

See Liothyronine; synthetic T_3 mostly used in myxoedema coma.

TRIMETHOPRIM

Antifolate antibiotic: inhibits dihydrofolate reductase.

Use: UTIs (rarely other infections).

CI: blood disorders (esp megaloblastic ↓Hb).

Caution: ↓folate (or predisposition to), porphyria, R/P/B/E.

SE: see Co-trimoxazole (Septrin), but much less frequent and severe (esp BM suppression, skin reactions). Also GI upset, rash, rarely other hypersensitivity.

Warn: those on long-term Rx to look for signs of blood disorder and to report fever, sore throat, rash, mouth ulcers, bruising or bleeding.

Interactions: ↑s phenytoin and digoxin levels. ↑s risk of arrhythmias with amiodarone, antifolate fx with pyrimethamine and toxicity with ciclosporin, azathioprine, mercaptopurine and methotrexate, W+.

Dose: 200 mg bd po (100 mg nocte for chronic infections or as Px if at risk; *NB*: risk of ↓folate if long-term Rx). *NB*: ↓dose if RF.

TRIMIPRAMINE

TCA; antagonises H_1, $5\text{-}HT_{2A}$ and α_1-adrenergic receptors, weak reuptake inhibitor of 5-HT, NA and DA.

Use: depression.

CI: recent MI (within 3 months), arrhythmias (esp HB), mania, porphyria, H/L (if severe).

Caution: phaeo, ↑T_4, chronic constipation, DM, epilepsy, Hx of bipolar disorder/psychosis, ↑intraocular pressure, risks of suicide, urinary retention, ↑prostate, glaucoma (angle-closure), L.

SE: antimuscarinic fx, **cardiac fx** (arrhythmias, HB, ↑HR, postural ↓BP, dizziness, syncope: **dangerous in OD**), ↑Wt, **sedation** (often ⇒ 'hangover'), seizures. Rarely mania, fever, blood disorders, hypersensitivity, Δ LFTs, ↓Na^+ (esp in elderly), agitation, confusion, NMS.

Warn: withdrawal fx within 5 days of stopping treatment, worse after use for 8 wks+; ↓dose gradually over 4 wk+; ↑ effects of alcohol.

Interactions: metab by P450; ☠ ↑risk of serotonin syndrome with MAOI, e.g. isocarboxazid, moclobemide, phenelzine, selegiline, tranylcypromine (avoid with/for 14 days after stopping MAOI) ☠; ↑risk of neurotoxicity with lithium; ↑levels with

bupropion, cinacalcet, dronedarone, fluvoxamine, fluoxetine, paroxetine, terbinafine; ↑fx of phenylephrine; ↓fx of adrenaline, ephedrine; some inhaled anaesthetics and sympathomimetics.
Dose: initially 50–75 mg po od at bedtime/in divided doses, ↑ to 150–300 mg od. Usual maintenance dose 75–150 mg od.

> ☠ Overdose is associated with high rate of fatality. TCA overdose ⇒ dilated pupils, arrhythmias, ↓BP, hypothermia, hyperreflexia, extensor plantar responses, seizures, respiratory depression and coma ☠.

TROPICAMIDE EYE DROPS
Antimuscarinic: mydriatic (lasts approximately 4 h), weak cycloplegic.
Use: dilated retinal examination. See also 'Dilating eye drops'.
CI: untreated acute angle-closure glaucoma.
Caution: ↑IOP* (inc predisposition to), inflamed eye (↑risk of systemic absorption).
SE: transient stinging and blurred vision and ↓accommodation. Rarely precipitation of acute angle-closure glaucoma (↑risk if >60 years, long sighted, FHx).
Warn: unable to drive until can read car number plate at 20 m (approximately 4 h).
Dose: 1 drop 1% solution 15–20 min before examination. 0.5% in children <1 year old. *NB:* rare cause of acute angle-closure glaucoma* (esp if >60 years or hypermetropic).

TRYPTOPHAN
Essential dietary amino acid, precursor of serotonin; ↑inhibitory action of serotonin on amygdaloid nuclei.
Use: treatment-resistant depression (with senior advice).
CI: Hx of eosinophilia myalgia syndrome (EMS).
SE: weakness, headache, dizziness, somnolence, blood dyscrasias, muscle ache, nausea, suicidal ideation, eosinophilia myalgia syndrome.

Monitor: signs of suicidal thoughts, esp on initiation and dose Δs.
Interactions: ☠ ↑risk of serotonin syndrome with MAOI, e.g. isocarboxazid, moclobemide, phenelzine, selegiline, tranylcypromine, and SSRI.☠
Dose: 1 g po tds, max 6 g od.

▼ **VALPROATE** See (Sodium) valproate and Semisodium valproate.

VALSARTAN/DIOVAN

Angiotensin II antagonist; see Losartan.
Use: HTN[1], MI with LV failure/dysfunction[2], heart failure[3].
CI: biliary obstruction, cirrhosis, **L** (if severe)/**P**/**B**.
Caution/SE/Interactions: see Losartan (inc warning about drugs that ↑K+).
Dose: initially 80 mg od[1] (*NB:* give 40 mg if ≥75 years old, LF, RF or ↓intravascular volume), 20 mg bd[2] or 40 mg bd[3], ↑ing if necessary to max 320 mg od[1] or 160 mg bd[2,3].

VANCOMYCIN

Glycopeptide antibiotic. Poor po absorption (unless bowel inflammation*), but still effective against *C. difficile***, as acts 'topically' in GI tract.
Use: serious Gram +ve infections[1] (inc endocarditis Px and systemic MRSA), AAC[2] (give po)**.
Caution: Hx of deafness, IBD* (only if given po), avoid rapid infusions (risk of anaphylaxis), **R**/**P**/**B**/**E**.
SE: nephrotoxicity, ototoxicity (stop if tinnitus develops), blood disorders, rash, hypersensitivity (inc anaphylaxis, severe skin reactions), nausea, fever, phlebitis/irritation at injection site.
Monitor: serum levels: keep pre-dose trough levels 10–15 mg/L; start monitoring after third dose (first dose if RF); *NB:* higher trough often recommended in osteomyelitis, endocarditis. Also monitor U&Es, FBC, urinalysis (and auditory function if elderly/RF).
Interactions: ↑nephrotoxicity with ciclosporin and aminoglycosides. ↑ototoxicity with loop diuretics. ↑s fx of suxamethonium.

Dose: 15–20 mg/kg bd/tds (max dose 2 g) ivi at 10 mg/min[1]; 125 mg qds po[2]. *NB:* ↓dose if RF or elderly.

NB: If ivi given too quickly ⇒ ↑risk of anaphylactoid reactions (e.g.↓BP, respiratory symptoms, skin reactions).

VARDENAFIL/LEVITRA

Phosphodiesterase type-5 inhibitor; see Sildenafil.
Use/CI/Caution/SE/Interactions: as sildenafil plus CI in hereditary degenerative retinal disorders, caution if susceptible to (or taking drugs that) ↑QTc, active PU or bleeding disorder and levels ↑ by grapefruit juice.
Dose: initially 10 mg approximately 25–60 min before sexual activity, adjusting to response (1 dose per 24 h, max 20 mg per dose). *NB:* halve dose if LF, RF, elderly or taking α-blocker.

VENLAFAXINE/EFFEXOR

Serotonin and noradrenaline reuptake inhibitor (SNRI): antidepressant with ↓sedative/antimuscarinic fx cf TCAs. ↑danger in OD/heart disease than other antidepressants.
Use: depression[1], generalised anxiety disorder, social anxiety disorder, panic disorder ± agoraphobia.
CI: conditions with very high risk of serious cardiac ventricular arrhythmia (e.g. significant LV dysfunction, NYHA class III/IV), uncontrolled HTN.
Caution: Hx of mania, seizures or glaucoma, L/R (avoid if either severe), H/P/B.
SE: GI upset, ↑BP (dose-related; monitor BP if dose >200 mg/day), withdrawal fx (common even if dose only a few hours late), rash (consider stopping drug, as can be first sign of severe reaction*), insomnia/agitation, dry mouth, sexual dysfunction, Wt Δ, drowsiness, dizziness, SIADH and ↑QTc.
Warn: report rashes*. Do not stop suddenly.
Monitor: BP if heart disease ± ECG.
Interactions: ☠ *never give with*, or ≤2 wk after, MAOIs. ☠ ↑s risk of bleeding with aspirin/NSAIDs, dabigatran and CNS toxicity

with selegiline. Avoid artemether/lumefantrine and piperaquine/artenimol. Mild **W+**.

Dose: immediate release: 37.5–187.5 mg bd po[1]; start low and ↑dose if required. Max in anxiety 225 mg/day in divided dose.

Effexor XL: MR od preparation available (initial dose 75 mg od; max in MDD 375 mg od, max in anxiety 225 mg od).

NB: Halve dose if moderate LF (PT 14–18 sec) or RF (GFR 10–30 mL/min).

VENTOLIN see Salbutamol; β-agonist bronchodilator.

VERAPAMIL

Ca^{2+} channel blocker (rate-limiting type): fx on heart ($\Rightarrow$ ↓HR, ↓contractility*) > vasculature (dilates peripheral/coronary arteries); i.e. reverse of the dihydropyridine type (e.g. nifedipine). Only Ca^{2+} channel blocker with useful antiarrhythmic properties (class IV).

Use: HTN[1], angina[2], arrhythmias (SVTs, esp instead of adenosine if asthma)[3].

CI: ↓BP, ↓HR (<50 bpm), second-/third-degree HB, ↓LV function, SAN block, SSS, AF or atrial flutter 2° to WPW, recent treatment with β-blocker, acute, **H** (inc Hx of)*.

Caution: AMI, first-degree HB, **L/P/B**.

SE: constipation (rarely other GI upset), **HF**, ↓BP (dose dependent), HB, headache, dizziness, fatigue, ankle oedema, hypersensitivity, skin reactions.

Warn: fx ↑d by grapefruit juice (avoid).

Interactions: ↑risk of AV block and HF with ☠ β-blockers ☠ disopyramide, flecainide, dronedarone, colchicine, fingolimod and amiodarone. ↑s hypotensive fx of antihypertensives (esp α-blockers) and anaesthetics. ↑s levels/fx of digoxin, theophyllines, carbamazepine, quinidine, ivabradine, dabigatran, tamsulosin and ciclosporin. Levels/fx ↓ by rifampicin and barbiturates. ↑risk of myopathy with simvastatin. Sirolimus ↑s levels of both drugs. Levels may be ↑ by clari-/erythromycin and ritonavir. Risk of VF with ☠ iv dantrolene ☠.

Dose: 120–160 mg tds po[1]; 80–120 mg tds po[2]; 40–120 mg tds po[3]; 5–10 mg iv (over 2 min [3 min in elderly] with ECG monitoring), followed by additional 5 mg iv if necessary after 5–10 min[3]. MR (od/bd) preparations available.[BNF] *NB:* ↓oral dose in LF.

VIAGRA see Sildenafil; phosphodiesterase inhibitor.

VITAMIN K see Phytomenadione.

VOLTAROL see Diclofenac; moderate-strength NSAID.

WARFARIN

Oral anticoagulant: blocks synthesis of vit K–dependent factors (II, VII, IX, X) and proteins C and S.
Use: Rx/Px of TE.
CI: severe HTN, PU, severe bleeding, haemorrhagic CVA, **P**.
Caution: recent surgery, bacterial endocarditis, 48 h post-partum, **L/R** (avoid if creatinine clearance <10 mL/min)/**B**.
SE: haemorrhage, rash, fever, diarrhoea. Rarely other GI upset, 'purple-toe syndrome', skin necrosis, hepatotoxicity, hypersensitivity.
Warn: fx are ↑d by alcohol and cranberry juice (avoid).
Dose: see BNF/SPC.

> *NB:* **W+** and **W−** denote significant interactions throughout this book: take particular care with antibiotics and drugs that affect cytochrome **P450** (see p. 341, refer 'Enzyme Interactions' heading in 'Basic Psychopharmacology' chapter) .

XALATAN see Latanoprost; topical PG analogue for glaucoma.

ZALEPLON

'Non-benzodiazepine' hypnotic; see Zopiclone.
Use/CI/Caution/SE/Interactions: see Zopiclone.
Dose: 10 mg nocte (5 mg if elderly). *NB:* halve dose if LF (avoid if severe), severe RF or elderly.

ZANTAC see Ranitidine; H antagonist.

ZESTRIL see Lisinopril; ACE-i.

ZIDOVUDINE (AZT)

Antiviral (nucleoside analogue): reverse-transcriptase inhibitor.
Use: HIV Rx (and Px, esp of vertical transmission).
CI: severe ↓NØ or ↓Hb (caution if other blood disorders), acute
porphyria, **B**.
Caution: ↓B12, ↑risk of lactic acidosis, **L/R/P/E**, lipodystrophy,
osteonecrosis, metabolic syndrome.
SE: blood disorders (esp ↓Hb or ↓WCC; monitor FBC), GI upset,
headache, fever, taste Δs, sleep disorders. Rarely hepatic/pancreatic
dysfunction, myopathy, seizures, other neurological/Ψ disorders,
rash and pruritus, metabolic syndrome (monitor Wt, lipids, glucose).
Interactions: levels ↑ by fluconazole, valproate, methadone and
probenecid. fx ↓ by tipranavir. ↑myelosuppression with ganciclovir,
co-trimoxazole. ↑risk of ↓Hb with ribavirin. ↓s fx of stavudine –
avoid use with stavudine.
Dose: see SPC/BNF.

ZIRTEK see Cetirizine; non-sedating antihistamine for allergies.

ZOLEDRONIC ACID/ZOMETA

Bisphosphonate: ↓s osteoclastic bone resorption.
Use: Px of bone damage[1] in advanced bone malignancy, damage or
Rx of ↑Ca^{2+} in malignancy[2], Rx of Paget's disease of bone[3], Rx of
osteoporosis (post-menopausal or in men)[4].
CI: **P/B**.
Caution: cardiac disease, dehydration*, ↓Ca^{2+}/PO$_4^{2-}$/Mg^{2+}.
L (if severe)/**R/H**.
SE: flu-like syndrome, fever, bone pain, fatigue, N&V. Also arthr-/
myalgia, ↓Ca^{2+}/PO$_4^{2-}$/Mg^{2+}, pruritus/rash, headache, conjunctivitis,
RF, hypersensitivity, blood disorders (esp ↓Hb), osteonecrosis
(esp of jaw; consider dental examination or preventive Rx before

starting drug) and atypical femur fractures (advise patients to report thigh/groin pain).
Monitor: Ca^{2+}, PO_4^{2-}, Mg^{2+}, U&E. Ensure patient adequately hydrated pre-dose* and advise good dental hygiene.
Dose: 4 mg ivi every 3–4 wk[1]; 4 mg ivi as single dose[2]. Also available as once-yearly preparation (Aclasta) 5 mg ivi over ≥15 min[3,4]. *NB:* ↓**dose in RF.**

ZOLMITRIPTAN/ZOMIG

$5\text{-}HT_{1B/1D}$ agonist for acute migraine.
Use/CI/Caution/SE/Interactions: as sumatriptan plus CI if Hx of CVA/TIA and in WPW or arrhythmias assoc with accessory cardiac conduction p'way.
Dose: 2.5 mg po (can repeat after ≥2 h if responded then recurs and can ↑doses to 5 mg if required). Max 10 mg/24 h (5 mg/24 h if moderate-to-severe LF). Available intranasally.[BNF/SPC]

ZOLPIDEM (TARTRATE)

'Non-benzodiazepine' hypnotic; see Zopiclone.
Use/CI/Caution/SE/Interactions: as zopiclone but CI in psychotic illness, P.
Dose: 10 mg nocte. *NB:* halve dose if LF (avoid if severe), severe RF or elderly.

ZOMORPH Morphine sulphate capsules (10, 30, 60, 100 or 200 mg), equivalent in efficacy to Oramorph but SR: 12-hrly doses.

ZOPICLONE

Short-acting hypnotic (cyclopyrrolone): potentiates GABA pathways via same receptors as benzodiazepines (although is not a benzodiazepine): can also ⇒ dependence* and tolerance.
Use: insomnia (not long term*).
CI: respiratory failure, sleep apnoea (severe), marked neuromuscular respiratory weakness (inc unstable MG), L (if severe**), B.

Caution: Ψ disorders, Hx of drug abuse*, muscle weakness, MG, R/P/E.

SE: *all rare:* GI upset, taste Δs, behavioural/Ψ disturbances (inc psychosis, aggression), hypersensitivity.

Interactions: levels ↑ by ritonavir, erythromycin and other enzyme inhibitors. Levels ↓ by rifampicin. Sedation ↑d by other sedative medications and alcohol.

Dose: 3.75mg–7.5 mg nocte, for up to 4 wk. *NB:* halve dose if LF (avoid if severe), severe RF or elderly.

ZOTON see Lansoprazole; PPI.

ZUCLOPENTHIXOL ACETATE/CLOPIXOL ACUPHASE

Thioxanthene antipsychotic; antagonises D_1/D_2 receptors, α_1-adrenoceptors and 5-HT_2 receptors.

Use: short-term management of psychosis or mania when an effect of 2–3 days is desirable.

CI: CNS depression, phaeo.

Caution: Parkinson's, ↑QTc, epilepsy, MG, phaeo, glaucoma (angle-closure), ↑prostate, severe respiratory disease, jaundice, blood disorders, ↑/↓thyroid, NMS, concurrent other antipsychotic prescription, H.

Class SE: EPSE, ↑prolactin and assoc Sx, sedation, ↑Wt, QT prolongation, VTE, blood dyscrasias, ↓seizure threshold, NMS.

SE: GI upset (D, discomfort), sexual dysfunction, rash, visual problems, ↓temperature, headaches.

Monitor: ECG may be required, esp if physical examination identifies cardiovascular risk factors/Hx of cardiovascular disease/patient is admitted as inpatient.

Interactions: metab by P450 (CYP2D6, CYP3A4); ↑fx of alcohol, barbiturates, CNS depressants, general anesthetics, anticoagulants; ↑risk of extrapyramidal effects (e.g. tardive dyskinesia) with metoclopramide, piperazine, antiparkinson medications; ↑risk of neurotoxicity with lithium; ↑risk of ↑QTc with class 1A and III antiarrhythmics (e.g. quinidine, amiodarone, sotalol), antipsychotics (e.g. thioridazine), macrolides (e.g.

erythromycin), antihistamines and quinolone antibiotics (e.g. moxifloxacin).
Dose: 50–150 mg im, then 50–150 mg after 2–3 days (one additional dose may be needed 1–2 days after first injection); max 400 mg in 2 wk/max four injections, max duration of treatment 2 wk – change to oral antipsychotic 2–3 days after last injection for maintenance treatment/to a longer-acting antipsychotic depot injection given concomitantly with last injection, administered into gluteal muscle/lateral thigh.

Do not confuse with zuclopenthixol decanoate.

ZUCLOPENTHIXOL DECANOATE/CLOPIXOL
See Zuclopenthixol acetate.
Use: maintenance in psychosis.
CI: CNS depression, phaeo, children.
Caution/SE/Monitor/Interactions: see Zuclopenthixol acetate.
Dose: test dose 100 mg im, administered into upper outer buttock/lateral thigh, followed by 200–500 mg after at least 7 days, then 200–500 mg every 1–4 wk, higher doses of >500 mg can be used, max 600 mg wkly; max single dose 600 mg at any time.

Do not confuse with zuclopenthixol acetate.

ZUCLOPENTHIXOL DIHYDROCHLORIDE/CLOPIXOL
See Zuclopenthixol acetate.
Use: psychosis.
CI: CNS depression due to any cause, e.g. alcohol, phaeo, withdrawn states.
Caution/SE/Monitor/Interactions: see Zuclopenthixol acetate.
Dose: initially 20–30 mg po od in divided doses, ↑ to 150 mg od, usual maintenance 20–50 mg od (max single dose 40 mg).

ZYBAN see Bupropion; adjunct to smoking cessation.

Disorders

PSYCHOSIS

DIAGNOSIS

Definition: Psychosis is a syndrome defined by positive symptoms, phenomena that are outside of normal experience, typically delusions, hallucinations and/or thought disorder. It may be secondary to another medical disorder or may be a primary psychiatric disorder. **Schizophrenia** is essentially a chronic idiopathic psychosis with a broad impairment of function with additional negative symptoms. These are typically loss of normal behaviours and motivation: affective flattening, alogia, avolition, anhedonia and attentional impairment (Andreasen, *Arch Gen Psychiatry* 1982; **39**(7):784–8).

Currently, it is impossible to predict for certain who will develop schizophrenia. However, in the **At Risk Mental State (ARMS)**, there are **attenuated psychotic symptoms** (Sx), which are predictive of a 20%–30% rate of full psychosis within 2 yr. **The Comprehensive Assessment of At Risk Mental State (CAARMS)** is used in the National Health Service (NHS) and Australia to identify ARMS. PACE (Personal Assessment and Crisis Evaluation) or COPS (Criteria of Prodromal Symptoms) are other scoring systems used to identify ARMS.

Even when full psychosis emerges, it is common in the first year to use the term **first episode (non-organic) psychosis (FEP)**, as it is initially unclear whether patients will develop schizophrenia or bipolar affective disorder (BPAD), or no enduring mental illness. FEP is particularly common within the 6 wks following childbirth and is termed **post-partum psychosis**. Following appropriate treatment, it is not uncommon for a significant recovery from FEP to occur, albeit often with some residual Sx. **Relapse**, however, is common. **Treatment-resistant schizophrenia** is usually defined as a failure to respond to two trials of antipsychotic medications, used at adequate doses for sufficient lengths of time.

Some patients with FEP do not ultimately fit a diagnosis of a schizophreniform illness. For some, this is because they are suffering from an **organic psychosis**, which may be due to drugs, epilepsy, neurodegenerative disease or many other medical disorders. **Delusional disorder** is characterised by a persistent delusion without other prominent features of schizophrenia (inappropriate affect, hallucinations, thought disorder). Psychosis can also be a feature of mania and severe depression; these **affective psychoses** are covered in the sections on BPAD and Depression.

TYPES OF MEDICATIONS

- First-generation antipsychotics (FGAs, aka 'typicals').
- Second-generation antipsychotics (SGAs, aka 'atypicals').
- Third-generation antipsychotics (TGAs, aka 'atypicals').

Class	Drug name	Route(s) po	im SA	im LA	Equiv po dose/mg[1]	Affinities[2] D2	Affinities[2] 5-HT2	Side effects EPSE	Side effects Met Syn	Side effects Other
FGA	Haloperidol	✔	✔	✔	10	+++	+	+++	+	
	Chlorpromazine	✔			600	+++	+++	++	++	Photosensitivity
	Sulpiride	✔			800	+++	−	+	+	
	Trifluoperazine	✔			20	+++	+	+++	+	
	Flupentixol	✔		✔	10	+++	+	++	+	
	Fluphenazine			✔	12	+++	+	+++	+	
	Zuclopenthixol[3]	✔		✔	50	+++	+	++	+	
SGA	Olanzapine	✔[4]	✔	✔	20	++	+++	+/−	+++	
	Risperidone	✔[4]		✔	6	+++	++	+	++	
	Paliperidone	✔		✔	9	+++	++	+	++	
	Quetiapine	✔			750	+	+	−	++	
	Amisulpride	✔			700	+++	−	+	+	
	Clozapine	✔	✔		400	+	+++	−	+++	See following
	Lurasidone	✔			120[5]	+++	+	+	+	
TGA	Aripiprazole[6]	✔[4]	✔	✔	30	+++	++	+	+	Akathisia

SA = short acting (for acute treatment).

LA = long acting (depot).

[1] Gardner et al., *Am J Psychiatry* 2010.

[2] Richtand et al., *Neuropsychopharmacology* 2007; Correll, *Eur Psychiatry* 2010; PDSP Ki Database (https://pdsp.unc.edu/databases/kidb.php).

[3] Studies on affinities not available; values quoted based on similarity to flupentixol.

[4] Available as quick dissolving/orodispersible preparation.

[5] Leucht & Samara, *Schizophr Bull* 2016. Given available formulations in the UK, this is approximately 111 mg.

[6] Partial agonist at D_2 and $5-HT_{1A}$. Antagonist at $5-HT_{2A}$.

All block D_2 receptors to varying degrees (dopamine antagonists); atypicals also antagonise 5-HT$_2$ receptors.

Three main DA brain systems account for many effects: nigrostriatal (movement), tuberoinfundibular (prolactin) and mesocorticolimbic systems (motivation and emotion).

Efficacy

Apart from clozapine, differences between antipsychotics are small. The following is a comparison of SGAs for overall Sx reduction (Leucht et al., *Lancet* 2013; **382**(9896): 951–62). All medications are compared relative to placebo (symptom reduction of zero).

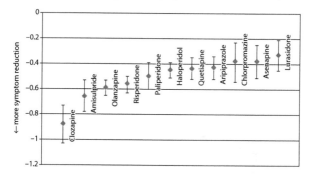

Depot antipsychotics (long-acting injections [LAIs])

Full adherence rates for oral antipsychotics after discharge from hospital are poor (Leucht & Heres, *J Clin Psychiatry* 2006; **67**(s5): 5–8):

10 days	1 yr	2 yr
75%	50%	25%

- Depot antipsychotics can improve adherence, provide consistent bioavailability and give regular contact with a nurse. However, there is a perceived stigma attached to depot injections.

- Depot injections do not allow rapid adjustments in dose. Ideally, the effective and tolerated doses should be established with oral medications before switching to a depot.
- Paliperidone is 9-hydroxyrisperidone, the active metabolite of risperidone. Patients who have been stabilised on oral risperidone are often switched to paliperidone LAI, as it has simpler pharmacokinetics than risperidone LAI.
- If medication consumption is supervised, orodispersible olanzapine/risperidone/aripiprazole may be an alternative option for improving adherence.
- Depot administration (full training required): See Feetam & White (Eds), *Guidance on the Administration to Adults of Oilbased Depot and other Long-Acting Intramuscular Antipsychotic Injections 5th Edition. 2016.**
  — Check injection sites and ask Re. SEs.
  — Two registered practitioners to check prescription.
  — Prepare injection according to SPC instructions.
  — Three possible injection sites: deltoid, gluteal, lateral thigh.

Licensed injection sites:

Drug	Deltoid	Gluteal	Lateral thigh
Aripiprazole	✔	✔	
Risperidone	✔	✔	
Paliperidone	✔	✔	
Olanzapine		✔	
Flupentixol		✔	✔
Zuclopenthixol		✔	✔
Other FGAs		✔	

  — Gluteal: Expose whole buttock with patient lying on front or side. To avoid sciatic nerve, inject in upper outer quadrant

---

* http://www.hpft.nhs.uk/media/1707/guidance-on-administration-of-oil-based-depot-and-long-acting-im-antipsychotic-injections-sept-2011.pdf [Accessed June 2018]).

of buttock aiming for gluteus maximus. Aspirate before injecting, and only proceed if no blood.
- Lateral thigh: Inject in the anterolateral aspect of the thigh halfway between the greater trochanter and the later condyle of the femur, aiming for vastus lateralis.
- Avoid injecting into moles/birthmarks, inflammation, oedema or scar tissue.
- To prevent depot leaking back from muscle to subcutaneous tissue, use the Z-track technique: Pull the skin sideways before the needle enters. Insert needle at 90°, deep enough to penetrate muscle (this depends on body habitus). Withdraw the needle and then release the skin, preventing tracking of the medication back through the site of needle entry.

CHOOSING A MEDICATION
At Risk Mental State (ARMS)
- Limited evidence for any intervention preventing the transition from ARMS to FEP.
- Do not prescribe antipsychotics to prevent transition to FEP.[NICE]
- However, patients with ARMS often have other mental health disorders including anxiety and depression. Prescribing should be appropriate to these individual presentations.

First episode (non-organic) psychosis (FEP)
- No significant difference in efficacy between FGAs and SGAs.
- Choose antipsychotic based on[BAP]:
  - Medication's side effect profile.
  - Patient's propensity for serious side effects (extrapyramidal side effects [EPSEs], metabolic syndrome).
  - Patient's preference.
  - Relevant medical history.
- Offer oral route first. A few centres offer depots.[BAP]
- Start at lower end of licensed dose range.[BAP]
- If a FGA is selected, use medium- or low-potency rather than high-potency drugs.[BAP]
- Specifically warn patients about weight (wt) gain before prescribing olanzapine in FEP.[NICE]

Relapsed psychosis

- Same principles apply as FEP when choosing an antipsychotic.[BAP]
- Higher doses of antipsychotics are often required, but use the minimum effective dose.[BAP]
- In addition, consider past experience of antipsychotics.[BAP]

Managing −ve Sx

- Consider whether −ve Sx might be due to +ve Sx, EPSEs or depression.
- More effective antipsychotics (see forest plot p. 185, refer graph under 'Efficacy' heading) tend to be best for −ve Sx.[BAP]
- Treat EPSEs.[BAP]
- Treat depression.[BAP]
- ↑Stimulation in environment.[BAP]
- Consider a selective serotonin reuptake inhibitor (SSRI), even if not depressed,[BAP] but check interactions (p. 341, refer 'Drug Interactions' in 'Basic Psychopharmacology' chapter).
- Cariprazine, a D_2/D_3 partial agonist, is a novel antipsychotic that has shown promise for −ve Sx.

Delusional disorder

(Fear, *Adv Psychiatr Treat* 2013; **19**(3): 212–20)

- Has a reputation for being difficult to treat, partly due to patients' poor insight.
- Often responds to standard antipsychotics +/− cognitive therapy.

Organic psychosis

- Treat the underlying disorder, but antipsychotics may become necessary.
- If medication-induced, consider withdrawal of causative agent. There is evidence for lithium in steroid-induced psychosis.

- If due to epilepsy, control of seizures or withdrawal of the offending anticonvulsant (e.g. levetiracetam, topiramate, zonisamide) is the mainstay of treatment. Benzodiazepines are preferred for psychotic agitation, though antipsychotics are occasionally used.
- If due to dementia and severe, antipsychotics may be used in low doses, but beware ↑stroke risk.
- In Parkinson's or Lewy body dementia, psychosis can be caused by pro-dopaminergic agents. Consider switching these. Otherwise, consider antipsychotic with low propensity for EPSEs, such as clozapine or quetiapine.
- In Huntington's, use atypicals to avoid worsening underlying bradykinesia (Jauhar & Ritchie, *Adv Psychiatr Treat* 2010; **16**(3): 168–75).
- In 22q11.2 deletion syndrome (DiGeorge syndrome), use antipsychotics starting at low doses and titrating slowly. Consider a prophylactic anticonvulsant if treating with clozapine, due to risks of seizures (Fung et al., *Genet Med* 2015; **17**(8): 599–601).

Post-partum psychosis
(Doyle et al., *Adv Psychiatr Treat* 2015; **21**(1): 5–14)
- Linked to BPAD, so treat as an affective psychosis.
- Give antipsychotic +/– mood stabiliser (avoid sodium valproate due to teratogenicity).
- Lithium prophylaxis may be indicated.
- Electroconvulsive therapy (ECT) is effective.

TREATMENT RESISTANCE
- Up to one-third of patients respond poorly to antipsychotics, deemed 'treatment resistant'.
- Clozapine has by far the best evidence,[BAP] but it has serious side effects and response can be slow (see box).

Clozapine response rates (Meltzer, Schizophr Bull 1992; 18(3): 515–542)

	6 wk	3 months	6 months
	30%	50%	60%–70%

- If clozapine response is poor, optimise therapy as follows:
  - Ensure compliance.
  - Check for ongoing substance misuse.
  - Ensure adequate plasma levels.
- Clozapine non-response (Lally & Gaughran, *Ir J Psychol Med* 2018; 27: 1–13):
  - Full multidisciplinary team assessment.
  - Reassess primary diagnosis and psychiatric co-morbidities.
  - Look for organic contributors.
  - Minimise other stressors.
  - Optimise clozapine to ensure plasma levels of 0.35–0.5 mg/L.
  - Consider trial of clozapine plasma levels of >0.5 mg/L with seizure prophylaxis.
  - Augment clozapine, e.g. with amisulpride, sulpiride, haloperidol or lamotrigine. If there is an affective component, augment with lithium.[BAP]
  - Psychological therapies such as cognitive behavioural therapy for psychosis (CBTp) and family work.
- Antipsychotic (including clozapine) + ECT can be useful if rapid effect required. ECT may be useful in stabilising a patient, such that they are able to tolerate clozapine titration.[BAP]
- High-dose antipsychotics (i.e. above BNF max): no convincing evidence for this strategy and it goes against many guidelines. Risk of sudden cardiac death is higher. Only use as a time-limited tentative trial after other options exhausted. May have a role in fast metabolisers.[BAP]
- Combined antipsychotics (other than with clozapine) → ↑SE, ↑drug interactions, ↓adherence and ↑mortality. Also, hard to work out which drug is having an effect. Only use as a time-limited tentative trial after other options exhausted.[BAP]

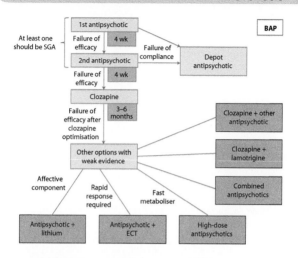

NON-PHARMACOLOGICAL MEASURES

A range of psychosocial interventions can be helpful in psychosis:

- Enhance medication adherence.
- ↓Expressed emotion among family members. (Behavioural Family Therapy)
- Patient support groups. (Mind, Rethink, Hearing Voices Network)
- Psychoeducation. (https://www.rcpsych.ac.uk/mental-health)
- Engagement in education and employment.
- Supported living.
- Care coordination.

> *CBT for psychosis*
> - Meta-analysis has shown small effect (pooled effect sizes −0.33). (Jauhar et al., *BJPsych* 2014; **204**(1): 20–9)
> - Some evidence in ARMS.
> - For established schizophrenia, CBT may be used *in addition* to antipsychotics to ↓ relapse, but is not optimal monotherapy.[NICE]

- Principles:
  - ↓Distress from +ve Sx.
  - ↓Behaviours that may be maintaining factors.
- Techniques:
  - Empathic and supportive stance to overcome paranoia.
  - Avoid both confrontation and collusion.
  - Normalise experiences.
  - Explore evidence for and against beliefs.
  - Teach helpful coping strategies.

STARTING MEDICATION

- Do baseline monitoring (see following).
- Generally start in 2°care.[NICE]
- Start at low dose and increase gradually based on clinical response (symptoms and side effects).[BAP]
- For clozapine, start at 12.5 mg od or bd on dy 1, then 25 mg od or bd on dy 2. If good tolerance, increase daily dose in increments of 25–50 mg, up to daily dose of 300 mg. If further increase required, increase by 50–100 mg weekly.[SPC]
- If considering olanzapine, discuss with the patient the higher risk of wt gain, which can occur soon after commencing treatment.[NICE]
- For FGAs, maintenance dose should be 300–600 mg chlorpromazine equivalent.[BAP]
- For SGAs, give same maintenance dose as that required during acute phase.[BAP]
- Carefully document changes in clinical presentation.[BAP]
- Early response can occur within 24 h of starting antipsychotic. Behaviour and emotional preoccupation change before psychotic conviction recedes.
- Achieve an adequate trial (i.e. 4 wk of adherence at the optimum dose).[BAP]
- +ve response at 2 wk predicts subsequent response (NPV=80%).
- Do not use initial loading doses ('rapid neuroleptization').[BAP] *NB*: However, paliperidone long-acting injectable has a recommended loading dose to avoid a long time to peak plasma concentration.
- Avoid combining antipsychotics (unless cross-titrating).[BAP]

SIDE EFFECTS

As a general rule, FGAs may cause EPSEs and hyperprolactinaemia, whereas SGAs may lead to metabolic syndrome. However, this is not exclusive, and there is some overlap. Patients may respond differently to different medications. For information on how to monitor side effects see section on Monitoring. See table on p. 184, refer table in 'Types of Medications' in 'Psychosis' section for antipsychotic-specific SEs.

FGAs	SGAs
Dystonia (muscle spasms)	Wt gain
Parkinsonism (rigidity, tremor, bradykinesia)	Dyslipidaemia
Akathisia (restlessness)	Impaired glucose tolerance
Tardive dyskinesia (abnormal movements)	Prolonged QT
↑Prolactin	
NMS	
Prolonged QT	

Clozapine

Some particular side effects (SEs):

- Neutropoenia and agranulocytosis (can be fatal)
- Myocarditis/cardiomyopathy
- ↑Saliva
- Constipation/gastrointestinal (GI) obstruction (can be fatal if perforates)
- Postural hypotension (common during titration, but often improves)
- Seizures (risk related to plasma levels)
- Pneumonia (also linked to other antipsychotics)

Vulnerabilities to side effects

Group	SE vulnerability
Women of reproductive age	↑Prolactin
FEP patients	↑Wt

(continued)

Group	SE vulnerability
Young men	Acute dystonia
Elderly	Postural hypotension
	QTc prolongation
	Tardive dyskinesia

Extrapyramidal side effects (EPSEs)

(Saifee & Edwards, *Pract Neurol* 2011; **11**(6): 341–8; Pringsheim et al., *Can J Psychiatry* 2018; **63**(11): 719–29)

- 'EPSEs' is an umbrella term for a range of iatrogenic side effects. These are dose related, usually in response to high-potency FGAs.
- EPSEs can be acute (acute dystonia, Parkinsonism, akathisia) or chronic (tardive dyskinesia, chronic dystonia).

EPSE	Features	Rx
Parkinsonism	Tremor (3–5 Hz), rigidity, bradykinesia	1. Consider switch or ↓dose
		2. Procyclidine up to 5 mg tds
Akathisia	Subjective restlessness, urge to move, tension when forced to stay still	1. ↓Dose
		2. Consider switch to clozapine, olanzapine or quetiapine
		3. Propranolol 80 mg
		4. Mirtazapine 15 mg
Dystonia (involuntary sustained muscle contraction)	Torticollis (neck), opisthotonus (backward arching), trismus (muscles of mastication), blepharospasm (eyelids forced shut), oculogyric crisis (eyes stuck in upward gaze), laryngeal dystonia (life threatening)	Acute: Procyclidine 5–10 mg im/iv stat; see p. 399, refer 'Acute Dystonia' in 'Emergencies' chapter Chronic: Trihexyphenidyl 1 mg, ↑ to 2–4 mg tds or procyclidine, as previously discussed; consider referral for Botox if focal

(*continued*)

EPSE	Features	Rx
Tardive dyskinesia	Orofacial dyskinesia (more common): tongue protrusion, lip smacking, sucking, chewing, grimacing Limb/trunk movements (rarer): shoulder shrugging, pelvis rotation, athetosis, choreiform movements	1. Consider switch to clozapine (↓dose of original antipsychotic does not tend to help) 2. Tetrabenazine 12.5 mg od, ↑slowly to 25–50 mg tds 3. Consider clonazepam, propranolol or baclofen
NMS	Rigidity, fever, altered consciousness	Stop antipsychotic and give benzodiazepines; see p. 386, refer 'Neuroleptic Malignant Syndrome' in 'Drug Toxicity Syndromes' in 'Emergencies' chapter

- Procyclidine:
  - Often effective as a Rx, but do not prescribe prophylactically.
  - Can add to anticholinergic burden (cognitive impairment, blurred vision, glaucoma, urinary retention, constipation, tachycardia).
  - Some patients request it because of its associated euphoria.

Metabolic syndrome

(Shiers et al., *Positive Cardiometabolic Health Resource: An Intervention Framework for Patients with Psychosis and Schizophrenia*. 2014 update. Royal College of Psychiatrists, London; Mizuno et al., *Schizophr Bull* 2014; 40(6): 1385–403)[BAP]
Metabolic syndrome consists of obesity, dyslipidaemia, hypertension (HTN) and impaired glucose tolerance.

Problem	Diagnosis	Treatment	
Weight gain	BMI >25 or wt gain >5 kg in 3 months	Consider switching antipsychotic (see table on p. 202, refer table in 'Swapping' section)	Metformin (off-license) → 3 kg ↓wt and ↑glucose tolerance
Impaired glucose tolerance	Fasting glucose ≥5.6 mmol/L or HbA1c 42–47 mmol/mol		Adding aripiprazole to clozapine/ olanzapine → 2 kg ↓wt
Dyslipidaemia	CVD risk of 10% using QRISK3 tool meets NICE threshold for statin	Diet	Atorvastatin 20 mg
HTN	Sys BP >140 or dia BP >90	Exercise	NICE CG127
DM	Fasting glucose ≥7.0 mmol/L, random glucose ≥11.1 mmol/L or HbA1c ≥ 48 mmol/mol	Smoking cessation	NICE NG28

Prolonged QTc

QT interval
- Time from ventricular depolarisation to end of repolarisation.
- Measure in lead II, V5 or V6.
- Measured as distance from start of Q-wave to end of T-wave.
- Corrected QT interval (QTc) can be calculated with *Bazett's formula*:

$$QTc = \frac{QT}{\sqrt{RR \text{ interval}}}$$

- If HR <60 or >100, better to use *Frederica's formula*:

$$QTc = \frac{QT}{RR^{1/3}}$$

Most antipsychotics have some effect upon the QT interval, increasing the risk of ventricular arrhythmias (especially torsade de pointes) and death. It can also be prolonged by electrolyte abnormalities ($\downarrow K^+$, $\downarrow Ca^{2+}$ or $\downarrow Mg^{2+}$) and congenital long QT syndromes.

Aripiprazole and lurasidone are considered the safest. Risks are increased if other cardiac risk factors are present, or when co-prescribed with other psychotropic or non-psychotropic medication that prolongs the QT interval. The following chart offers suggested management.

QTc	Management[MPG]
♂ <440 ms ♀ <470 ms	Normal QTc. No action unless abnormal T-wave morphology.
♂ 440–500 ms ♀ 470–500 ms	Repeat electrocardiogram (ECG). Consider $\downarrow$dose or switching. Check K^+, Ca^{2+}, Mg^{2+}. Consider referral to cardiologist.
>500 ms	Stop drug. Check K^+, Ca^{2+}, Mg^{2+}. Consult cardiologist.
Abnormal T-wave morphology	Consider $\downarrow$dose or switching. Consult cardiologist.

QTc-prolonging drugs (QT interval and drug therapy, Drug Ther Bull 2016)

- Antipsychotics
- TCAs
- Anti-arrhythmics (e.g. amiodarone, sotalol)
- Macrolides (e.g. clarithromycin, erythromycin, azithromycin)
- Quinolones (e.g. ciprofloxacin, moxifloxacin)
- Triazoles (e.g. fluconazole, ketoconazole)
- Antimalarials (e.g. quinine, chloroquine)
- Antihistamines (e.g. promethazine, hydroxyzine)
- Methadone

Free tool to check drugs at https://crediblemeds.org

↑Prolactin

(Gupta et al., *BJPsych Adv* 2017; **23**(40): 278–86)

- Measure prolactin in low stress environment, ≥2 h after waking and ≥1 h after eating.
- Two forms of prolactin: free prolactin (active) and macroprolactin (inactive).
  - If ↑prolactin, check macroprolactin levels, as this may be causing **pseudohyperprolactinaemia**, which is not clinically significant.
- Often asymptomatic.
- Sequelae include gynaecomastia, galactorrhoea, sexual dysfunction, subfertility and osteoporosis.
- Weigh risks of ↑prolactin against risks of switching antipsychotic.

Prolactin level (mIU/L)	Sx	Management
400–2000	–	If benefits of antipsychotic outweigh risk, continue to monitor prolactin.
2000–3000	+	Consider: ↓dose, switch antipsychotic, add aripiprazole, add DA agonist (cabergoline or bromocriptine) but may worsen psychosis, endocrinology r/f.
	+/–	
>3000 or visual field defect	+/–	Consider other causes of ↑prolactin. Consider magnetic resonance imaging (MRI) pituitary.

Depot side effects

- 15%–20% get inflammation and induration at injection site, causing pain that is usually mild
→ Rx: ↑dose interval

MONITORING

Antipsychotics require the following monitoring.

Test	Baseline	1 month	2 months	3 months	6 months	Annual	Notes
BMI[BAP]	✓	✓	✓	✓	✓	✓	
BP[BAP]	✓			✓	✓	✓	NICE also suggests pulse
ECG[1, BAP]	✓						
Bloods							
HbA1c[BAP]	✓			✓	✓	✓	Consider using plasma glucose to measure immediate effects
Lipids[BAP]	✓			✓	✓	✓	Can use random lipids if fasting not possible
Prolactin (Gupta, *BJPsych Adv* 2017)	✓			✓		✓	Also if symptomatic or considering pregnancy

[1] Perform a baseline ECG if

- Medication is high risk for QT prolongation (e.g. pimozide, sertindole), high-dose medication used, acute parenteral administration or combination with other QT-prolonging drugs.
- Family history of long QT syndrome.
- Personal history of CVD, electrolyte abnormalities, central nervous system (CNS) disorders or systemic disease.
- Admitted as inpatient.[NICE]

Perform serial ECGs if

- Abnormality on baseline ECG.
- Sx of CVD (e.g. syncope, palpitations, chest pain).
- High-dose antipsychotics prescribed.
- Electrolyte abnormalities.

Full blood count (FBC), renal function and liver function tests (LFTs) are also often performed at baseline and annually to assess general health and drug metabolism.

In addition, when reviewing person, enquire about

- Efficacy: Symptoms, behaviour, cognition
- Compliance
- Side effects: ↑prolactin, EPSEs, anticholinergic
- Substance misuse (alcohol, drugs, smoking)

Clozapine

- Monitor white cell count (WCC) and differential to detect neutropoenia and agranulocytosis[SPC]
  - Baseline
  - Every week for the first 18 wk
  - Every 2 wk between weeks 18 and 52
  - Every 4 wk after 1 yr
  - For 4 wk after stopping clozapine
  - Also, remind patient to immediately seek medical assistance if they have any signs of an infection.
- Acting on WCC:[SPC]

WCC ($\times 10^9$/mm)	Absolute neutrophil count (ANC) ($\times 10^9$/mm)	Action
≥3.5	≥2	Continue clozapine with standard monitoring
≥3 and <3.5	≥1.5 and <2	Continue clozapine with twice-weekly monitoring
<3	<1.5	Stop clozapine immediately and do not re-challenge; consider second confirmatory sample, but stop clozapine after first sample

Plasma levels

- Useful for clozapine. Once titration is complete, measure plasma levels and adjust dose accordingly. Usual range is 350–500 microgram/L, but some respond at lower levels. Norclozapine is a clozapine metabolite, and its levels are also sometimes measured.
  - Clozapine:norclozapine ratio is normally ~1.25. A ↓ratio may be caused by enzyme induction or recent non-compliance. An ↑ratio may be due to enzyme inhibition, incorrect sampling time or saturation of clozapine metabolism.
- For other antipsychotics, main use is determining concordance, but dose-plasma level relationship is usually not strong enough to determine partial concordance.

STOPPING

- Consensus guidelines recommend continuing an antipsychotic for ≥6 months to 2 yr after a psychotic episode. Patients should be informed of a high risk of relapse if they stop antipsychotics within 1–2 yr of psychotic episode.[NICE]
- Controversies with some arguing for both longer and shorter durations.

The decision to stop must be assessed on a case-by-case basis, based upon:

- Patient/carer wishes after an informed discussion
- Ongoing psychotic symptoms
- Severity of current adverse effects
- Previous patterns of illness
- Previous response to cessation
- Social circumstances (support and stressors)
- Patient/carer insight into relapse indicators
- Risk of harm to self/others

Withdrawal must be **gradual** (preferably over months) to avoid relapse and discontinuation symptoms of headache, insomnia, nausea, etc. Rebound psychosis is most common with clozapine.

SWAPPING

If intolerable side effects, adverse reactions or poor response, then consider switching to an alternative antipsychotic:

- Consider the risk of destabilisation of illness and adverse effects of the new drug.
- Gradually cross-taper over 2–4 wk.
- Avoid abrupt discontinuation, especially of clozapine (unless for serious adverse effect).
- If switching from oral to depot, gradually reduce oral dose after giving depot.

The following table lists circumstances when a switch may be necessary, with recommended drugs.

Acute EPSEs	Aripiprazole, olanzapine, quetiapine, clozapine
Raised prolactin	Aripiprazole, quetiapine, ziprasidone
Postural hypotension	Amisulpride, aripiprazole, lurasidone
QT prolongation	Aripiprazole, lurasidone
Sedation	Amisulpride, aripiprazole, risperidone, sulpiride
Sexual side effects	Aripiprazole, quetiapine
Tardive dyskinesia	Clozapine
Wt gain	Amisulpride, aripiprazole, haloperidol, lurasidone, ziprasidone
Dyslipidaemia	Aripiprazole, ziprasidone

SPECIAL GROUPS
Children

- Psychosis is less common in children.
- Children are more susceptible to EPSEs and sedation.
- If considering olanzapine, discuss the higher risk of wt gain.[NICE]
- Good options: aripiprazole, olanzapine, risperidone, quetiapine, paliperidone.[MPG]

Elderly

- When antipsychotics have been used in dementia, they have been associated with ↑risk of CVA, so caution is required.
- Lower doses are used.

Pregnancy

- Choice of antipsychotic in pregnancy should be guided by past treatment response. There is increasing evidence for SGAs and no clear difference in risk between FGAs and SGAs.[BAP]
- Consider even when women of childbearing potential are not planning pregnancy; ≥50% of pregnancies are unplanned.
- If woman on antipsychotic struggling to become pregnant, consider switching to a drug with a lower propensity to ↑prolactin.[BAP]
- Unclear whether antipsychotics as a group pose an increased risk of major malformations.
- If they do, it is likely to be small (odds ratio [OR] 1.21–1.45) and non-specific. Risk of cardiovascular malformations may ↑from 1% to 1.5%.
- Pregnancy → impaired glucose tolerance → ↑risk of gestational diabetes mellitus (DM) if combined with SGA. SGAs (especially olanzapine and clozapine) should be prescribed with caution, and enhanced monitoring is recommended.[BAP]
- Late pregnancy exposure can occasionally cause neonatal EPSEs.[BAP]
- Newer drugs (e.g. aripiprazole, lurasidone) have less evidence and warrant additional caution.[BAP]
- There are concerns about folate deficiency in women with schizophrenia resulting in neural tube defects. Recommend high-dose folic acid supplementation (5 mg od) in 3 months before and after conception.[BAP]
- For a woman stabilised on an antipsychotic:[BAP]
  - Consider that switch risks destabilising illness without any benefit for foetus.

- If switching, consider risks of antipsychotic as well as previous response.
- If established on clozapine, benefits of continuation likely to outweigh risks.
- Depots may be continued.

Breastfeeding

Relative Infant Dose (RID)

$$RID = \frac{Infant\ dose/kg/day}{Maternal\ dose/kg/day}$$

<10% of maternal dose is generally considered acceptable

- Olanzapine is a good option overall.[MPG]
- Breastfeeding on clozapine is contraindicated, as can cause agranulocytosis in the infant.[BAP]
- The RID for quetiapine, chlorpromazine and olanzapine is <2%, but it is significantly higher for sulpiride, haloperidol and risperidone.
- Consider infant's physical health when starting an antipsychotic in a breastfeeding woman.[BAP]
- Monitor for sedation and EPSEs in infant.[BAP]

Renal impairment[BNF]
- Haloperidol and olanzapine are good options.[MPG]
- Most antipsychotics undergo extensive hepatic metabolism with little unchanged drug being excreted in the urine. Only sulpiride, amisulpride and paliperidone rely heavily on renal excretion. (NB: Risperidone is also metabolised to paliperidone.) These are, therefore, best avoided in renal impairment.
- Other antipsychotics are likely to be safe, but check individual monographs.
- Anticholinergic SEs may result in further urinary retention.
- Start with lower doses and titrate more slowly.

Hepatic impairment[BNF]

- Sulpiride, amisulpride and paliperidone are safer, as they undergo negligible hepatic metabolism. Haloperidol has reasonable clinical experience in low doses.[MPG]
- Phenothiazines (chlorpromazine, fluphenazine, trifluoperazine) are hepatotoxic.
- Antipsychotics may precipitate coma in liver failure.
- Clozapine should be avoided.
- Check individual monographs.

Physical health problems

- **Long QT syndrome** (congenital or due to other medications): Avoid antipsychotics that prolong the QT interval. Aripiprazole and lurasidone are safer. See p. 196, refer 'Prolonged QTc'.
- **Epilepsy:** Antipsychotics are generally safe and even clozapine has been used successfully. Titrate slowly and monitor seizure frequency.
- **Diabetes:** SGAs are likely to worsen T2DM. Typicals and aripiprazole are good options.

Persistent aggression

Valproate augmentation of an antipsychotic has some very limited evidence but should be avoided in women of child-bearing potential.[BAP]

Co-morbid depression

(Upthegrove, *Adv Psychiatr Treat* 2009; **15**(5): 372–9)

- Monitor for coexisting mental health problems (including depression, anxiety and substance misuse), especially in early treatment.[NICE]
- Depression is common (40% post-psychotic phase, 80% in longitudinal studies). Strong predictor of suicidal behaviour and poor functional outcome.
- Consider switching antipsychotic if prescribed haloperidol.

- Antidepressant co-prescribing is effective in the treatment of co-morbid major depression: most evidence for SSRIs (Gregory et al., *Br J Psychiatry* 2017; **211**(4): 198–204).
- Generally, good safety evidence for co-prescribing antidepressant with antipsychotic (Tiihonen et al., *Arch Gen Psychiatry* 2012; **69**(5): 476–83) with no higher risk for mortality but significantly decreased risk of completed suicide. Increased QTc monitoring may be needed.
- Avoid citalopram and escitalopram with antipsychotics, as risk of QTc prolongation[MHRA].

Co-morbid substance misuse[BAP]

- Smoking: NRT, bupropion and varenicline all have good evidence. NRT is safest, as there is some controversial evidence about psychological SE (including suicidal ideation) with bupropion and varenicline.
- In alcohol abuse, clozapine has some evidence for reducing substance misuse.

FURTHER INFORMATION

Barnes et al., 'Evidence-based guidelines for the pharmacological treatment of schizophrenia: recommendations from the British Association for Psychopharmacology', *J Psychopharmacol* 2011; **25**(5): 567–620.

Cooper et al., 'BAP guidelines on the management of weight gain, metabolic disturbances and cardiovascular risk associated with psychosis and antipsychotic drug treatment', *J Psychopharmacol* 2016; **30**(8): 717–48.

BIPOLAR AFFECTIVE DISORDER

DIAGNOSIS

BPAD is a relapsing and remitting psychiatric disorder. For a diagnosis to be made, there must be at least one episode of (hypo) mania and at least one depressive episode. **BPAD-I** is characterised by **mania** + depression, whereas **BPAD-II** is characterised by **hypomania** + depression.

Features of mania: **DIG FAST**

* **D**istractibility
* **I**rresponsible and disinhibited behaviour
* **G**randiosity
* **F**light of ideas
* **A**ctivity ↑
* **S**leep ↓
* **T**alkativeness

Mania can be accompanied by **psychotic features,** usually grandiose delusions, second-person auditory hallucinations or thought disorder. **Hypomania** exhibits the features of mania, but to a mild degree such that there is no severe occupational or social dysfunction. A **mixed episode** has features of both depression and mania.

Differential diagnosis:

Psychiatric	Organic
• **Emotionally unstable personality disorder (EUPD)** (impulsivity, chronic emptiness, emotional instability, self-destructive behaviour)	• **Hyperthyroidism** (↑HR, tremor, proptosis, diarrhoea; Investigation [Ix]: thyroid function tests [TFTs])
• **Attention deficit hyperactivity disorder (ADHD)** (developmental trajectory, anger, overactivity, mood instability)	• **Cushing's disease** (purple striae, facial plethora, buffalo hump, glucose intolerance; Ix: 24 h urinary cortisol, dexamethasone suppression test)
	• **Drug-induced psychosis** (especially cocaine, amphetamines, synthetic cannabinoids; resolves within five half-lives of drug)
• **Cyclothymia** (depression and mild elation not meeting threshold for BPAD)	• **Prescribed medications** (corticosteroids, antidepressants, DA agonists, anabolic steroids, thyroid hormones, chloroquine)
• **Schizoaffective disorder** (features of schizophrenia and a mood disorder)	• **Stroke** (especially R limbic system; vascular RFs, acute onset, unilateral neuro deficits; Ix: computerised tomography [CT] head)
• **Depression** (no [hypo]mania)	• **MS** (especially orbitofrontal lesions; F>M, diplopia, paraesthesia, asymmetrical upper motor neurone [UMN] signs; Ix: MRI brain)
• **Delirium** (altered consciousness, disorientation, intercurrent illness)	• **Brain tumour** (especially frontal; subacute, headache worse in mornings/coughing, papilloedema, focal UMN signs; Ix: CT/ MRI brain)

Differentiating BPAD and EUPD
BPAD and EUPD are often confused and may be co-morbid.

	BPAD	EUPD
Duration of mood episodes	Consistent for a few days or longer	Very labile
Distinctiveness of episodes	Mood episodes can be distinguished from baseline	Less distinguishable from background
Impulsivity	Present only in (hypo)manic episodes	Continually present
Triggers for episodes	Often none obvious	Tend to be present, though reaction can be out of proportion
Grandiosity and euphoria	Often present in (hypo)mania	Not a feature
Frequent self-harm	Uncommon	Common
Failure to co-operate	Not a feature when euthymic	Affects many areas of life

TYPES OF MOOD STABILISING DRUGS

Drug	Pharmacology	Side effects				
		Sedation	GI Sx	↑wt	Stevens-Johnson syndrome (SJS)/ toxic epidermal necrolysis (TEN)	Teratogenicity
Lithium	Modulates multiple cellular signalling cascades	+	+	++	−	Some cardiac risk described but not replicated
Valproate	Inhibits GABA transaminase ⇒ ↑synaptic GABA	++	++	++	−	+++
Lamotrigine	Stabilises sodium channels	−	−	−	++	+
Carbamazepine	Stabilises sodium channels	+	++	++	++	++

− not described, + low risk, ++ medium risk, +++ high risk.
Source: Schmidt & Schachter, *BMJ* 2014; **28**(348): g254.

Oxcarbazepine and eslicarbazepine have a similar mechanism to carbamazepine but are occasionally used for their slightly different SE profile and lower potential for drug-drug interactions.

See Psychosis section for details of antipsychotics.

Formulations

Lithium, valproate and carbamazepine are all available in various formulations. For clarity, the brand should always be prescribed alongside the drug name and formulation, e.g. sodium valproate 500 mg MR tablets (Epilim Chrono).

Lithium

- Lithium is available as two compounds: **lithium carbonate**, as a tablet, and **lithium citrate**, as a liquid.
- The two main brands in use in the United Kingdom are **Priadel** and **Camcolit**. Brands should be kept the same where possible, as equivalent bioavailability cannot be guaranteed.
- For tablets, lithium carbonate can be prescribed as **Priadel MR**, **Camcolit IR** or **Camcolit MR**.
- For liquid, lithium citrate can be prescribed as **Priadel liquid** or **Li-Liquid** (both **IR**). There is no liquid MR formulation. State strength of liquid and dose to be taken.
- Lithium citrate and lithium carbonate doses are markedly different – see table below.
- Conversion:

Lithium citrate liquid		Equivalent lithium carbonate tablet dose
Formulation	Dose	
Priadel liquid	520 mg (5 mL)	204 mg (≈200 mg)
Li-liquid*	509 mg (5 mL)	200 mg

* Li-liquid is also available as 1018 mg in 5 mL.

- IR formulations (liquid and tablets) are taken bd.
- MR formulations (tablets) have the advantage of od dosing and ↓nephrotoxicity.

Valproate

Chemical form	Brand	IR formulation	MR formulation	Liquid	License for BPAD	License for epilepsy
Sodium valproate	Epilim	✔	✔	✔		✔
	Episenta		✔		✔	✔
Valproic acid	Convulex	✔				✔
Semisodium valproate	Depakote	✔			✔	

- Valproate is available in three chemical forms:
  - **Sodium valproate** (Epilim and Episenta).
  - **Valproic acid** (Convulex).
  - **Semisodium valproate** (Depakote).
- Semisodium valproate has equimolar quantities of sodium valproate and valproic acid.
- Despite the restricted licenses, Epilim Chrono (the MR) form is often used to improve compliance in BPAD.
- The stated doses on different valproate formulations should be bioequivalent, but monitor response carefully if switching. Available doses of tablets are often different; e.g. Epilim Chrono has 200 mg, 300 mg and 500 mg tablets, whereas Depakote comes as 250 mg and 500 mg tablets.

CHOOSING A MEDICATION

Most evidence is for bipolar I disorder, so caution is required with extrapolation to bipolar II.

Treatment of mania and mixed episodes

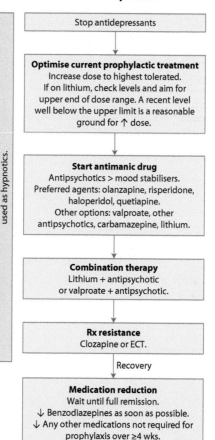

Benzodiazepines for tranquillisation and restoring sleep. Z-drugs may also be used as hypnotics.

Stop antidepressants

Optimise current prophylactic treatment
Increase dose to highest tolerated.
If on lithium, check levels and aim for
upper end of dose range. A recent level
well below the upper limit is a reasonable
ground for ↑ dose.

Start antimanic drug
Antipsychotics > mood stabilisers.
Preferred agents: olanzapine, risperidone,
haloperidol, quetiapine.
Other options: valproate, other
antipsychotics, carbamazepine, lithium.

Combination therapy
Lithium + antipsychotic
or valproate + antipsychotic.

Rx resistance
Clozapine or ECT.

Recovery

Medication reduction
Wait until full remission.
↓ Benzodiazepines as soon as possible.
↓ Any other medications not required for
prophylaxis over ≥4 wks.

BAP

- Strongly consider inpatient admission[BAP] and ensure a calming environment with reduced stimulation.[NICE]
- Medications are necessary; psychotherapy is not an alternative.[BAP]
- Antipsychotics are the preferred option.[NICE] They are not merely sedative and are more effective than anticonvulsants or lithium.[BAP] If the first antipsychotic is poorly tolerated, offer an alternative antipsychotic.[NICE]
- Olanzapine and haloperidol have the advantage of having a short-acting im formulation.[BAP]
- Avoid antipsychotics with a high propensity to EPSEs, as BPAD patients are more sensitive than SZ patients.[BAP]
- Lithium has the advantage that it is the most effective long-term treatment, but titration means that its effect is usually much slower than other agents in mania.[BAP]
- If using ECT, bear in mind that benzodiazepines and anticonvulsants ↑seizure threshold, so ↓dose of medications or higher starting voltages likely to be required.
- Medication should be reduced slowly. There is evidence for benefits from continuing an antipsychotic at 6 months but not at 1 yr.[BAP]
- Mixed episodes should be treated similarly to manic episodes. Antipsychotics may be used. Antidepressants should be avoided. ECT is an option.[BAP]

Treatment of depression

- Evidence base is poor with controversies over the use of antidepressants.
- BAP recommend lamotrigine as first-line pharmacotherapy, as shown in algorithm p. 211, refer diagram under 'Treatment of mania and mixed episodes' heading, but NICE recommends olanzapine + fluoxetine combination or quetiapine monotherapy as first line.
- Lamotrigine may be added on to existing therapy.[BAP] Interestingly, in one trial, the addition of folate to lamotrigine reduced its effect.
- Evidence for lithium is limited, but it is likely to be effective and may be considered.[BAP] If patient already taking lithium, check plasma level and ensure adequate dose.[NICE]

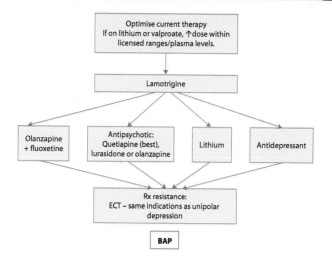

Antidepressants in BPAD

- If antidepressants are used in bipolar I disorder, they should be given with lithium, valproate or an antipsychotic.[BAP]
- Antidepressants are sometimes used as monotherapy in bipolar II disorder, but titration should be slow and patients should be closely monitored for hypomania.[BAP]
- SSRIs seem to be less likely to cause a manic switch than TCAs and SNRIs. When combined with a mood stabiliser, they are unlikely to cause mania.[BAP]
- Bipolar depression can remit more quickly than unipolar depression. Consider tapering down an antidepressant after 12 wk in remission.[BAP]
- Avoid in patients with mixed features, rapid cycling or as monotherapy.[BAP]
- Overall, lamotrigine is a better option.[BAP]

Long-term prophylaxis

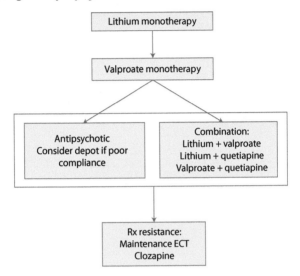

Role of lithium
- Overall, the best option for relapse prevention with strong evidence[BAP, NICE]
- Prevents mania and (to a lesser extent) depression
- Reduces suicide rates
- Early use of lithium ⇒ better long-term outcome
- But intermittent lithium Rx can cause rebound mania, so patients must be able to take it consistently for ≥2 yr.[BAP]

- A within-patient trial is often used to guide therapy, i.e. if a patient responds well to an acute anti-manic agent, this may be continued long term.[BAP,NICE] This is a valid strategy but results in disproportionate use of antipsychotics over lithium in long term.[BAP]
- Antipsychotics have the advantage that many are available as depots.[BAP] They can also be helpful if there are features of non-affective psychosis. The only depot with randomised controlled trial (RCT) support is risperidone. Since the pharmacokinetics of risperidone LAI make it hard to use, paliperidone palmitate is a good option. Naturalistic studies suggest depot medication prevents re-admission more effectively than oral equivalent.
- In general, there is a hierarchy for preferred medications: lithium > valproate > olanzapine > lamotrigine > quetiapine > carbamazepine.[BAP]
- However, when considering which agent, consideration should be given to which pole affects the patient most:[BAP]

Prevention of mania	Prevention of depression
Lithium	Lithium
Olanzapine	Lamotrigine
Quetiapine	Quetiapine
Risperidone LAI	Lurasidone
Valproate	Any treatment that has been effective in acute
Carbamazepine	depression for the patient

Rapid cycling BPAD
- Defined as ≥4 episodes/yr.
- Treat in the same way as BPAD in general.[BAP/NICE]
- Clozapine (with mood stabilisers) may be used in treatment-resistant cases.[BAP]
- Thyroid disorders may contribute. Reduce/discontinue any antidepressants that might be contributing.[BAP]

Early signs of relapse
- Consider acute prescriptions of antipsychotics or benzodiazepines if patient shows early signs of relapse (e.g. insomnia).[BAP]
- With appropriate education and support, some patients can have 'rescue packs' prescribed and dispensed in advance to use if they experience signs of relapse.[BAP]

Rescue packs
- Suitable for patients with a good understanding of their illness.[BAP]
- To be used by patient if they spot warning signs of mania.
- Options:
  - Higher doses of current medications.
  - Benzodiazepines or Z-drugs to assist sleep.
  - Antipsychotics.

- If clozapine has been required in the manic episode, it may be continued as prophylaxis.[BAP]
- If antidepressants are used, they should be combined with a mood stabiliser or antipsychotic.[BAP]
- Valproate should not be offered to women of childbearing potential (see p. 223, refer 'Valproate and Pregnancy' box).

Prophylaxis in BPAD-II
Consider lamotrigine or quetiapine monotherapy.[BAP]

- Because of interactions with carbamazepine, it should be used in combination with caution.[BAP]
- Oxcarbazepine and eslicarbazepine use has been extrapolated from carbamazepine without strong evidence, based on their chemical similarities.[BAP] Their side effect burden sometimes means they are better tolerated.

NON-PHARMACOLOGICAL MANAGEMENT

- Evidence for psychological therapy for bipolar depression is poorer than for unipolar depression. There have been large failed trials using CBT.[BAP]
- The most important non-pharmacological intervention is psychoeducation.[BAP]
  - Can be delivered in a group setting.[BAP]
  - Best early in the illness.[BAP]
  - http://beatingbipolar.org is a good resource.
- Other psychological therapies with some evidence in relapse prevention:
  - Family focussed therapy.
  - CBT (showed initial promise, but no benefit in larger RCTs).
  - Interpersonal social rhythm therapy (relies on ensuring regular sleep and daily activities; good early evidence).
- Group cognitive remediation may improve longer-term cognitive outcomes.[BAP]
- Consider developing an advanced directive with the patient specifying which treatments they would prefer when they are unwell.[BAP]

Psychoeducation: Key points

- Sx: Depression and (hypo)mania
- Medications: SEs, compliance, not stopping suddenly
- Pregnancy: Risks of relapse and medications
- Drugs: Avoid recreational drugs; alcohol only in moderation
- Family and friends: Involve in care if possible
- Relapse indicators: Know yours; sleep disturbance is common
- Sleep hygiene and regular routine: Some apps can help
- Life decisions: Avoid while manic[NICE]

STARTING

- **Lithium:** Start at 400 mg in one or two divided doses and adjust dose every 5–7 days aiming for plasma levels of 0.6–0.8 mmol/L (levels of 0.8–1.0 mmol/L may be more effective but risks are higher if continued in long term). Once levels are stable, switch to *nocte* dosing, as bd may ↑nephrotoxicity.[BAP] MR formulation often preferred. Restart at previous dose after periods of non-adherence, if no evidence of reduced renal function.

- **Valproate:** Sodium valproate has an MR formulation (Epilim Chrono), so may be given once daily (at night). Otherwise, valproate formulations should be prescribed bd. Faster loading may be used in acute mania.

- **Lamotrigine:** Titration is very important to avoid SJS/TEN. Rate of titration (see monograph) depends on whether it is being co-prescribed with any enzyme inhibitors (e.g. valproate) or inducers (e.g. carbamazepine). Valproate inhibits lamotrigine metabolism, so if given together lamotrigine dose should be halved.[BAP]
  - If a patient has not been taking lamotrigine for ≥5 half-lives, it should be re-titrated as if starting for the first time. Half-life is 33 h in a healthy person with no other medications, but is higher with enzyme inhibitors and lower with enzyme inducers.[SPC]

- **Carbamazepine:** Potent enzyme inducer, so check interactions carefully (see monograph and p. 342, refer table in 'Basic Psychopharmacology' chapter). It also induces its own metabolism, so within a few weeks of Rx clearance can ↑threefold. Dose adjustments are recommended to ensure therapeutic efficacy. Titration is not as essential as with lamotrigine, but it is recommended to reduce the initial sedation.

SIDE EFFECTS

- Prolonged release formulations can ↓some SEs.
- Lithium toxicity can occur as an emergency (see p. 389, refer 'Lithium Toxicity' section in 'Drug Toxicity Syndromes' in 'Emergencies' chapter).

Side effect	Medications	Mx
Hypothyroidism (2%–3%. F > M. Best marker is ↑TSH)	Lithium	• If slightly ↑TSH with normal T_4, monitor. Usually transient. • Treat with levothyroxine if symptomatic, ↓T_4 or TSH > 10. Check thyroid autoantibodies. • r/f to endo if complicated.
Hyperparathyroidism (dyspepsia, renal stones, osteoporosis)	Lithium	• Usually mild and asymptomatic, just monitor PTH and calcium. • If severe or symptomatic, consider withdrawing Li. • If Li needs to be continued, r/f to endo for consideration of cinacalcet or parathyroidectomy.
Postural tremor (*NB: cerebellar* tremor on lithium suggests toxicity)	Lithium, valproate	• ↓dose, MR formulation. • Propranolol 30–100 mg/day in divided doses (if not asthmatic).
SJS/TEN (lamotrigine > carbamazepine)	Lamotrigine, carbamazepine	• Patient should contact psychiatrist or GP immediately if any rash. • In early rash, hard to distinguish between serious and benign, so always stop lamotrigine.[BAP] • If rash is trivial and resolves on its own, lamotrigine may be re-introduced at a slower rate.[BAP] • If rash is widespread, mucosal, heavily involving the face or accompanied by fever or sore throat, all possible causative agents should be stopped. Consideration should be given to never retrying lamotrigine, or using extreme caution if it is.[BAP]

(*continued*)

Side effect	Medications	Mx
Nephrogenic diabetes insipidus (polyuria, nocturia, polydipsia)	Lithium	• If no impact on function, monitor. • If impairing, measure 24 h urine volume and osmolality. • Fluid restriction contra-indicated.[BAP] • ↓dose, MR formulation or switch. • Consider amiloride, but monitor urea and electrolytes (U&Es).[BAP] • Consider renal r/f.
CKD (20% overall, but CKD 5 only in 1%; risk factors: chronic Rx, Li toxicity, co-morbidities)	Lithium	• Monitor Li levels at ≤2 month intervals. • Keep levels at lower end of range. • Avoid other nephrotoxins. • If eGFR <60, consider stopping Li but balance risks and benefits.
↑LFTs	Valproate	Stop valproate if[NICE]: • 3× upper limit of normal. • Continuing to rise or • Symptomatic.
Haematological abnormalities	Carbamazepine (↓neutrophils), valproate (↓Plt), lamotrigine (↓neutrophils)	Monitor, but more important that clinicians and patients are aware of Sx (neutropoenia → fever, sore throat, rash, mouth ulcers; ↓Plt → bruising). Encourage patient to seek urgent medical attention[BAP] and perform FBC if Sx occur.

Source: Ferrier et al., *BJPsych Adv* 1995; **1**(4): 102–8; Canning et al., *Men Heal Clin* 2012; **1**(7): 174–6; Ferrier et al., *BJPsych Adv* 2006; **12**(4): 256–64; Gupta et al., *BJPsych Adv* 2013; **19**(6): 457–66.

MONITORING

- Many medications used in BPAD are associated with adverse metabolic side effects, but not all of the poor cardiovascular outcomes in BPAD are due to medications.

- If prescribed an antipsychotic, follow guidance in the Psychosis section (p. 198, refer 'Monitoring' heading in 'Psychosis' section of this chapter).
- In general, drug plasma levels are taken at trough (i.e. just before the next dose is given). Lithium is the exception: levels are generally taken 12 h post-dose, regardless of the regimen.[MPG]

Drug	Baseline	Follow-up	Annual
All patients (regardless of medications)[BAP]	BP BMI HbA1c/glucose Lipids		BP BMI HbA1c/glucose Lipids
Lithium[1,BAP]	U&Es TFTs Calcium	Li levels: 5–7 days post-dose increase. When stable, 3-monthly intervals for 1 yr, then 6-monthly thereafter.	U&Es TFTs Calcium
Valproate[BAP]	FBC LFTs Pregnancy test (if relevant)	LFTs within 6 months	
Lamotrigine[NICE]	FBC U&Es LFTs		
Carbamazepine[1,BAP]	FBC U&Es LFTs HLA-B1502 genetic screening[2,MHRA]	Rpt FBC, U&Es and LFTs within 2 months	

[1] Can be pro-arrhythmogenic, so some sources also recommend a baseline ECG if any established cardiac disease or risk factors for it.

[2] In individuals of East Asian origin, as this predicts SJS/TEN.

Lithium

- More frequent monitoring is necessary if patients are physically unwell or taking drugs that alter lithium levels (e.g. diuretics, ACE-i, NSAIDs).[BAP]
- Toxicity can be present with normal Li levels. Levels >2 mmol/L are associated with life-threatening toxicity.

STOPPING

- Relapse does still occur after years of remission. General advice is for prophylaxis indefinitely.[BAP]
- Discontinuing is safer in patients who meet all of the following criteria[BAP]:
  - Currently completely well
  - No mood episodes for 4 yr
  - No serious risks in previous depression or mania
  - No rapid cycling
- Before stopping medications, discuss risks and benefits.
- If stopping any medication, ↓dose over ≥4 wk, preferably longer.[BAP]
  - Abrupt lithium discontinuation → 50% risk of mania in 12 wk. Only stop abruptly in medical emergency or overdose.
- Put crisis plan in place for relapse.[BAP]
- Antidepressants should be stopped abruptly in mania, but should otherwise follow the schedules on p. 238, refer table in 'Depression' section of this chapter. If used in rapid cycling BPAD, a more rapid taper should be used than with unipolar depression.[BAP]

SWAPPING

- Lithium, valproate, lamotrigine and carbamazepine can each be used in combination with the exception of lithium + carbamazepine, which increases neurotoxicity.[BNF] Antipsychotics may also be combined with mood stabilisers. The main SE to be aware of is cumulative sedation.
- Therefore, best practice is usually to titrate up the new drug before reducing the old to minimise risk of relapse.

SPECIAL GROUPS
Children
- Start at lower doses, but be prepared to increase to higher doses relative to body mass.
- Harder to diagnose BPAD. Requires monitoring over a period of time by an experienced clinician.[BAP]
- In mania, use aripiprazole first line.[BAP, NICE] Other options are olanzapine, quetiapine and risperidone.[BAP]
- In bipolar depression, extrapolate from adult guidelines, but bear in mind that antidepressants may more easily induce a switch to mania in children.[BAP] Offer a structured psychological intervention (CBT or interpersonal therapy [IPT]) lasting ≥3 months.[NICE]
- Risk of disruption to education and emotional development may incline clinicians towards prophylaxis.[BAP]

Elderly
- 10% of BPAD develops in >50s.
- Carbamazepine and valproate can ↓bone mineral density, resulting in ↑risk of fractures.
- Consider lower doses and slower titration.[BAP]

Pregnancy

> *Valproate and pregnancy*[MHRA]
> - Highly teratogenic, causing congenital malformations in 10% and serious developmental disorders in 30%–40%.
> - Valproate should not be prescribed for women or girls of child-bearing potential unless other treatments are ineffective or not tolerated.
> - Valproate must not be used in any woman or girl able to have children unless she has a pregnancy prevention programme in place (including highly effective contraception, e.g. IUD or implant).
> - It is important that women do not stop taking valproate without first discussing with their doctor.

- Valproate should not be prescribed for pregnant women with BPAD.
- See risk materials produced by the MHRA, including checklist for prescribers and patient information booklet (https://www.gov.uk/drug-safety-update/valproate-medicines-epilim-depakote-pregnancy-prevention-programme-materials-online).

- Post-partum psychosis often develops into BPAD, and BPAD often relapses in the post-partum period. Depression and manic episodes in the post-partum period are also common.
- Pregnancy is not protective against relapse and giving birth often precipitates it.
- Mood stabilisers may cause birth defects, but risks of untreated illness are also substantial.
- Balance the risks of medications against the benefits of relapse prevention. Often mood stabilisers are still required in pregnancy, but valproate is contraindicated.[BAP]
- Most of teratogenicity is in first trimester.
- Antipsychotics, antidepressants, lamotrigine and lithium have low risks of teratogenicity.[BAP]
  - If the patient requires an antidepressant during pregnancy, be mindful of manic switch if the mood stabiliser is withdrawn.
- Offer an antipsychotic as prophylaxis in BPAD if woman becomes pregnant and is stopping lithium, or if the woman plans to breastfeed.[NICE]
- **Carbamazepine** should be avoided in women who are considering pregnancy.[NICE] Risk of major malformation ~6%.
- **Lamotrigine** may be used during pregnancy as risk of major malformation does not seem significantly elevated above baseline (from data in epilepsy), but serum levels should be checked frequently during gestation and the postpartum period.[NICE]
  - Lamotrigine concentrations can drop by 50% in second and third trimesters.

- **Lithium** may increase the risk of cardiac malformations (0.05%–0.1%, especially Ebstein's anomaly), but the absolute risk is still low. Dose often needs to be adjusted in pregnancy and levels closely monitored, especially in third trimester and immediately following birth.[NICE]
- **Valproate:** See box p. 223, refer box entitled 'Valproate and Pregnancy'.
- Consider neonatal effects of the psychotropic and ensure enhanced monitoring after birth.[BAP]
- ECT is an option for severe mania.[BAP]

Breastfeeding

- Women should decide whether to breastfeed after a discussion of risks and benefits.[BAP]
- In general, breastfeeding should be encouraged, except in women taking lithium, carbamazepine or clozapine.[NICE]
- **Lithium** is a relative contraindication (CI) to breastfeeding, due to narrow therapeutic index with an RID (see box on p. 204, refer box entitled 'Relative Infant Dose') of 40%.[BAP]
- An advantage of bottle-feeding is that it allows parents to share nocturnal feeding, improving the woman's sleep.[BAP] Another option is expressed breast milk.

Renal impairment

- If possible, avoid lithium. Enhanced monitoring is necessary.[MPG]
- Valproate, carbamazepine and lamotrigine with slow titration are good options.[MPG]

Hepatic impairment

- Valproate should be avoided due to potential hepatotoxicity.
- Lithium is the best option, but careful monitoring is required.[MPG]

Physical health problems

- Check interactions (p. 341, refer 'Drug Interactions' in 'Basic Psychopharmacology' chapter). Carbamazepine is a notorious enzyme inducer. Valproate inhibits metabolism of a few drugs.
- **MS:** Patients often reduce fluid intake due to urethral sphincter disturbance. Lithium requires a good fluid intake, so should be avoided in these patients. Antipsychotics are good options.[MPG]

- **Epilepsy**: Liaise with neurologist to find medications that can treat both disorders. In general, valproate is good for generalised seizures, while lamotrigine and carbamazepine are preferred for focal seizures.
- **HIV**: Avoid carbamazepine due to risk of neutropoenia and potential failure of antiretrovirals (ARVs).[MPG]

Further information

Goodwin et al., 'Evidence-based guidelines for treating bipolar disorder: revised third edition recommendations from the British Association for Psychopharmacology', *J Psychopharmacol* 2016; **30**(6): 495–553.

DEPRESSION

DIAGNOSIS

- Depression is a syndrome characterised by the following clinical features:
  - Depressed mood
  - Energy low (anergia)
  - Pleasure lost (anhedonia)
  - Retardation or agitation
  - Eating ↑/↓(appetite or wt)
  - Sleep ↑/↓
  - Suicidal ideation
  - I'm a failure (loss of confidence)
  - Only me to blame (guilt)
  - No concentration
- Differential diagnosis:

Psychiatric	Organic
• BPAD (screen for mania and hypomania; screening Ix: MDQ or HCL-16)	• Hypothyroidism (fatigue++, ↓HR, cold intolerance, constipation; Ix: TFTs) • Anaemia (fatigue, breathlessness, chest pain; Ix: FBC)

(continued)

Psychiatric	Organic
• Anxiety disorders (see p. 243, refer 'Anxiety Disorders' section) • Acute stress reaction (hours–days) • Adjustment disorder (clearly related to life event) • EUPD (impulsivity, chronic emptiness, emotional instability, self-destructive behaviour) • Dysthymia (less severe than depression but lasting ≥2 yr) • Substance misuse (screen for EtOH and drugs) • Negative symptoms of schizophrenia (screen for psychosis)	• B12/folate deficiency (glossitis, peripheral neuropathy, diarrhoea; Ix: FBC, B12/folate levels) • Dementia (can be hard to distinguish from depressive pseudodementia; Hx of gradual cognitive decline; Ix: Mini-Mental State Examination [MMSE]) • Obstructive sleep apnoea (OSA) (excessive daytime sleepiness, nocturnal apnoeic episodes; Ix: Epworth Sleepiness Scale) • Cushing's disease (purple striae, facial plethora, buffalo hump, glucose intolerance; Ix: 24 h urinary cortisol, dexamethasone suppression test) • Drugs (esp. tetrabenazine, steroids, baclofen, ß-blockers, opioids) • Addison's (postural hypotension, skin pigmentation, $\downarrow$Na$^+$, $\uparrow$K$^+$; Ix: serum cortisol, short Synacthen test) • Parkinson's (tremor, rigidity, bradykinesia) • Hypercalcaemia (renal stones, abdominal groans, pain in bones)

- For a new diagnosis of depression, the following Ix are appropriate: FBC, U&E, LFTs, bone profile, TFTs. Consider other Ix as previously discussed if suggested by clinical picture.
- Depression may be categorised by severity based on number of symptoms, intensity and functional impairment. The following types of depression may also be considered:
  - Melancholic depression: unreactive mood, diurnal variation (worse in morning), early morning wakening, psychomotor agitation/retardation, $\downarrow$wt/appetite.
  - Atypical depression: mood reactivity, $\uparrow$wt/appetite, hypersomnia, leaden paralysis, fatigue. F > M.
  - Psychotic depression: severe depression with hallucinations or delusions that are generally mood congruent.

TYPES OF ANTIDEPRESSANT DRUGS[BAP(ADAPTED)]

| Class | Drug | Action | Side effects | | | | | | | Lethality in overdose |
			Anticho-linergic	Sedation	Insomnia/agitation	Postural ↓BP	Sexual dysfunction[a]	↑Wt	Other	
SSRI	Citalopram	SRI	−	−	+	−	++	−	Nausea, ↑QTc	Low
	Escitalopram	SRI	−	−	+	−	++	−	Nausea, ↑QTc	Low
	Sertraline	SRI	−	−	+	−	++	−	Nausea	Low
	Fluoxetine	SRI	−	−	++	−	++	−	Nausea, rash	Low
	Fluvoxamine	SRI	−	−	+	−	+	−	Nausea	Low
	Paroxetine	SRI	+	+	+	−	+++	+	Nausea	Low
SNRI	Duloxetine	SRI+NRI	−	−	+	−	++	−	Nausea, sweating	?Low
	Venlafaxine	SRI>NRI	−	−	+	−	++	−	Nausea, HTN, sweating	Mod
Tricyclic antidepressant (TCA)	Clomipramine	SRI+NRI	++	++	+	++	++	+	Cardiac fx	Mod
	Amitriptyline	NRI>SRI	++	++	−	++	+	++	Cardiac fx	High
	Dosulepin	NRI>SRI	++	++	−	++	+	++	Cardiac fx	High
	Imipramine	NRI>SRI	++	+	+	++	+	++	Cardiac fx	High
	Nortriptyline	NRI	+	+	+	+	+	−	Cardiac fx	Low
	Lofepramine	NRI	+	−	+	+	+	−	Cardiac fx, sweating	Low
	Doxepin	SRI+NRI	++	++	−	++	+	+	Cardiac fx	High
	Trimipramine	SRI+NRI	++	+++	−	++	+	++	Cardiac fx	High

(continued)

			Side effects							Lethality in overdose
Class	Drug	Action	Anticholinergic	Sedation	Insomnia/ agitation	Postural ↓BP	Sexual dysfunction^a	↑wt	Other	
Receptor antagonists	Mirtazapine	5-HT$_2$+5-HT$_3$+α$_2$ ant	-	++	-	-	-	+++		Low
	Mianserin	5-HT$_2$+α$_1$+α$_2$ ant	+	++	-	-	-	-		Low
	Trazodone	5-HT$_2$+α$_1$ ant > SRI	-	++	-	++	-	+	Priapism	Low
Monoamine oxidase inhibitor (MAOI)	Phenelzine	Irreversible MAO-A/B	+	+	++	++	++	++	HTN crisis, oedema	High
	Tranylcypromine	Irreversible MAO-A/B	+	+	++	++	++	++		High
	Isocarboxazid	Irreversible MAO-A/B	+	+	++	++	++	++		High
Other	Moclobemide	Reversible MAO-A	-	-	+	-	-	-		Low
	Vortioxetine	SRI + 5-HT$_{1A}$ ag, 5-HT$_{1B}$ pa, 5-HT$_{1D/3/7}$ ant	-	-	-	-	+/-	-	Nausea	?
	Reboxetine	NRI	+	-	+	-	+	-		Low
	Bupropion	NRI+DRI	-	-	+	-	+	-	↓Seizure threshold	?Mod
	Agomelatine	MT ag and 5-HT$_{2x}$ ant	+	+	+	-	-	-	Monitor LFTs	?Low

Note. ant, antagonist; DRI, dopamine reuptake inhibitor; MAO, monoamine oxidase inhibitor; NRI, noradrenaline reuptake inhibitor; pa, partial agonist; SRI, serotonin reuptake inhibitor.

CHOICE
Depressive episode

- Effect size for antidepressants is greater for more severe and longer-lasting depression.
- First-line antidepressant should usually be an SSRI.[NICE]
- Consider[BAP]:
  - Side effect profile, given patient preferences and co-morbidities.
  - Lethality in overdose, given suicide risk.
  - Drug interactions.
  - Prior response of patient and family members.

Most effective antidepressants[BAP]

- **Sertraline**
- **Escitalopram (20 mg)**
- **Mirtazapine**
- **Venlafaxine (≥150 mg)**
- **Amitriptyline**
- **Clomipramine**
- **Vortioxetine***

* Released since guideline publication and included on the basis of expert advice.

- Use SEs to your advantage:
  - Sedating antidepressants for patients with insomnia
  - Activating antidepressants for somnolent patients
  - Antidepressants that ↑Wt for cachectic patients
- If patient also has an anxiety disorder (see p. 243, refer 'Anxiety Disorders' section in this chapter), pick an antidepressant that also treats the anxiety disorder.
- Consider ECT if urgent response required (e.g. depressive stupor, high risk of suicide, extreme distress and ↓fluid intake), psychotic features present or previous good response.[BAP]
- Avoid St John's wort due to potential for interactions and differing preparations.[BAP,NICE]
- Dosulepin should generally be avoided,[NICE] due to very high risk of death in overdose.

Psychotic depression

- Antidepressant + antipsychotic is better than monotherapy with either.[BAP]
- TCAs are possibly more effective than SSRIs.
- ECT is an option.[BAP]

Pseudobulbar affect

(Ahmed & Simmons, *Ther Clin Risk Manag* 2013)

- Affective lability with inappropriate laughter or crying.
- Occurs in MS, MND, dementia and CVA.
- Use low doses of an SSRI or TCA, e.g. fluoxetine 20 mg OD, citalopram 20 mg OD, sertraline 50 mg OD, amitriptyline 20–100 mg ON, nortriptyline 20–100 mg ON.

TREATMENT RESISTANCE

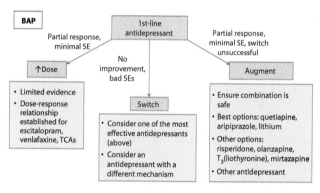

- Assess risks and benefits of further treatment against continued depression.[BAP]
- Address social factors (e.g. occupational issues, financial problems, social isolation, abusive relationships).[BAP]
- Assess for co-morbid disorders, e.g. BPAD or psychosis.[BAP]

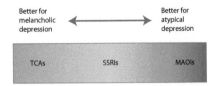

- If a patient discontinues an SSRI due to lack of efficacy, switching to a different class is slightly more effective than switching to another SSRI.[BAP]
- Flupentixol and amisulpride (unlicensed) are antipsychotics with some possible antidepressant actions and are occasionally used.
- Some combinations of antidepressants can be extremely dangerous and risk serotonin syndrome. See 'Possible antidepressant combinations' box on p. 233 for safe options.
- Modafinil may be used in partial responders to SSRIs who are troubled by persistent somnolence or fatigue,[BAP] but it may worsen anxiety.
- For patients who relapse while on an antidepressant, most episodes will be self-limiting within 3 months. ↑Dose of antidepressant is effective in most.[BAP]

Starting an MAOI
- Warn of dietary restrictions (on p. 237, refer box 'Food to avoid with MAOIs').
- Avoid co-prescription with any serotonergic or noradrenergic medications (including antidepressants, sympathomimetics and some opioids). Many other medications are cautioned.
- Advise patient to inform any prescriber that they are taking an MAOI.
- Advise patient to discuss with pharmacist before taking an over-the-counter (OTC) nasal decongestant.
- Moclobemide is safer than irreversible MAOIs and requires a less strict diet, but is possibly less efficacious.
- If diet not tolerated, selegiline, mainly an MAO-B inhibitor with some MAO-A inhibition, can be used without dietary restriction at lower doses, although it is not widely available in the United Kingdom.

- Due to their complex interactions, MAOIs should be used with care.
- The combination of venlafaxine + mirtazapine is sometimes termed 'California Rocket Fuel'.

Possible antidepressant combinations

- All combinations risk serotonin syndrome
- None of the evidence for combinations is especially strong

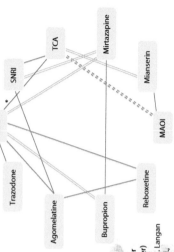

— Evidence for safety

═ Evidence for safety and efficacy

═ ═ ═ Evidence for efficacy but caution required. Start MAOI and TCA together at low doses and gradually titrate up.

* Beware of pharmacokinetic interactions (see p. 341, refer 'Drug Interactions' in 'Basic Psychopharmacology' chapter)

(Rojo et al, Acta Psychiatr Scand Suppl 2005; 112(s428): 25–31. Langan et al, Ther Adv Psychopharmacol 2011; 1(6): 175–80; Sühs et al, Brain Behav 2015; 5(4): e00318.)

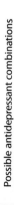

ECT in depression
- Indications: Urgent response required, psychotic features, previous good response.
- Some antidepressants (especially TCAs) can ↓seizure threshold.
- Acute efficacy +++, but relapse common, so start antidepressant.
- Maintenance ECT only if response >> antidepressants. Regularly assess risks and benefits.

NON-PHARMACOLOGICAL MEASURES
- CBT and antidepressants are similarly efficacious in acute Rx, but CBT may better prevent relapse.
- CBT, IPT and behavioural activation can all be used as monotherapy in mild-moderate depression. For severe depression, do not use psychotherapy monotherapy.[BAP]

CBT for depression
1 Collaborative formulation with patient using five areas: situation, thoughts, moods, behaviour, biology. Emphasise connections.
2 Behavioural activation: Monitor activities with diary and demonstrate how lack of pleasurable activities → ↓mood. Schedule new activities that give pleasure and sense of achievement.
3 Cognitive reformulation: Identify automatic thoughts. Discuss evidence for and against thoughts. Develop modified perspectives.

STARTING
- Prescribe antidepressant if depression is moderate-severe or lasts ≥2 yr.[BAP]
  - Consider antidepressant if depression with previous history of moderate-severe episode or current episode lasts ≥2–3 months.[BAP]
- Rule out BPAD by screening for mania/hypomania.

- Patient education: Nature of disorder, time to efficacy, possibility of suicidal thoughts on starting Rx, SEs, duration of Rx and problems with discontinuing.
- If ↑risk of suicide, consider providing prescriptions weekly or fortnightly. Instalment prescriptions can also be provided.
- If titrating up (e.g. TCAs), increase dose every 3–7 days.
- 35% of improvement occurs within first week, but very dramatic response suggests placebo and may not be sustained.[BAP]
- If augmenting with an antipsychotic, doses are usually lower than for treatment of psychosis (see individual monographs). However, lithium augmentation should still aim for plasma levels >0.6 mmol/L.[BAP]

Are antidepressants addictive?
- **Common Q from patients.**
- **Antidepressants can cause a withdrawal syndrome *but* they are not addictive.**
- **There is no tolerance, craving, compulsion or euphoria.**

SIDE EFFECTS
- Cardiac arrhythmias:
  - Citalopram and escitalopram prolong the QTc. These should be avoided in patients with congenital long QT syndrome or in those taking other medications that prolong the QTc (see p. 197, refer box 'QTc prolonging drugs').
  - TCAs prolong the PR interval, QRS complex and QT interval. They are unsuitable for those with pre-existing cardiac disease.
- Serotonin syndrome is an acute and potentially life-threatening reaction to antidepressants involving autonomic dysfunction, neuromuscular disturbance and altered mental status (see p. 389, refer 'Serotonin Syndrome' in 'Drug toxicity syndromes' in 'Emergencies' chapter).
- SSRIs can ↑risk of bleeding by inhibiting platelet aggregation. See under special groups for appropriate actions.

- General management of SEs:
  - Dose reduction +/− slower retitration
  - Switch to drug with lower propensity to this SE
  - Lifestyle modifications (e.g. sleep hygiene, diet, exercise)
- Specific management:

Side effect	Rx
Dry mouth	Sipping water regularly, sugar-free gum, OTC saliva substitutes (e.g. BioXtra, Salivese, Xerotin).
Drowsiness	Distinguish from hypersomnolence of depression. Dose sedating drugs in evening or at night. Consider modafinil,[BAP] but beware worsening co-morbid anxiety.
Nausea	Usually transient. Provide reassurance.[BAP]
Paradoxical anxiety/agitation in first 1–2 wk of Rx	Explanation and reassurance. Consider short course of benzodiazepine[BAP] (e.g. diazepam 2 mg tds for 7–10 days).
Male sexual dysfunction	For erectile dysfunction, consider sildenafil or tadalafil.[BAP]
Female sexual dysfunction	Bupropion or sildenafil.[BAP]
Hyponatraemia (Kirby & Ames, *Int J Geriatr Psychiatry* 2001; Goh, *Am Fam Physician* 2004) • Early features: headache, fatigue, loss of appetite, insomnia, muscle cramps • Late features: N&V, confusion, seizures, coma, death	If asymptomatic and Na$^+$ ≥130 mmol/L, monitor. Otherwise, try to discontinue antidepressant. If euvolaemic, fluid-restrict (e.g. 1–1.5 L/day). If dehydrated, may need iv hypertonic saline. If antidepressant needs to be continued, consider demeclocycline or tolvaptan with endocrinology input.

MAOI tyramine ('cheese') effect (Shulman et al., *CNS Drugs* 2013; 27(10): 789–97)

- Causes a hypertensive crisis.
- Occurs in patients on MAOIs in combination with foods high in tyramine.
- Risk is lower on moclobemide.

- Effect can also occur in patients who take the OTC nasal decongestants pseudoephedrine and phenylephrine with an MAOI.

Food to avoid with MAOIs
- **Alcohol (especially beer)**
- **Beans**
- **Cheese**
- **Yeast extracts (Marmite)**
- **Processed meat**

For details, see the Sunnybrook MAOI Diet

MONITORING
- After starting an antidepressant, arrange a follow-up appointment in 1–2 wk. (This in itself may be therapeutic.)
- Thereafter, assess as clinically indicated.
- Assess:
  - Rx response
  - SE
  - Suicide risk
- Agomelatine has been associated with hepatotoxicity, but no fatalities. LFTs should be measured before starting (or increasing the dose) and then at 3 wk, 6 wk, 3 months and 6 months.[SPC]
- Plasma level monitoring is *rarely* used, but has the following roles[BAP]:
  - Detecting non-concordance.
  - Finding fast metabolisers.
  - Determining effects of interactions.
  - Supporting diagnosis of TCA toxicity.

STOPPING
- Highest risk of relapse is in 6 months after stopping antidepressant.
- For a single episode of depression, continue for 6–9 months after remission.[BAP]
- If multiple episodes, continue for ≥1 yr. If high risk of relapse, consider long-term Rx.[BAP]

- Antidepressants ↓relapse risk by 70%, but should be kept at the treatment dose.[BAP]
- Speed of discontinuation[BAP]:

Situation	Rate of discontinuation
Serious adverse effect	Abrupt or rapid
Mild adverse effect	4 wk
Planned withdrawal after long-term prophylaxis	Several months

> *Risk of relapse*
> The following are associated with high risk of relapse on stopping an antidepressant:
>
> - Short time from previous episode
> - Chronic depression
> - Severe episode
> - Rx resistance
> - Psychosis
> - Physical co-morbidity

Antidepressant withdrawal syndrome

- Can occur following withdrawal from any antidepressant

Risk factors	Features	Rx
- Abrupt discontinuation - Short half-lives (e.g. venlafaxine, paroxetine, fluvoxamine), but agomelatine has very low rates - High doses - Rx ≥ 9 wk	**FINISH** - **F**lu-like Sx - **I**nsomnia (with vivid dreams) - **N**ausea - **I**mbalance - **S**ensory disturbances (tingling, electric shocks) - **H**yperarousal (irritability, anxiety)	- Explanation and reassurance (usually effective) - Re-start antidepressant and slowly taper down - For SSRIs/SNRIs, can switch to fluoxetine (long half-life); continue fluoxetine until Sx subside, then stop abruptly

SWAPPING

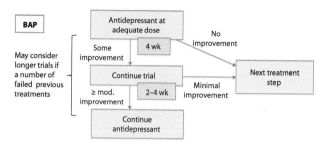

- If switching to a drug of the same class (usually to another SSRI) or one that would be compatible in a combination, switch abruptly. This simplifies the process for the patient and avoids discontinuation Sx.[BAP]
- To avoid pharmacodynamic interactions, when switching to/from an MAOI, taper down and then leave 2–3 wk before starting the new drug.[MPG]
- Fluoxetine has a long half-life. If switching from fluoxetine to an MAOI, leave 5–6 wk drug free before starting the MAOI. If switching from fluoxetine to another antidepressant, usually leave 4–7 days drug free. Cautious cross-tapering may be performed when switching from fluoxetine to agomelatine, mirtazapine or trazodone.[MPG]

SPECIAL GROUPS
Children
- If depression is mild, use watchful waiting for 4 wk before starting treatment.[NICE]
- Antidepressants are not first line. Consider if severe or recurrent.[BAP, NICE] Only offer with concurrent psychological therapy.[NICE]

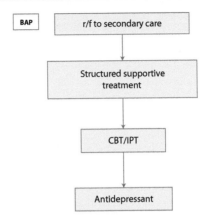

- Antidepressants may be associated with ↑suicidal ideation and behaviours. To avoid agitation on initiation of medications, titrate slowly and monitor carefully.
- SSRIs are the only antidepressants that should generally be used.[BAP] Fluoxetine appears to be most effective. Its long half-life can compensate for slightly erratic compliance.
- If age <13 yr, antidepressant effect is small and not statistically significant, compared to a high placebo response. Evidence is not established, but use of fluoxetine may be considered.[NICE]
- Start with low doses based on age and weight and titrate up. However, children have faster metabolisms, so often require higher final doses relative to their weight than adults.
- Monitor carefully after starting an antidepressant, e.g. weekly contact for first 4 wk.[NICE]

Elderly
- Drug clearance can be lower, so lower doses are often required.
- Response can take longer, and a longer duration of treatment may be required to prevent relapse.

- In Rx-resistant depression, best evidence is for augmenting with lithium. Some evidence for venlafaxine and selegiline.[BAP]
- Often at risk of falls, so try to avoid drugs that cause postural hypotension.
- If sedation is required, mirtazapine is a good option.
- SSRI-induced hyponatraemia is more common.

Pregnancy

- No current classes of antidepressants are absolutely contraindicated. Most safety evidence exists for SSRIs. Sertraline is often preferred.
- Antidepressants are associated with no impact on miscarriage rate, a small impact on gestational age (0.45 wk earlier), small ↓in Apgar scores (0.37 at 1 min) and a small ↓in birth wt (74 g but non-significant if control group is women with depression) (Ross et al., *JAMA Psychiatry* 2013; 70(4): 436–43).
- Antidepressant withdrawal syndrome has been observed in neonates.
- On discovering pregnancy, avoid abrupt discontinuation of antidepressant.[BAP]
- Weigh risks and benefits. If depression is mild, consider tapering down antidepressant and discontinuing. If moderate-severe, consider continuing or switching to an antidepressant with better safety evidence.[BAP] Also consider severity of past episodes and any prior postpartum episodes.
- There is an increased risk of persistent pulmonary hypertension of the newborn for offspring of women on SSRIs in pregnancy (absolute risk 3:1000 versus 2:1000 in general population). Consider weaning off antidepressants near term to avoid this.[BAP]

Breastfeeding

- High risk of postpartum depression in those who have been depressed in pregnancy, so usually best to continue an antidepressant if they have been on one in pregnancy.[BAP]

- In general, continue with same antidepressant used in pregnancy rather than switching.
- Sertraline is also preferred in breastfeeding and has a low RID (see p. 204, refer box 'Relative Infant Dose'), although paroxetine may also be used.

Renal impairment
- Citalopram and sertraline are reasonable choices.[MPG]
- TCAs can usually be given at normal doses, except dosulepin (Phipps & Turkington, *Adv Psychiatr Treat* 2001; 7(6): 426–32).
- ↑QTc prolongation is common in renal failure, so monitor carefully if citalopram or TCAs are used.
- Doses often require reduction (see individual monographs).

Hepatic impairment
- Prescribe fewest number of medications possible, starting at low doses and increasing slowly. Avoid medications with extensive metabolism and those with prominent sedation.
- Sertraline and mirtazapine are good options, but reduce dose.[MPG] See individual monographs.
- SSRIs can be used at low doses, but avoid fluoxetine due to long half-life.[MPG]
- Anticholinergic SEs of TCAs can worsen hepatic encephalopathy.
- MAOIs can be hepatotoxic, so should be avoided.

Physical health problems
- Depression more common in presence of medical disorders, but antidepressants may be less effective.
- SSRIs are usually first line, as better tolerated.[BAP]
- Check interactions (p. 341, refer 'Drug Interactions' in 'Basic Psychopharmacology' chapter). Citalopram and escitalopram are least prone to interactions.
- **Cardiac failure or arrhythmia**: Avoid TCAs as proarrhythmogenic and ↑risk of MI. Check QTc before prescribing citalopram/escitalopram.[BAP]

- **Acute coronary syndrome:** Best evidence for SSRIs (especially sertraline), mirtazapine and bupropion.[BAP]
- **Bleeding disorders:** Avoid SSRIs.[BAP]
- **Patients on aspirin, NSAIDs or anticoagulants:** Either avoid SSRIs or add in a PPI to reduce risk of GI bleed.[BAP]
- **Diabetes:** SSRIs are preferred. Fluoxetine is useful for T2DM, as it is associated with Wt loss.
- **Epilepsy:** SSRIs are generally considered safe (and may actually be protective) but should be titrated more slowly. Other options are mirtazapine, venlafaxine and moclobemide. Avoid clomipramine and bupropion, as they ↓seizure threshold. Check interactions with anticonvulsants.
- **Stroke:** Due to their effect on Pt aggregation, SSRIs can be protective post-ischaemic stroke, but ↑bleeding risk post-haemorrhagic stroke. If ischaemic, SSRIs may be used. Otherwise, there is evidence for nortriptyline.

Further information

Cleare et al., 'Evidence-based guidelines for treating depressive disorders with antidepressants: a revision of the 2008 British Association for Psychopharmacology guidelines', *J Psychopharmacol* 2015; **29**(5): 459–525.

ANXIETY DISORDERS

DIAGNOSIS

The drugs in this chapter have substantial overlap with those used in depression, so this chapter should be read in conjunction with the previous section.

Anxiety disorders are common and varied. The algorithm that follows shows a diagnostic screening approach.

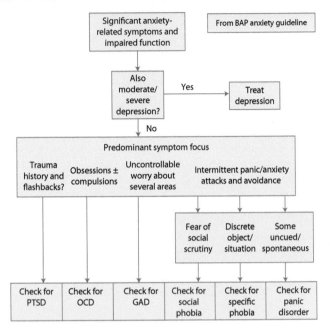

Source: Diagnosis algorithm reprinted from David S Baldwin et al., 'Evidence-based pharmacological treatment of anxiety disorders, post-traumatic stress disorder and obsessive-compulsive disorder: a revision of the 2005 guidelines from the British Association for Psychopharmacology', *J Psychopharmacol* 2014; **28**(5), 1–37, SAGE Publishing, https://doi.org/10.1177/0269881114525674.

- 'Organic' causes:
  - Drug use (caffeine, amphetamines, cocaine, β-agonists, theophylline)
  - Drug withdrawal (alcohol, benzodiazepines)
  - Cardiac arrhythmia (FHx, ischaemic heart disease [IHD], syncope, Sx with exercise; Ix: ECG, 7-day Holter monitor)
  - ↑thyroid (↑HR, tremor, proptosis, diarrhoea; Ix: TFTs)
  - Phaeochromocytoma (palpitations, HTN, headaches; Ix: 24 h urinary metanephrines)
  - ↓Ca^{2+} (muscle spasms, seizures, arrhythmia; Ix: bone profile)
  - Porphyria (rash, blisters, red urine, abdominal pain, vomiting; Ix: urinary porphobilinogen is good screen)
- For a new diagnosis of an anxiety disorder, the following Ix are often appropriate: FBC, U&E, LFTs (including γ-GT), bone profile, TFTs. Consider other Ix as previously mentioned if suggested by clinical picture.

TYPES OF ANXIOLYTIC DRUGS

Most drugs used for anxiety disorders are also used in depression and are listed with their SEs on p. 228, refer 'Types of Antidepressant Drugs' table.

Side effects

Class	Drug	Action	Sedation	Insomnia/ agitation	Postural ↓BP	↑wt	Other	Lethality in overdose
Gabapentinoids	Gabapentin	VGCC ant	+	−	−	+	Nausea	Low
	Pregabalin	VGCC ant	++	−	+	+	Dizziness, nausea, ankle swelling	Low
Other	Buspirone	5-HT$_{1A}$ pa	−	++	−	−	Nausea	?Mod

Note: pa, partial agonist; VGCC ant, voltage-gated calcium channel antagonist.

MEDICATIONS LICENSED FOR ANXIETY DISORDERS[BNF]

	GAD	Panic disorder	Specific phobia	Social anxiety disorder	PTSD	OCD
Citalopram		✓				
Escitalopram	✓	✓		✓		✓
Sertraline		✓		✓	✓	✓
Fluoxetine						✓
Fluvoxamine						✓
Paroxetine	✓	✓		✓	✓	✓
Duloxetine	✓					
Venlafaxine	✓			✓		
Clomipramine			✓			✓
Trazodone	✓					
Moclobemide				✓		
Pregabalin	✓					
Buspirone	✓					
Chlordiazepoxide[1]	✓					
Clonazepam[1]		✓				
Lorazepam[1]	✓	✓				
Oxazepam[1]	✓					

[1] Benzodiazepines are not generally recommended treatments for anxiety[NICE]: they do provide short-term relief, but tend to be ineffective in the long term and cause dependence. Benzodiazepines are covered in more detail on p. 280, refer section entitled 'Sleep Disorders and Agitation'.

Some recommended medications (as follows) for anxiety disorders are not licensed for these purposes, despite good evidence from randomised placebo-controlled trials. They can be prescribed off-label (see p. 357, refer 'Off-license Prescribing' in 'Miscellaneous' chapter for RCPsych/BAP position statement on unlicensed applications of licensed drugs in psychiatric practice).

CHOOSING A MEDICATION

> *Recreational drugs*
> - Many people with anxiety symptoms and disorders 'self-medicate'.
> - Ask Re. use of alcohol, cannabis and street benzodiazepines.
> - Consider dual diagnosis with a substance misuse disorder.

- For mild disorders, supportive care with patient education and support groups (e.g. Anxiety UK, Obsessive Action) may be sufficient.
- If moderate-severe depression is also present, treat the depression first.[BAP] Anxiety may improve with resolution of depression.
- Pharmacological and psychological therapy are probably similarly effective in acute illness, but should usually be offered separately in the initial stages of treatment.[BAP]
- SSRIs should be considered first-line therapy,[BAP, NICE] and sertraline is preferred for GAD (although it is not licensed for that condition).[NICE]
- SNRIs are effective but are somewhat less well tolerated than SSRIs.
- Benzodiazepines should generally be avoided or limited to short-term use ('crisis management').[BAP] Avoid in PTSD, as they tend to be ineffective and risks outweigh benefits.
- Antipsychotics have efficacy in some circumstances, but their SE profile limits their role. They are usually prescribed in low doses, except in PTSD.
- Propranolol and atenolol are often prescribed in primary care for somatic Sx of anxiety, but there is little evidence to support their use.[BAP]
- Pregabalin has evidence for a dose-response relationship. Response may be seen within the first wk.
- General principles of Rx resistance[BAP]:
  - ↑Dose is a good strategy with pregabalin, but evidence with SSRIs/SNRIs is inconsistent.
  - In OCD, consider high doses of SSRIs (even beyond licensed maximums).

- Switch to an alternative Rx.
- Augment SSRI/SNRI with pregabalin or antipsychotic (but depends on disorder).
- Some herbal remedies have evidence for efficacy (Kava/*Piper methysticum*, *Passiflora* extracts, L-lysine and L-arginine), but they are less efficacious than standard Rx and Kava can be hepatotoxic. Overall, they are not recommended.[BAP]
- Clomipramine seems to be the most effective TCA for anxiety disorders, possibly due to its high serotonin reuptake inhibition.

BAP guidance summary

Disorder[BAP]	First line	Second line	Other
PTSD	Some SSRIs (paroxetine, sertraline) Trauma-focused CBT EMDR	Venlafaxine	Augment with olanzapine, risperidone or prazosin
OCD	All SSRIs CBT Exposure therapy Cognitive therapy	Clomipramine	Augment SSRI/clomipramine with risperidone, olanzapine, aripiprazole, quetiapine (or ondansetron) Augment SSRI with ondansetron or topiramate
GAD	Some SSRIs (escitalopram, paroxetine, sertraline) CBT Applied relaxation	SNRI Pregabalin	Agomelatine, quetiapine, imipramine, buspirone, hydroxyzine, trazodone Benzodiazepines in patients who prove resistant to multiple treatment approaches and who remain significantly distressed by impairing anxiety symptoms

(continued)

Disorder[BAP]	First line	Second line	Other
Social anxiety disorder	Some SSRIs (escitalopram, fluoxetine, fluvoxamine, paroxetine, sertraline) CBT with exposure	Venlafaxine, phenelzine, moclobemide, gabapentin, pregabalin, olanzapine Augment SSRI with buspirone Benzodiazepines in patients who prove resistant to multiple treatment approaches and who remain significantly distressed by impairing anxiety symptoms	
Specific phobia	Exposure-based psychological Rx[1]	SSRI (paroxetine, escitalopram)	
Panic disorder	All SSRIs CBT	Some TCAs (clomipramine, imipramine, lofepramine), venlafaxine, reboxetine	Gabapentin, valproate Benzodiazepines in patients who prove resistant to multiple treatment approaches and who remain significantly distressed by impairing anxiety symptoms
Health anxiety	(Mindfulness-based) CBT, stress management[1]		

[1] There is evidence for some forms of psychotherapy for all of the anxiety disorders listed here, but for these disorders it is generally preferred to pharmacotherapy.

NON-PHARMACOLOGICAL MEASURES

Psychological therapy is very important in anxiety disorders. Most evidence-based treatments focus on a broadly cognitive-behavioural model, but it is adapted to individual disorders. For an overview of CBT and other psychotherapy techniques, see p. 319, refer 'Psychological Therapies' in 'Non-pharmacological Treatments' chapter.

In anxiety disorders, CBT-based interventions typically include some of the following elements. These can be adapted and extended in specific disorders.

1 Objectifying thoughts (they are just thoughts, not facts).

2 Gradual exposure to anxiety-provoking situations and response prevention.

3 Divide worries into problems that you can change and those you cannot.

4 For problems that you can change, come up with a plan to deal with them. For those that cannot be changed, do not worry about them, as there is nothing you can do.

5 Relaxation and mindfulness techniques.

In specific phobias, these techniques are used with an emphasis on **graded exposure**, in which the feared stimulus is gradually introduced in a supportive environment. In OCD, a similar technique called **exposure and response prevention (ERP)** is used; in this the person is exposed to the anxiety-provoking situation until they can do it without a compulsion developing.

Routine 'psychological debriefing' after exposure to traumatic events is not helpful in preventing PTSD.[BAP]

Relaxation exercise
Use this acutely to calm down a very anxious patient or teach them to do this on their own.

1 Take slow deep breaths in and out.
2 Tense the muscles in your legs. Hold for 5 sec. Release. Notice the relaxation.
3 Tense the muscles in your arms. Hold for 5 sec. Release.
4 Tense the muscles in your face. Hold for 5 sec. Release.
5 Feel the release of muscle tension all over your body.

STARTING

- Medications for anxiety (particularly antidepressants) can often worsen nervousness and agitation in the first 1–2 wk before they start to have an effect, so warn patients about this and see them more frequently during this period.[BAP] Consider adding short course of benzodiazepine (e.g. diazepam 2 mg tds for 7–10 days).
- Due to heightened anxiety when starting antidepressants, patients with anxiety disorders may benefit from slower titration, but balance this against a delay in reaching a therapeutic dose.

- Pregabalin can be started immediately at a treatment dose of 150 mg daily in two to three divided doses. If required, it can be increased in steps of 150 mg after 7 days up to 600 mg daily total. However, many patients will benefit from more gradual dose titration.
- Gabapentin requires more complex titration. Day 1: 300 mg od. Day 2: 300 mg bd. Day 3: 300 mg tds.

MONITORING

Routine care: clinical efficacy and SEs.

See p. 237, refer 'Monitoring' section in 'Depression' section of 'Disorders' chapter.

SIDE EFFECTS

- Heightened anxiety when starting antidepressants is common:
  1 Provide explanation and reassurance.
  2 Slow down medication titration.
  3 Short course of benzodiazepine (e.g. diazepam 2 mg tds for 7–10 days).
- Gabapentinoids can cause euphoria and dependence. They can be misused or diverted. Those who have a history of substance misuse are at particular risk. To avoid misuse (Public Health England*, 'Advice for prescribers on the risk of the misuse of pregabalin and gabapentin', 2014):
  – If drug is ineffective for target Sx, stop it.
  – If dependence suspected, control access to medication (limited amount prescribed, no replacement prescriptions). Consider planned withdrawal.
- Gabapentinoids can cause respiratory depression, especially in those with RFs (e.g. COPD, concurrent use of opioids).

STOPPING

- For anxiety disorders, there is evidence for benefit of continuing the medication for 6–18 months following remission. Beyond this, evidence is unclear.BAP

---

* https://assets.publishing.service.gov.uk/government/uploads/system/uploads/attachment_
  data/file/385791/PHE-NHS_England_pregabalin_and_gabapentin_advice_Dec_2014.pdf

- ↓Dose over 3 months to ↓ discontinuation or rebound Sx.[BAP]
- Gabapentinoids can safely be tapered down over 1 wk, but more gradual discontinuation is preferred (Public Health England*, 'Advice for prescribers on the risk of the misuse of pregabalin and gabapentin', 2014):
  - Gabapentin: ↓daily dose by up to 300 mg every 4 days.
  - Pregabalin: ↓daily dose by 50–100 mg/wk.

SWAPPING

- In anxiety disorders, response can take longer and may require up to 12 wk (though usually onset of effect is seen within 4 wk).[BAP]
- For more guidance, see p. 239, refer 'Swapping' heading in 'Depression' section of 'Disorders' chapter.

SPECIAL GROUPS
Children

- Diagnosis is difficult, as fear and worry can be part of normal development, but anxiety disorders are also common in CAMHS. Less research, so therapeutic options are less certain.
- Psychological Rx should be first line.[BAP]
- Use medications for non-responders with much caution and careful monitoring.[BAP]
- SSRI therapy can be effective in GAD, social anxiety, separation anxiety, PTSD and OCD. Fluoxetine is a good option.[BAP] Benzodiazepines are not recommended.
- The balance of risks and benefits favours SSRIs for anxiety more than for depression.[BAP]

Elderly

- Use same treatment options as with younger adults, but be aware of renal impairment, co-morbidity, cognitive impairment, risk of falls, hypotension and sedative effects.[BAP]

Pregnancy

- Anxiety disorders sometimes improve.

---

* https://assets.publishing.service.gov.uk/government/uploads/system/uploads/attachment_data/file/385791/PHE-NHS_England_pregabalin_and_gabapentin_advice_Dec_2014.pdf

- If possible, psychological treatments are good options, but medications are sometimes needed.[BAP]
- If medications are used, SSRIs should generally be first line.[BAP]
- Early studies associated benzodiazepines with congenital malformations, but more recent evidence has not replicated this. They should generally be avoided near term due to risk of a neonatal withdrawal syndrome and/or 'floppy infant syndrome'.[UKTIS]
- There is little information of the use of gabapentinoids in pregnancy. Studies are too small to draw definite conclusions. For pregabalin, animal and cohort studies have suggested ↑risk of major malformation. Gabapentin has not so far shown an ↑risk of major malformation.[UKTIS]
- Weigh potential risks and benefits of medications.[BAP]

Breastfeeding
- There is no CI to breastfeeding in women taking gabapentinoids.[BNF]

Renal impairment
- Gabapentinoids are renally excreted with negligible metabolism.
- Therefore, ↓dose in renal impairment.

Hepatic impairment
- Metabolism of gabapentinoids is not expected to be altered.[SPC]

Physical health problems
- **Epilepsy:** Gabapentinoids have anticonvulsant properties (licensed for focal seizures), so may safely be used in epilepsy. However, they should be withdrawn slowly to avoid precipitating seizures.

Further information
Baldwin et al., 'Evidence-based pharmacological treatment of anxiety disorders, post-traumatic stress disorder and obsessive-compulsive disorder: a revision of the 2005 guidelines from the British Association for Psychopharmacology', *J Psychopharmacol* 2014; 28(5): 1–37.

DEMENTIA

Definition: Dementia is a progressive neurodegenerative disorder characterised by cognitive decline and ↓function (i.e. ↓activities of daily living [ADLs]) +/− behavioural/psychological changes. Approximately 60% Alzheimer's disease (AD), 20% vascular dementia (VaD), 15% dementia with Lewy bodies (DLB) and 5% other (e.g. fronto-temporal dementia [FTD]).

There is increasing emphasis on recognising pre-dementia syndromes, e.g. mild cognitive impairment (MCI), to enable prediction of, and ultimately reduce/reverse, disease progression.

Differential diagnosis: Important to consider +/− exclude other causes, especially if treatable (see box).

Other/treatable causes of dementia
Causes I AVOIDED

I	Infection: **Syphillis and HIV** (rarely others[1])
A	Alcohol-related brain damage (including Korsakoff's)
V	Vasculitis: Including sarcoid, systemic lupus erythematous
O	Other autoimmune: Limbic encephalitis/channelopathies, e.g. anti-NMDAR Abs
I	Intracranial: Tumour, NPH[2], subdural, injury (including repetitive minor = 'dementia pugilistica')
D	Deficiencies: **B12** (also B1 and B6) and Excesses: Copper (Wilson's), toxins[3] (e.g. lead)
E	Endocrine: ↓T4 (also ↓/↑ cortisol, ↓/↑ PTH, ↑ Ca²⁺)
D	Depression and other 'functional' (psychogenic) causes, i.e. dissociative or anxiety related

[1] Viruses (especially HSV), Whipple's disease (*Tropheryma whipplei* ⇒ GI/rheum/neuro disease), Lyme disease (*Borrelia* spp) TB and fungi, Creutzfeldt-Jakob disease (CJD)

[2] NPH = normal pressure hydrocephalus (suspect if gait +/− urinary dysfunction)

[3] Also includes drugs (especially anticholinergics) (see box on drugs that can commonly cause/worsen cognitive impairment).

Should be routinely excluded (Ix = HIV/syphilis serology, brain scan, B12, T4) – other causes normally only require investigation if suggestive features from history or neuro +/− psych exam. Rapid (<6 months) or young (<65 yr) onset should alert to previously discussed causes or rarer more rapid degenerative disorders (e.g. prion disease, CADASIL, etc.)

MILD COGNITIVE IMPAIRMENT (MCI)

'Pre-dementia' stage (on cognitive decline 'continuum'); objective cognitive impairment, but help with ADLs not yet needed – see box for details.

MCI definition *(Langa & Levine, JAMA 2014)*
- Concern of cognition changes from patient, knowledgeable informant or skilled clinician observing patient
- Objective evidence of impairment (from cognitive testing) in at least one cognitive domain including memory, executive function, attention, language, or visuospatial skills
- Preservation of independence with ADLs (but may show ↓efficiency/↑errors)
- No significant ↓in social or occupational functioning (i.e. not demented)

There are currently no evidence-based treatments. AChE-i and Vit E do not ↓risk of AD[BAP].

However, the following is recommended:

1 Follow-up (e.g. 6 months)
2 Control/optimise vascular risk factors (stop smoking, control ↑BP/diabetes/dyslipidaemia/AF)
3 ↑Mental/physical activity
4 ↓Heavy alcohol/illicit drug use
5 Optimise vision, hearing and sleep-disordered breathing
6 ↓(Ideally stopping) any medications that can ↓cognition (see box)

Drugs that can commonly cause/worsen cognitive impairment

Anticholinergics (common action of many drug classes):

- Bronchodilators – e.g. atropine, ipratropium (also amino/theophylline)
- Antihistamines/antiemetics – e.g. cyclizine, cinnarizine, prochlorperazine
- Sleeping tablets – e.g. promethazine
- Allergies – e.g. cetirizine, loratadine, chlorphenamine
- Antispasmodics – e.g. hyoscine, procyclidine
- Bladder stabilizers – e.g. oxybutynin
- Tricyclic antidepressants – e.g. amitriptyline, lofepramine, dosulepin, trazadone

Other

- Opioids
- Benzodiazepines
- Antihypertensives – diuretics (e.g. furosemide), α-agonists
- Antiarrhythmic – e.g. digoxin
- Steroids – especially high dose and/or potency
- Chemotherapy – e.g. asparginase, cytosine, chlorambucil, ifosfamide, vinblastine/vincristine

ALZHEIMER'S DISEASE (AD)

Pathology: amyloid plaques and neurofibrillary tangles $\Rightarrow$ neuronal loss and brain atrophy, especially medial temporal lobe (e.g. hippocampus) in early stages. Neocortical cholinergic neuronal loss predominates.

Diagnosis: largely clinical but excluding other causes important (see box on Other/treatable causes of dementia). Medial temporal lobe atrophy is highly suggestive. Biomarkers are of increasing diagnostic utility (especially CSF markers [$\downarrow A\beta_{1-42}/\uparrow$tau] and amyloid [positron emission tomography, PET] imaging) and may allow detection of prodromal/preclinical disease. See box for research diagnostic criteria.

NIA diagnostic guidelines for AD (McKhann et al., Alzheimers Dement. 2011)

Probable AD is diagnosed when the patient meets criteria for dementia and has the following characteristics:

A Insidious onset over months to years.

B Clear history of worsening cognition.

C Initial and most prominent deficits in one of the following:

    a Amnesia, including impairment in learning and recall of recently learned information.

    b Non-amnestic presentations: word-finding, visuospatial function, executive function.

D Do not apply the diagnosis in the presence of substantial cerebrovascular disease, non-dementia core features of dementia with Lewy bodies, prominent features of frontotemporal dementia or evidence for another disease or medications that could substantially affect cognition.

Treatment

Trials generally use the following:

- 1° outcome = MMSE or cognitive scale of AD Assessment Scale (ADAS-cog; total score = 70)
- Staging by MMSE: normal = 27–30, mild = 21–26, moderate = 10–20, severe = 0–9 (NICE 2011)
- NB: MMSE is screening tool and not diagnostic.

1 **Cognitive treatments**

    Currently two classes (see Table 2.1 for key comparisons):

    — **Cholinesterase inhibitors (AChE-i):** donepezil, rivastigmine and galantamine

      - All recommended for mild-mod AD (MMSE > 10)[NICE/BAP] although cognitive improvement over placebo small as are improvements in ADLs.
      - Switch to another drug if first not tolerated/effective.[BAP]
      - Benefits may persist in severe AD (e.g. Howard et al, *NEJM* 2012).

Table 2.1 Doses, side effects (SEs) and cautions of cognitive treatments

	Donepezil	Rivastigmine	Galantamine	Memantine
Dose range	5–10 mg od	1.5–6 mg bd (or 4.6–9.5 mg/24 h patch[1])	4–12 mg bd (or 8–24 mg XL od)	5–20 mg od
Side effects	Commonly nausea, diarrhoea, vomiting, headache; also sleep disturbance, dizziness, ↓HR			Somnolence, dizziness
Cautions	Stop if: GI ulceration or ↓HR (e.g. heart block or other drugs that ↓HR)			Hepatic impairment, seizures/epilepsy

[1] Can ↑dose to 13.3 mg/24 h after 6 months in patient who have a meaningful cognitive deterioration and/or fn decline while on 9.5 mg/24 h.

- **NMDA receptor antagonists:** memantine
  - Recommended for moderate-severe AD (MMSE <21) *if cannot take/tolerate AChE-i*[NICE/BAP]; benefits on cognition, ADLs and behaviour.

NB: Benefits of giving both AChE-i and memantine unclear,[BAP] but recent meta-analysis suggests improved cognition, behavioural disturbance, ADLs and global function for moderate-severe AD (Matsunaga et al, *Int J Neuropsychopharmacol* 2014; EFNS Guidelines, 2015). Consider adding memantine in moderate-severe disease.[NICE] All three licensed AChE-i have similar efficacy. Interrupting treatment course of AChE-i may ⇒ rapidly ↓and unrecoverable efficacy. Failure to respond and/or intolerance to one agent does not preclude a response/tolerability with another. Tolerability may be affected by dose or speed of titration.

2 **Other pharmacological treatment**

Optimise vascular risk factors and other factors. The following all currently lack evidence to justify use[BAP]: Latrepirdine (antihistamine), Ginkgo biloba, hormone replacement therapy (HRT), statins, folate + vitamin B12, vitamin E, multivitamins, omega-3 fatty acids, huperzine A,

> **NICE Guidance on AChE-i**
> - Donepezil, galantamine and rivastigmine for mild to moderate AD.
> - Memantine for moderate AD if intolerant of AChE-i, or severe AD.
> - Consider memantine in addition to an AChE inhibitor if they have moderate disease.
> - Offer memantine in addition to an AChE inhibitor if they have severe disease.
> - Treatment must only be initiated following specialist advice.
> - Carer's view should be sought.
> - Do not stop AChE inhibitors in people with Alzheimer's disease because of disease severity alone.
> - Patients require regular review by a specialist team.
> - Start with medication at lowest acquisition cost but take into account tolerance, adherence and the possibility of interactions and dosing profiles.
>
> Clinicians should not rely solely on cognition scores in situations where any physical, sensory or learning disability or communication difficulty could influence the clinical picture. However, an alternative AChE inhibitor could be prescribed if it is considered appropriate when taking into account adverse event profile, expectations about adherence, medical co-morbidity, possibility of drug interactions and dosing profile.

saffron and cerebrolysin. *NB: Some have significant side effects, and this should be factored into decisions to prescribe/ recommend.*

3 **Non-pharmacological treatment**

Group cognitive stimulation and activities to promote well-being tailored to person's preferences are recommended.[NICE]

4 **Treatments in development**

There is a concerted effort to target disease progression. No drugs are currently licenced, but the following are the most promising agents.

Anti-amyloid

Immunotherapy: Active immunisation (Aβ 1-42 vaccination) research suspended as can ⇒ meningoencephalitis. Passive immunization (e.g. monoclonal Ab against amyloid, e.g. *bapineuzumab* and *solanezumab*) under investigation but trials in established dementia have not been positive; potential for disease modification if given early (at pre-clinical dementia stage) is currently under investigation.

* *Secretase inhibitors (e.g. semagacestat):* targets buildup of Aβ fragments. Currently no evidence of efficacy.

Anti-tau

* *Tau kinase inhibitors:* (↓tau hyperphosphorylation), tau aggregation inhibitors, microtubule stabilisation; under investigation, no current clear evidence of efficacy.

Neuroprotective/restorative

* Anti-inflammatory agents: e.g. NSAIDs, anti-oxidants and nerve growth factor; under investigation, no current clear evidence of efficacy.

VASCULAR DEMENTIA (VaD)

Pathology: Cerebrovascular disease, ranging from large infarcts and haemorrhages to deep white matter changes associated with ischaemia resulting in a similar clinical picture to AD.

Diagnosis: See box on 'NINDS-AIREN' diagnostic criteria for VaD. *NB: VaD unlikely w/o focal neurological signs (e.g. gait disturbance) or cerebrovascular lesions on neuroimaging, and if early and progressive memory loss is the most prominent feature.*

Treatment:

* There are no licenced treatments for VaD in the United Kingdom.
* Managing underlying cardiovascular risk factors is primary intervention (especially BP, lipid profile, diabetes, smoking, diet, exercise, etc.).

> **'NINDS-AIREN' diagnostic criteria for VaD** (Román et al., 1993
> Neurology 43[2]:250–60)
>
> 1 Dementia: Impairment in memory and two other cognitive
>   domains
> 2 Evidence of cerebrovascular disease: On examination or
>   brain imaging
> 3 A relationship between the two aforementioned
>   conditions, or a relationship inferred by:
>   a   Symptoms within 3 months of a stroke
>   b   Abrupt ↓ in cognition
>   c   Fluctuating stepwise cognitive deterioration
> 4 Clinical features of VaD: Gait disturbance, falls, urinary
>   incontinence, pseudobulbar palsy, personality/mood
>   changes

- AChE-i and memantine not recommended, as although can improve cognition, global improvements not seen and adverse events common.[BAP]
- Clinically distinguishing VaD from AD can be challenging as the disorders can coexist, and it can be hard to distinguish age-related vascular MRI changes from VaD diagnosis. *Those with mixed VaD and AD may benefit from AChE-i or memantine.*[BAP]

DEMENTIA WITH LEWY BODIES (DLB)

Pathology: Lewy bodies ⇒ ↓dopaminergic and cholinergic neurons ⇒ variable levels (and relative temporal onset) of cognitive, movement and neuropsychiatric disorders.

Diagnosis: See box for consensus diagnostic criteria. Dementia occurs before, or concurrently, with parkinsonism; if Parkinson's disease diagnosis ≥1 yr before dementia then called Parkinson's disease dementia (PDD).

Consensus criteria for probable and possible DLB (McKeith et al., Neurology 2005; 65(12): 1863–72)

Central feature – essential for any (possible or probable) diagnosis

- *Progressive cognitive decline* affecting social or occupational function.

NB: ↓Memory may not occur in early stages but usually evident with progression.

↓Attention, executive function and visuo-spatial ability may be especially prominent.

Core features
- *Fluctuating cognition* – pronounced variations in attention and alertness
- *Recurrent visual hallucinations* – typically well formed and detailed
- *Parkinsonism* – triad of tremor, rigidity and bradykinesia

Suggestive features
- REM sleep behaviour disorder
- Severe neuroleptic sensitivity
- ↓DA transporter uptake in basal ganglia on single-photon emission computed tomography (SPECT) or PET imaging

Supportive features (commonly present, but unproven diagnostic specificity)

- Repeated falls and syncope
- Transient, unexplained loss of consciousness
- Severe autonomic dysfunction e.g. orthostatic hypotension, urinary incontinence
- Hallucinations in other modalities
- Systematised delusions
- Depression
- Relative preservation of medial temporal lobe structures on structural imaging
- Generalized ↓ uptake on SPECT/PET perfusion scan with ↓occipital activity

- Abnormal (↓ uptake) MIBG myocardial scintigraphy
- Prominent slow wave activity on electroencephalogram with temporal lobe sharp waves

Diagnosis of DLB less likely if:

- Cerebrovascular disease evident from focal neurological signs or brain imaging
- Other physical illness present/brain disorder could account in part for symptoms
- Parkinsonism only appears for first time at stage of severe dementia

Probable diagnosis = Central + 2 Core (or 1 Core + 1 Suggestive)
Possible diagnosis = Central + 1 Core (or 1 Suggestive)

Treatment:
- AChE-i: Can ↓cognitive and neuropsychiatric symptoms[BAP] and all agents equally effective.[BAP] There is high-quality evidence for rivastigmine and donepezil in Lewy body dementias.
- Memantine: Can ↓cognitive symptoms and ⇒ global improvements.[BAP]
- Should be patient focused, depend on symptom severity and patient/carer wishes.[BAP]
- Start/↑ drugs cautiously: Treating one symptom can worsen others (e.g. antipsychotics can ↑parkinsonism, and antiparkinsonian drugs can ↑psychosis).

FRONTOTEMPORAL DEMENTIA (FTD)

Heterogeneous group of syndromes associated with degeneration/atrophy of prefrontal and anterior temporal lobes ⇒ behaviour changes and ↓executive function.
   Pathology: Tau or TDP-43 protein (present in >90% of cases).
   Diagnosis: Two main variants:

1 Frontal (fvFTD): Behavioural
2 Temporal (tvFTD): Language impairment

Includes Pick's disease, primary progressive aphasia and semantic dementia. Corticobasal degeneration (CBD) and progressive supranuclear palsy (PSP) are related 'tau-opathies' (aka 'Pick complex').

Treatment: No specific agents licensed. Treatment is symptomatic and prognosis poor.

* AChE-i and memantine not recommended[BAP] and may cause agitation.
* SSRIs have mixed evidence of improved behavioural (but not cognitive) symptoms.[BAP]
* Disease-modifying therapies (targetting Tau pathology) currently under investigation.

BEHAVIOURAL AND PSYCHOLOGICAL SYMPTOMS OF DEMENTIA (BPSDs)

BPSD = non-cognitive neuropsychiatric symptoms in dementia (see box). Approximately 75% of dementia cases have ≥1 BPSD symptom; number/severity of symptoms variable.

Spectrum of BPSD symptoms

Common

* Aggression
* Agitation or restlessness
* Anxiety
* Depression
* Sleep disturbance
* Apathy

Other

* Psychosis: Delusions, hallucinations
* Repetitive vocalisation, cursing and swearing
* Shadowing (following others, e.g. carer, closely)
* Sundowning (behaviour worsens after 5 p.m.)
* Wandering
* Non-specific behaviour disturbance, e.g. hoarding

Ensure other causes considered/treated (e.g. delirium, pain). Patients (and carers/families) should be involved in decision-making.

Treatment is divided into pharmacological and non-pharmacological therapies; non-pharmacological approaches should generally be considered first.

Non-pharmacological therapies

Behavioural analysis/intervention: 'ABC' (Antecedent-Behaviour-Consequence) charts to identify modifiable environmental, social or autobiographical factors.

Psychoeducation: For patients, carers and families (↓s anxiety/↑s empathetic care). Mild-moderate depression and/or anxiety in mild-moderate dementia may benefit from psychological therapy.[NICE]

Environment: Music and ↑calm/comfort/familiarity (= 'Snoezelen') Personalised activities to promote engagement, pleasure and interest (↓s distress/agitation/aggression)[NICE] (Livingston Lancet 2017).

Complementary therapies: e.g. aromatherapy

Pharmacological therapies

NB: start at low dose, ↑ slowly and review regularly with low threshold to ↓/stop

Antipsychotics: *NB: significant risks; ↑ all-cause mortality and cerebrovascular events.* FGAs can ↑ arrhythmias, and SGAs can ↑ VTE and ⇒ aspiration pneumonia. Can ↓ aggression and psychosis. Currently only risperidone licensed; should be used cautiously in all dementias, especially in DLB (only under specialist supervision) when severe sensitivity reactions can occur; use in short courses (<6 weeks) for persistent aggression or psychosis causing severe distress in moderate-severe AD when non-pharmacological approaches exhausted, or if risk of harm to self or others. Can also ⇒ xs sedation, confusion, EPSEs and may accelerate cognitive decline. Antipsychotics should only be offered if patient is at risk of harming themselves/others, or they experience agitation/psychotic Sx that are causing them severe distress.

Cognitive treatments

- AChE-i recommended for non-cognitive, distressing or challenging symptoms when non-pharmacological approaches exhausted or antipsychotics inappropriate/ineffective.[NICE]
- Memantine may be useful in AD (and possibly also VaD) but evidence for efficacy limited.

Benzodiazepines

NB: *avoid if possible or use with great caution as can ⇒ cognitive decline, falls & hip fractures in elderly.* Can ↓ anxiety.

Antidepressants

Can counteract negative fx of depression on cognition, but overall limited evidence of efficacy and only recommended if treating pre-existing depression.[NICE] Sedating drugs (e.g. trazodone) may also ⇒ ↓irritability/agitation, and SSRIs may ↓agitation. TCAs should be avoided as ↑risk of falls/confusion due to anticholinergic fx – other drugs causing anticholinergic fx should also be avoided (or ↓dose) where appropriate.

Mood stabilisers

Currently insufficient evidence to support use, but may be justified if other treatments ineffective/not tolerated. Valproate is best avoided.

SUMMARY

Table 2.2 summarises the pharmacological management of each form of dementia.

Table 2.2 Antidementia drugs – summary of recommendations for cognitive treatments

Disorder		AChE-i	Memantine
MCI		–	–
AD	Mild	✔	–
	Moderate	✔	✔
	Severe	–	✔
VaD		–	–
FTD		–	–
LBD/PDD		✔	✔

Key: ✔ = recommended, – = not recommended, AD = Alzheimer's disease, FTD = fronto-temporal dementia, LBD = Lewy body dementia, MCI = mild cognitive impairment, PDD = Parkinson's disease dementia, VaD = vascular dementia.

Notes: MMSE staging: mild = 21–26, moderate = 10–20, severe = 0–9.

Further information

O'Brien et al., 'Clinical practice with anti-dementia drugs: a revised (third) consensus statement from the British Association for Psychopharmacology', *J Psychopharmacol* 2017; **31**(2): 1–22.

ATTENTION DEFICIT HYPERACTIVITY DISORDER (ADHD)

DIAGNOSIS

ADHD is a **neurodevelopmental** disorder and starts in childhood, although in 20%–40% it persists to adulthood and is sometimes not diagnosed until this point, particularly when co-morbid with mood, anxiety and substance misuse disorders. It may also be missed in the older adult population. It has three core features: **hyperactivity, impulsivity** and **inattentiveness**. These must be persistent and impairing with difficulties demonstrated across at least **two settings** (e.g. school, home, work), so history should be obtained from multiple sources.

ADHD may be classified as predominantly inattentive, predominantly hyperactive-impulsive or combined (meeting criteria for both).

It is associated with several organic developmental syndromes: Turner's syndrome, fragile X syndrome, Williams' syndrome, PKU and foetal alcohol syndrome. There is a wide differential diagnosis, but special Ix are not indicated unless there is a particular suspicion of another disorder. There is a high co-morbidity with anxiety disorders, substance misuse and autism.

Differential diagnosis[1]:

Psychiatric	Organic
• **Anxiety** (hyperactivity is driven by psychomotor agitation, exaggerated startle response, anxious cognitions)	• **Learning disability** (Ix: neuropsychological testing shows impaired IQ rather than inattention)
• **Substance misuse** (must assess in absence of recreational drugs; Ix: urine drug screen)	• **Lead toxicity** (old furnishings or upbringing in developing world, peripheral motor neuropathy, bradycardia; Ix: serum lead)
• **Depression** (low mood driving poor engagement)	• **Iron deficiency anaemia** (irritability + classic signs of pallor, koilonychia, angular stomatitis; Ix: FBC, iron studies)
• **EUPD** (impulsivity, chronic emptiness, emotional instability, self-destructive behaviour)	• **Hyperthyroidism** (↑HR, tremor, proptosis, diarrhoea; Ix: TFTs)
• **Conduct disorder** (persistent rule breaking involving aggression, property damage, lying or theft)	• **Sensory impairment** (auditory or visual; Ix: hearing and eye tests)
• **Oppositional defiant disorder** (similar to conduct disorder but milder)	• **Absence seizures** (distinct episodes of staring lasting 10–20 sec, sometimes accompanied by eyelid flickering)
• **BPAD** (distinct episodes of qualitatively different manic behaviour)	• **Medications** (especially β-agonists, antihistamines, antiepileptics)
• **Autism** (FHx, stereotyped behaviours/interests, impaired social skills, rigid routines)	• **Frontal lobe injury** (traumatic brain injury, SOL or degenerative disease resulting in disinhibition, poor executive function and primitive reflexes; Ix: Frontal Assessment Battery)

[1] These may also be comorbid with ADHD.

TYPES OF MEDICATIONS

	Drug	Mechanism	$t_{1/2}$ (h)	SEs	
Stimulants	Methylphenidate	DARI, NARI	IR: 2.5 MR: 3.5	Abuse potential, insomnia	↑HR, ↑BP, N&V, abdominal pain, ↓appetite, ↓wt, ↓growth
	Dexamfetamine	DARI, NARI	11		
	Lisdexamfetamine	DARI, NARI	1+11[1]		
Other	Modafinil (specialist only)	DARI (weak)	14	Insomnia	
	Atomoxetine	NARI [2]	5	Somnolence, suicidal ideation	
	Bupropion (specialist only)	NDRI	14	Insomnia, GI Sx, agitation, anxiety, tremor	
	Guanfacine MR	α_2 agonist	17	↓HR, ↓BP, somnolence, nausea, ↑wt	
	Clonidine	α_2 agonist	4		

[1] 1 hr as an inactive form before being converted to dexamfetamine.

[2] Causes ↑DA in prefrontal cortex.

METHYLPHENIDATE FORMULATIONS

Methylphenidate may be prescribed in XL forms, which contain varying ratios of IR and MR drug:

	IR (%)	MR (%)
Concerta XL	22	78
Equasym XL	30	70
Medikinet XL	50	50

Not all the methylphenidate in Concerta XL is bioavailable; hence, 18 mg Concerta XL ≡ 15 mg methylphenidate. The IR portion gives a rapid effect, while the MR continues this over a longer period of time. If switching from an IR form, be aware that an 'equivalent' dose might result in less effectiveness in the morning; e.g. switching from methylphenidate IR 5 mg tds to Concerta XL

18 mg OM (which contains only 4 mg methylphenidate IR) would effectively underdose a patient by 20% in the morning.

CHOOSING A MEDICATION

- Consider the preferences of patient (+/− carers) when considering which interventions to provide.[BAP]
- Consider factors such as schools (which may not keep medication for daytime use).
- These medicines may affect driving, and stimulants are controlled substances for which there are severe penalties for impaired driving.
- Effect sizes in adults are smaller than those in children.
- In adults and children, environmental modifications should be implemented and reviewed before medications are considered.[NICE]
  - If there is little improvement, consider medications.[BAP]
- For adults, lisdexamfetamine or methylphenidate may be given as first-line medications.[NICE] Lisdexamfetamine is licensed in adults; not all other products are licensed in adults.
- **MR** methylphenidate is less liable to be abused than **IR**, is easier to take and may be more appropriate for schoolchildren (as medication is not taken at schooltime), so is preferred.[BAP]
- **Lisdexamfetamine** is a pro-drug, which is metabolised to the active dexamfetamine, but it may be less liable to abuse than dexamfetamine.[BAP]
- **Guanfacine** may safely be given in combination with stimulants and atomoxetine.
- Stimulants and atomoxetine are cautioned in the presence of established or suspected cardiac disease.[BAP]

Drug	Time to efficacy	Abuse potential	Other notes	Drug interactions
Methylphenidate IR	Immediate	High		MAOIs – may cause hypertensive crisis (avoid concomitant use and for 14 days after stopping MAOI)
Methylphenidate MR	Immediate	Medium	Some products licensed in adults	Fluoxetine/paroxetine/CYP2D6 inhibitors – may increase levels of dexamfetamine and lisdexamfetamine
			Can be abruptly stopped if necessary	
Lisdexamfetamine	Immediate	?Low	Licensed in adults	Serotonin syndrome (theoretical) – caution with serotonergics
Dexamfetamine	Immediate	High	Avoid abrupt withdrawal	Antipsychotics antagonise stimulants
Atomoxetine	2 weeks at an effective dose	None	Second line	Avoid MAOIs, as per stimulants
			Probably less effective than stimulants	Fluoxetine/paroxetine increase atomoxetine levels – slower titration
				Strong caution with noradrenergic agents (venlafaxine, mirtazapine, imipramine)
				May prolong QT interval
Guanfacine	Requires often prolonged titration; rapid at an effective dose	None	Third line	CYP3A4/5:
			Can be given with stimulants	Inducers (phenytoin, CBZ, modafinil, rifampicin, St John's wort) may reduce efficacy
			Requires retitration if two or more doses missed	Inhibitors (clarithromycin, ciprofloxacin) may increase exposure and reduce tolerability

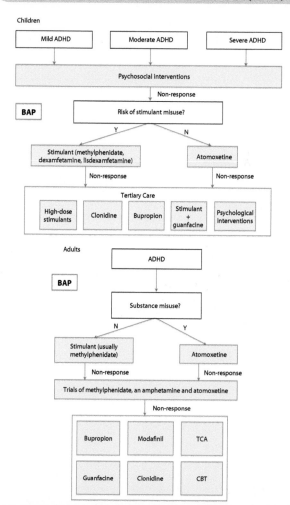

TREATMENT RESISTANCE
- Review diagnosis, patient motivation, co-morbidities and compliance.
- Combinations of medications are commonly used, but there is no robust evidence for this strategy and there are limited data on adverse events, which are probably more common.[BAP]
- Stimulants and α_2 agonists have complementary SEs making them an attractive choice, but the combination has not yet established sufficient evidence.[BAP]

NON-PHARMACOLOGICAL MEASURES
- Substance misuse common in ADHD and may complicate assessing efficacy of therapy. Liaise with drug and alcohol services.[BAP]
- All patients should be encouraged to implement personalised environmental modifications, e.g. alterations to seating arrangements, ↓noise, ↓distractions, headphones, frequent breaks and providing written instructions.[NICE]
- For children, provide parents and teachers with evidence-based information about ADHD.[BAP] Parental training: can be helpful in improving parenting and reducing oppositional behaviour,[BAP] but they do not help with ADHD Sx.
- Educational interventions: teach child problem-solving or self-control strategies; assist teachers in adapting environment or teaching styles.
- Dietary interventions have shown some early promise, but the studies have numerous limitations.[BAP] Do not advise dietary elimination as part of standard care, but if there seems to be a link, recommend keeping diary tracking diet and Sx; if the diary shows a relationship, refer to a dietician.[NICE]
- CBT in adults can be helpful by encouraging memory aids, time scheduling and 'stop and think' techniques.[BAP]

STARTING

* Assess abuse or diversion potential for stimulants, including from relatives and carers.[BAP] Use of psychostimulants is becoming increasingly popular for 'cognitive enhancement' in schools and universities.
* Conduct a structured dose titration, increasing doses according to effectiveness and tolerability.[BAP]
* ↑Dose until optimal control of Sx. If SEs limit titration, consider switch.[BAP]
* Methylphenidate and dexamfetamine: titrate to optimal dose over 4–6 wk.[BAP]
* Atomoxetine, guanfacine and lisdexamfetamine: ↑dose weekly.[BAP]
* Atomoxetine is metabolised by CYP2D6. In slow metabolisers, SEs are more pronounced, so slower titration is required. Suspect if intolerant to other drugs metabolised by CYP2D6 (see p. 341, refer 'Drug Interactions' in 'Basic Psychopharmacology' chapter).[BAP]

SIDE EFFECTS

SE	Notes	Rx
HTN (stimulants, atomoxetine)	↑BP by average of 1–4 mm Hg, but in a few can be up to 10 mm Hg	• ↓Dose • Drug holiday
↑HR (stimulants, atomoxetine)	Average just 1–2 bpm	• Monitor
Postural hypotension (clonidine, guanfacine)	Definition: ↓sys BP of 20 mm Hg or ↓dias BP of 10 mm Hg	• Standing up slowly • ↑Fluid and salt intake • Be careful with hot drinks and baths

(continued)

SE	Notes	Rx
↓Growth rate and weight loss (stimulants)	Cause small reduction Monitor weight: <ul><li>Every 3 months for children 10 yr or younger</li><li>At 3, 6 months then 6 monthly for 11+</li><li>Every 6 months for adults</li></ul> Monitor height every 6 months for all CAMHS	<ul><li>Take first dose after breakfast</li><li>High-energy nutritious snacks</li><li>Drug holidays</li><li>Refer to paed endocrinology if extrapolating from growth charts gives a final ht below predicted</li><li>Consider switch if refractory to above management</li></ul>
Insomnia (stimulants)	Also common in unmedicated ADHD	<ul><li>Sleep hygiene</li><li>Switch from stimulant to atomoxetine</li><li>Melatonin (see p. 283, refer 'Types of Medications' heading in 'Sleep Disorders and Agitation' section of 'Disorders' chapter</li></ul>
Abuse or drug diversion (stimulants)	To experience euphoria, must be snorted or injected; prescription stimulants do not seem to result in higher rates of subsequent substance misuse	<ul><li>Monitor at times of high risk, e.g. starting university[BAP]</li><li>Switch to atomoxetine</li><li>Involve substance misuse services</li></ul>
Suicidal thoughts (atomoxetine)	Rare	<ul><li>Monitor carefully</li><li>Consider switch</li></ul>
Tics (stimulants)	Rare (evidence is mixed about role of stimulants in producing tics)	<ul><li>Consider if drug induced</li><li>Assess if benefit of treatment outweighs impairment caused by tics</li></ul>

Source: Graham et al., *Eur Child Adolesc Psychiatry* 2011; **20**(1): 17–37.[NICE]

Use the following formula to calculate predicted height:
Predicted Height

$$\text{♂ predicted ht (cm)} = \frac{ht_{father} + ht_{mother} + 13}{2}$$

$$\text{♀ predicted ht (cm)} = \frac{ht_{father} + ht_{mother} - 13}{2}$$

MONITORING

- This is crucially important to outcomes and requires the use of structured tools, e.g. those used in the Dundee ADHD Clinical Care Pathway (Coghill & Seth, *Child Adolesc Psychiatry Ment Health* 2015; **9**(52): 1–14). Ascertaining progress merely with vague questions is not sufficient.
- Baseline assessment: ht, wt, pulse, BP, auscultation of heart and lungs, ECG (if cardiac disease, FHx of cardiac disease or abnormal cardiac exam), suicide/self-harm risk, stimulant abuse risk.[BAP]
- For atomoxetine, establish if there is any pre-existing liver disease, but in its absence, LFTs are not necessary.[BAP]
- Review efficacy at least annually[BAP] – use structured tools as previously noted.

STOPPING

- Continue medications as long as they are considered clinically useful, reviewing at least annually. Use the effects of any missed doses or drug holidays to aid this review.[BAP]
- Assess when transitioning from child to adult services to check whether medication still required.[BAP]
- Clonidine and guanfacine should be gradually tapered down to avoid rebound HTN. Atomoxetine may be stopped abruptly. The situation is less clear with stimulants, but drug holidays are possible with effective abrupt temporary discontinuation (Shier et al., *J Cent Nerv Syst Dis* 2013; **5**: 1–17).

Drug holidays
- Purposes: (1) assess whether meds still required, (2) allow SE alleviation and catch-up growth (e.g. in school holidays) or (3) to accommodate a patient's preference to feel normal off meds.
- Duration varies between 2 days at the weekends to several months over a holiday.
- Less used in adults, as demands on concentration more constant.
- Limited evidence, but it tends to be favourable.
  (Graham et al., *Eur Child Adolesc Psychiatry* 2011; **20**(1): 17–37)

SWAPPING

- After structured titration with dose increases as indicated by effectiveness and tolerability, a medication trial at an adequate dose should be 6 wk.[NICE]
- There is no guidance on swapping, and cross-tapering is not appropriate. Start next treatment when the previous has been stopped.

PRESCRIBING IN SPECIAL GROUPS
Children

- First-line Rx: Information and support, including advice on parenting and liaison with school.[NICE]
- Children <5 yr: Do not prescribe medications without specialist (ideally tertiary) input.[NICE]
- Children ≥5 yr: Offer medications if Sx are causing significant impairment in >1 domain after environmental modifications.[NICE]
- MR methylphenidate is preferred in practice, as it is easy to take and is thought to be the better-tolerated stimulant.
- Whenever meds are used, it should be part of a package that includes behavioural, psychological and educational interventions.[BAP]
- For children who have benefited from medications but have impairment in >1 domain, consider course of CBT.[NICE]

Elderly

(Torgerson et al., *Neuropsychiatr Dis Treat* 2016; 8(12): 79–87)

- ADHD less common with age, but Rx may still be helpful.
- Prior to prescribing meds, need thorough physical assessment to exclude co-morbidities.
- Titrate slowly.
- Be aware there is no safety data for older adults.

Pregnancy

- Adolescents and young women with ADHD may engage in more risky sexual behaviour, so are at risk of unplanned pregnancies.
- No evidence that ADHD gets better or worse during pregnancy.
- Medications used in ADHD have been associated with some harm in animals, but there is no robust evidence in humans, though numbers of infants exposed are very small.[BAP]
- Methylphenidate does not appear to be linked to congenital malformations, although it is possible that it is associated with ↑risk of miscarriage (although this may be due to confounders).[BAP]
- If stimulants taken near to birth, neonatal withdrawal is likely.[BAP]
- Low birth weight has been reported with dexamfetamine; therefore, this is also likely with lisdexamfetamine.
- Benefits of continuing medications (↓maternal impulsive behaviour) should be weighed against risks to foetus.[BAP]

Breastfeeding

- Methylphenidate is likely to be safe, but is best taken after the morning feed.[BAP]
- Atomoxetine and amphetamines are cautioned.[BAP]
- Modafinil and bupropion should be avoided.[BAP]

Physical health problems

- **Cardiac disease:** Methylphenidate and atomoxetine are cautioned but may be used if slowly titrated and carefully monitored.[BAP]

— Any concerns on baseline monitoring, or premature cardiac mortality in first-degree relatives, should warrant a cardiology opinion.

- **Epilepsy:** ADHD more common. Stimulants and atomoxetine are cautioned but can be used with careful monitoring. Avoid bupropion (Graham et al., *Eur Child Adolesc Psychiatry* 2011; **20**(1): 17–37).

Further information

Bolea-Alamañac et al., 'Evidence-based guidelines for the pharmacological management of attention deficit hyperactivity disorder: update on recommendations from the British Association for Psychopharmacology', *J Psychopharmacol* 2014; **28**(3): 1–25.

SLEEP DISORDERS AND AGITATION

DIAGNOSIS

Insomnia is impaired sleep (in terms of onset, maintenance or waking) despite adequate opportunity (consider shift work, newborn babies, excessive light, lack of a comfortable bed, etc) resulting in an impairment of daytime functioning. It increases the risk of HTN, depression, anxiety and road traffic accidents. **Sleep latency** refers to the time between going to bed and sleep commencing.

In **circadian rhythm disorder** the individual's sleep-wake cycle is out of sync with what is required of them. This often occurs in shift work, but other forms are **jet lag disorder** (worse when traveling eastwards), **delayed sleep-phase syndrome** (onset of sleep and waking are consistently later than normal) and **non-24-h sleep-wake rhythm disorder** (sleep and waking times become progressively later).

Parasomnias cover a wide range of sleep disturbances and can occur in REM (nightmare disorder, REM sleep behaviour disorder) or non-REM (sleep terrors, sleepwalking) sleep. **Night terrors** (pavor nocturnus) are distinguished from nightmares by autonomic arousal and a lack of recollection. **Somnambulism** (sleepwalking) can involve familiar activities such as washing or making tea; it can be precipitated by drugs such as alcohol, hypnotics and lithium. **REM behaviour disorder** (RBD) is characterised by vivid dreams and failure of the normal skeletal muscle paralysis during REM sleep, resulting in acting out of dreams; it is associated with Lewy body disorders. **Restless legs syndrome** (RLS) is characterised by an irresistible urge to move one's legs, usually while trying to sleep; it is associated with renal impairment, iron deficiency anaemia, pregnancy and many psychotropic drugs (e.g. SSRIs, SNRIs, TCAs, mirtazapine and antipsychotics).

  Agitation is not a diagnosis in itself and is seen in psychiatric disorders such as psychosis, mania, EUPD and ASPD. Agitated individuals may pose a risk to themselves and others.

Causes of insomnia:

Psychiatric	Organic
~½ have underlying psychiatric disorder	• **Pain** (especially MSK)
• **Acute stress** (occupational, relational)	• **Restless legs syndrome**
• **Depression** (early morning wakening)[1]	• **Orthopnoea** (↑pillows to sleep due to breathlessness lying flat)
• **Anxiety**	• **Paroxysmal nocturnal dyspnoea** (waking up breathless in the middle of the night)
• **Stimulant use** (caffeine, cocaine, amphetamines)	• **Parkinson's disease** (tremor, rigidity, bradykinesia)
• **Sedative withdrawal** (benzodiazepines, Z-drugs, alcohol)	• **Hyperthyroidism** (↑HR, tremor, proptosis, diarrhoea; Ix: TFTs)
	• **Prescribed medications** (β-agonists, methylphenidate, arousing SSRIs)

---

[1] Insomnia is a risk factor for depression, not simply a symptom of it.

Screening for other sleep disorders[BAP]:

Disorder	Qs
Obstructive sleep apnoea (OSA)	• Are you a very heavy snorer? • Do you ever wake up choking? • Does your partner say that you sometimes stop breathing at night? • Do you feel very sleepy during the day? • Do you wake up with a headache?
Restless legs syndrome (RLS)	• Do you have a sense of discomfort in your legs, or elsewhere in your body, that is worse at night, worse at rest and temporarily relieved by movement?
Periodic limb movements in sleep (PMLS)	• Do your legs twitch and can't stay still in bed? • Do you wake from sleep with jerky leg movements?
Narcolepsy	• Do you feel very sleepy during the day and find yourself falling asleep in inappropriate situations? • Do you have collapses or extreme muscle weakness triggered by emotion, for instance when you're laughing? (cataplexy)
Circadian rhythm sleep disorder	• Do you tend to sleep well but just at the 'wrong times' and are these times regular?
Parasomnias	• Do you have unusual behaviours associated with your sleep that trouble you or are dangerous? • Do you have unpleasant experiences before, during or after sleep, such as nightmares, paralysis or feeling, seeing and hearing things that aren't there? (Nightmare disorder is the sleep disorder most consistently associated with suicide.)

Source: Adapted from Wilson et al., *J Psychopharmacology* 2010; **24**(11):1577–1600.

Investigations for sleep disorders may include a collateral history (e.g. from a bed partner), a sleep diary or polysomnography. The **Epworth Sleepiness Scale** is a useful way of screening for excessive daytime sleepiness: 0–5 is low-normal, 6–10 is high-normal, 11–12 is mild, 13–15 is moderate and 16–24 is severe.

TYPES OF MEDICATIONS

Class	Drug	Action	Equivalent po dose[1]	$T_{\frac{1}{2}}$ (h)[1]
Benzodiazepines	Alprazolam[2]	GABA-A PAM	0.5 mg	6–12
	Chlordiazepoxide		25 mg	5–30
	Clonazepam		1 mg	18–50
	Diazepam		10 mg	20–100
	Flurazepam		15–30 mg	40–250[3]
	Loprazolam		1–2 mg	6–12
	Lorazepam		1 mg	10–20
	Lormetazepam		1–2 mg	10–12
	Nitrazepam		10 mg	15–38
	Oxazepam		30 mg	4–15
	Temazepam		20 mg	8–22
Z-drugs	Zaleplon	GABA-A PAM with α_1 subtype		2[4]
	Zolpidem	specificity		2
	Zopiclone			5–6
Antihistamines	Diphenhydramine	H_1 ant		2–9
	Hydroxyzine			14–20
	Promethazine			5–14
Antidepressants	Amitriptyline	NRI>SRI		16–40
	Doxepin	SRI+NRI		8–24
	Mirtazapine	$5\text{-}HT_2 + 5\text{-}HT_3 + \alpha_2$ ant		20–40
	Paroxetine	SRI		~24
	Trazodone	$5\text{-}HT_2 + \alpha_1$ ant > SRI		5–13
	Trimipramine	SRI+NRI		23
Antipsychotics	Olanzapine	$D_2 + 5\text{-}HT_2$ ant		30–50
	Quetiapine	$D_2 + 5\text{-}HT_2$ ant		7
Other	Melatonin	$MT_1 + MT_2$ ag		4[5]

[1] Derived from authorative sources, inc.[MPG] and Ashton, 'Benzodiazepines: how they work and how to withdraw' (aka 'The Ashton Manual) 2002. Available from https://benzo.org.uk/manual.

[2] Cannot be prescribed on the NHS but is sometimes prescribed privately and used recreationally.

[3] Active metabolite.

[4] Half-life from Tmax is one hour. Tmax occurs 1hr after ingestion

[5] MR formulation (Circadin) has $T_{\frac{1}{2}}$ of 4 h, but IR form is <1 h.

CHOOSING A MEDICATION

Insomnia

- Short-acting benzodiazepines and Z-drugs are effective.[BAP] Z-drugs, temazepam, loprazolam and lormetazepam are recommended options for short-term use.[NICE]
- Initial treatment with a benzodiazepine or Z-drug should not normally extend beyond 2^{NICE}–4^{BAP} wk.
- $T_{1/2}$ is very important:
  - Benzodiazepines with shorter half-lives have a better SE profile. If $T_{1/2} > 6$ h, hangover effects likely.[BAP]
  - For initial insomnia, drugs with short $T_{1/2}$ are good. For mid- or late-insomnia, longer $T_{1/2}$ is better.[BAP]
  - All hypnotics reach T_{max} very quickly, so should be taken in the bedroom to avoid patients falling asleep prematurely. The exception is nitrazepam, where T_{max} is variable.
  - Due to their short $T_{1/2}$, **zolpidem** and **zaleplon** are not useful for early morning wakening or for maintaining sleep throughout the night.[BAP]
  - Zaleplon can, however, be taken up to 5 h before time of desired waking.[BAP]
- Consider the presence of substance misuse, when deciding on whether to prescribe drugs that can cause dependence.[BAP]
- Melatonin MR is effective if age >55 yr. It ↓s sleep latency and ↑s sleep quality.[BAP]

Antihistamines

- Sedating antihistamines have some limited evidence for short-term use in insomnia.[BAP]
- Can be a useful strategy in patients where risk of dependence is high[BAP] and for difficulties with sleep maintenance (as they have longer half-lives).

Antidepressants

- If depression is present, treat the depression appropriately with antidepressants at a therapeutic dose for depression.[BAP]

- Antidepressants used for insomnia are generally prescribed at lower doses than would be required for depression. Often the antihistamine action is the primary mechanism.
- There is some evidence for the antidepressants in the previous table, but they often have SEs ++ due to wide receptor actions.[BAP]
- TCAs are cautioned because of their toxicity in overdose even when low doses are prescribed.[BAP]

Antipsychotics

- Olanzapine and quetiapine seem to improve sleep but should not be used first-line due to high SE burden.[BAP]
- In patients taking antipsychotics for psychosis or BPAD, sleep tends to improve on switching from a typical to an atypical drug. Quetiapine tends to improve insomnia in SZ and BPAD.

Circadian rhythm disorders

- Melatonin is an effective treatment for jet lag disorder, delayed sleep phase syndrome, and free-running sleep disorder, but timing is critical.[BAP]
- Melatonin is effective in blind people with free-running sleep disorder.[BAP]
- Light therapy is effective for delayed sleep phase syndrome,[BAP] but timing is critical and may be best done in specialist centres.

Parasomnias

- Weak evidence.
- ↓Triggers (e.g. frightening films, recreational drugs, late-night meals).[BAP]
- Ensure safety of patient and others, e.g. by separate sleeping arrangements, locking doors/windows, sleeping on ground floor.
- For NREM parasomnias, there is some evidence for clonazepam and antidepressants.

- For REM sleep behaviour disorder, use melatonin (3–12 mg) or clonazepam.
- Nightmares in the context of PTSD respond well to prazosin and may also be improved by trazodone.

Agitation

- For acute transient agitation, see section on rapid tranquilisation (p. 373, refer 'Rapid Tranquilisation' section in 'Emergencies' chapter).
- If agitation is longer lasting, a benzodiazepine with a longer half-life may be helpful for use in an inpatient setting.
- Clonazepam po up to 1–2 mg qds, diazepam po up to 10 mg tds or lorazepam up to 1 mg qds may be used.
- Level of sedation and interaction with other sedative medication should be carefully monitored.

NON-PHARMACOLOGICAL MEASURES

- Advise the person not to drive if they feel sleepy, but they do not need to inform the Driver and Vehicle Licensing Agency (DVLA) unless a primary sleep disorder is diagnosed.[NICE]
- Light therapy is a treatment for delayed sleep phase syndrome.
  - Requires exposure to bright light for 30–120 min depending on properties of the lamp.

Sleep hygiene techniques

- Exercise (but not near bedtime)
- Reduce caffeine, nicotine and other stimulants
- Reduce alcohol (helps with falling asleep but impairs sleep quality)
- Set a regular routine, getting up at the same time every day
- Take a warm bath before bed
- Avoid screens before bedtime
- If kept awake by worries, write down a plan for when you will deal with them

Source: nhs.uk

CBT for insomnia (CBTi)
- Individual or group. Also available in self-help books and online.
- Takes longer to work than medications, but the effects are more durable. With the exception of a single study, research shows that the effect of medication is lost once the medication is discontinued. However, the benefits of CBT endure long after the active therapy ends.
- Identifies a vicious cycle of racing thoughts → inability to sleep → further agitation in striving to sleep → further inability to sleep.
- Behavioural techniques: Rising at the same time every day, avoiding napping, going to bed later so that the time in bed closely matches the actual time asleep, changing the association with the bedroom by banning all activities from the bedroom aside from sleep and sex, and leaving the bedroom if one does not fall asleep to ensure there is almost no time spent awake in the bed.
- Cognitive techniques: Replace negative thoughts about sleep (e.g. 'I can't function without 8 h of sleep', 'My insomnia will never improve') with more positive ones ('There are other factors that affect how well I function in the day', 'Other people with insomnia have got better, so there is a good chance I will too').

STARTING
- Warn patients of risk of tolerance and dependence.
- Use lowest effective dose for the shortest period necessary.[NICE]
- Explain that this is a one-off prescription.[NICE]
- Do not issue further prescriptions without seeing the patient.[NICE]
- Intermittent doses may decrease the likelihood of tolerance and dependence. This can be on a PRN basis as required. It is a good strategy if insomnia is intermittent and patients can predict when they are going to have insomnia.[BAP]

SIDE EFFECTS
- Benzodiazepines → ataxia, anterograde amnesia, dysarthria, confusion, dependence, falls (in elderly).

- SEs less severe for Z-drugs than benzodiazepines.
- Road traffic accidents are more common in people the day after taking benzodiazepines or zopiclone, although sleep deprivation impairs driving performance as well.
  - The impairment in driving with benzodiazepines is similar to that when using alcohol.
  - If a patient is taking a medication that may impair driving performance, they should contact the DVLA.
- Benzodiazepines occasionally cause paradoxical excitement or disinhibition; this is more common in the elderly.
- Benzodiazepine dependence is more likely with drugs that have shorter half-lives.
- Benzodiazepine overdose can cause respiratory depression (see p. 382, refer 'Benzodiazepine Overdose' section in 'Emergencies' chapter).
- Melatonin does not impair memory, and its SE burden is favourable.

MONITORING

- Review patient within 2 wk of starting a hypnotic.[NICE]
- If a patient is on long-term benzodiazepines, r/v every 3–6 months to consider weaning down.[BAP]

STOPPING

- In general, even patients who have been on benzodiazepines for some time should be withdrawn gradually over a long period of time, unless there are significant risks.[BAP]
- Benzodiazepines should not be withdrawn rapidly due to a withdrawal syndrome, which can result in life-threatening seizures. Sx are agitation, insomnia, nausea, vomiting, muscle cramps, hyperhidrosis, depersonalisation and hyperaesthesia. This lasts longer following withdrawal from medications with a longer $T_{1/2}$, but usually persists for ~1 month.
- Risk factors for benzodiazepine continuation: substance misuse history, depression, dependent personality disorder, physical illness.
- One method to see if hypnotics are still providing any benefit is to periodically taper and assess Sx.[BAP]

- Benzodiazepine withdrawal may be monitored with the Clinical Institute Withdrawal Assessment Scale – Benzodiazepines (**CIWA-B**).
- Tips for tapering benzodiazepines:
  - Discuss with patient: Lack of patient involvement may result in illicit purchasing.
  - Switch to a benzodiazepine with a longer $T_{1/2}$ (see following section on Swapping).[BAP]
  - Taper off over 2 wk (short-term use) or several months (long-term use).[BAP]
  - Consider offering PRN benzodiazepines if Sx are intermittent.[BAP]
  - CBT alongside benzodiazepine withdrawal can help.[BAP]
- Suggested taper schedule[MPG]:

Current dose of diazepam	Recommended ↓in daily dose every 1–2 wk
>50 mg	10 mg
30–50 mg	5 mg
20–30 mg	2 mg
<20 mg	1 mg

SWAPPING

- Switching to a benzodiazepine with a long $T_{1/2}$ (e.g. diazepam or clonazepam) can be helpful when weaning a patient down, as this may ↓withdrawal Sx.
- Use the table on p. 283, refer 'Types of Medications' heading in this section to check dose equivalence, but err on the side of caution if giving high doses.

SPECIAL GROUPS
Children

- Behavioural treatment with sleep hygiene is usually effective.[BAP]
- Melatonin is a good first-line medication for initial insomnia or delayed sleep phase syndrome. It has an evidence base in autism, ADHD and learning disability.[BAP]

- Antihistamines only work in the context of behavioural treatments, but they may be useful adjuncts or short-term agents.[BAP] Some children may show paradoxical excitement due to the anticholinergic actions.[SPC]
- Clonidine is sometimes used, but it has a narrow therapeutic window.

Elderly
- CBTi is effective.[BAP]
- Melatonin MR has an evidence base for treatment up to 13 wk if age >55 yr (though frequently prescribed for longer), so it should be the first-line medication. [BAP]
- Benzodiazepines and Z-drugs have a complex relationship to risk of falls. The sedation and ataxia may ↑risk of falls, so use a medication with a short $T_{1/2}$.[BAP] However, insomnia may also be a RF for falls due to wandering; hypnotics may even ↓this risk.

Learning disability
- Insomnia is common and may be linked to some genetic syndromes (e.g. Smith-Magenis).
- Behavioural techniques and patient/carer education can be helpful.
- Melatonin is effective in this group for insomnia.[BAP]

Pregnancy
- Insomnia common due to nausea, back pain, urinary frequency, foetal movements, gastro-oesophageal reflux, pruritus and cramping. RLS is also very common.
- In mild cases of insomnia or RLS reassurance that some sleep disruption in pregnancy is normal and may well resolve in post-partum period is often sufficient; however, more severe insomnia should be monitored closely and addressed.
- Minimise discomfort by treating pain and using pillow supports.[BAP]
- CBTi is reasonable, but no specific evidence base.[BAP]
- If medications needed, zolpidem and diphenhydramine (ideally avoid in third trimester) are best options. Discuss risks and benefits.[BAP]

- For RLS, DA agonists are contraindicated. Iron and folate supplementation are often effective, even if patient is not deficient. ↓ caffeine. Mild to moderate exercise in evening with stretching and massage helpful.[BAP]

Breastfeeding

- Z-drugs are preferred to benzodiazepines, as they tend to have shorter $T_{1/2}$ and only small amounts pass into breast milk. Use intermittent dosing for a short period of time. There is no particular preference for one Z-drug over another,[UKDILAS] but if all other factors are equal, general advice is to use a drug with a short $T_{1/2}$.
- Discourage co-sleeping when mother has taken a hypnotic.[UKDILAS]

Menopause

- ↑Rates of insomnia and OSA after menopause.
- General management of insomnia may be followed, but if perimenopausal, consider HRT.[BAP]

Renal impairment

- Benzodiazepines and Z-drugs are hepatically metabolised, so are relatively safe, although longer-acting benzodiazepines may show accumulation of active metabolites. Use short-acting drugs, start low and go slow. Risk of excessive sedation in renal impairment.

Hepatic impairment

- Rule out hepatic encephalopathy as a cause of sleep disruption.
- All benzodiazepines and Z-drugs are hepatically metabolised and precipitate coma, so they should be used with great caution. Best options are Z-drugs, lorazepam, oxazepam or temazepam.

Further information

Baldwin et al., 'Benzodiazepines: risks and benefits. A reconsideration', *J Psychopharmacol* 2013; **27**(11): 967–71.

Wilson et al., 'British Association for Psychopharmacology consensus statement on evidence-based treatment of insomnia, parasomnias and circadian rhythm disorders', *J Psychopharmacol* 2010; **24**(11): 1577–1600.

SUBSTANCE MISUSE

DIAGNOSIS

Substance misuse is a serious medical disorder, as well as being highly co-morbid with psychiatric disorders; for instance, up to 60% of people with schizophrenia smoke tobacco. Various treatment targets exist for different aspects, such as acute intoxication, harmful use, substitution, detoxification, relapse prevention and associated complications.

Acute intoxication can result in life-threatening risk to self through severe respiratory depression (see p. 380, refer 'Drug Toxicity Syndromes' section in 'Emergencies' chapter for emergency Mx of opioid and benzodiazepine overdose) but can sometimes endanger others if it provokes an episode of drug-induced psychosis (see p. 303, refer Stimulants (cocaine, amphetamine, methamfetamine, mephedrone, pipradrols)). **Harmful use** covers substance use that damages mental or physical health. **Substitution** involves giving medication with a similar mechanism of action but slower kinetics than drugs of abuse. **Detoxification** is medically assisted withdrawal from dependence on a substance in order to avoid symptoms, which are often very unpleasant and, in the case of alcohol and benzodiazepines, can result in life-threatening seizures. Relapse rates after withdrawal from drugs and alcohol are high, so **relapse prevention** strategies are important.

> *Features of dependence (PC LOWE)*
> **Persistence despite harm, Cravings, Loss of control, Other
> activities neglected, physiological Withdrawal, Evidence of
> tolerance.**

In terms of associated complications, **Wernicke's encephalopathy** is a medical emergency due to thiamine deficiency. The classic triad of confusion, ataxia and ophthalmoplegia is rarely seen, so a high index of suspicion is needed for subclinical presentations, and patients at risk should be identified. Untreated, a proportion of patients progress to **Korsakoff's syndrome**, a form of irreversible alcohol-related brain disorder that is characterised by anterograde and retrograde amnesia, often accompanied by confabulation.

> *Units of alcohol*
> - 1 'unit of alcohol' = 10 mL of pure ethanol (8 g), i.e. 250 mL of 14% wine = 3.5 units
> - As a rough guide:
>   - **Beer**: 440 mL can = 2 units (4 if super-strength); 1 pint = 2.5–3 units
>   - **Wine**: Small glass (175 mL) = 2 units; bottle (750 mL) = 10 units
>   - **Spirits**: 25 mL measure = 1 unit; 70 cL bottle = 30 units

TYPES OF MEDICATIONS

Disorders	Drug (mechanism)	Mechanism	Important SEs
Alcohol disorders	Acamprosate	Anti-glutamatergic - reduces NMDA function	Nausea, diarrhoea, pruritic rash
	Nalmefene	μ/δ opioid ant; κ opioid p.a.	Insomnia, dizziness, headache, nausea
	Disulfiram (Antabuse)	Inhibits aldehyde dehydrogenase	Only if alcohol ingested – N&V, flushing, headache, ↑HR, ↓BP
Opioid disorders	Naltrexone	μ/δ/κ opioid ant	Nausea, sedation, headache, abdominal pain
	Methadone[1]	μ opioid ag	Constipation, abdominal pain, sedation, QTc prolongation
	Buprenorphine (Subutex)	μ opioid partial ag; δ/κ opioid ant	Constipation, nausea, diarrhoea, headache
	Buprenorphine + naloxone (Suboxone)[2]	μ opioid partial ag; δ/κ opioid ant + μ/δ/κ opioid ant	
	Lofexidine (limited availability)	α2adr ag	Dry mouth, hypotension, sedation
Nicotine disorders	Nicotine replacement therapy (NRT)	nAChR ag	Skin irritation (patches), watery eyes (nasal spray), insomnia, headache
	Bupropion	NDRI + nAChR ant	Insomnia, headache, dry mouth, nausea, HTN, seizure risk
	Varenicline	nAChR p.a.	Nausea, insomnia, vivid dreams, headache

[1] Methadone should be prescribed as a 1 mg/1 mL oral solution, as the tablets are easily crushed for injection. BAPMPG

[2] ... when taken repeatedly, or buprenorphine (naloxone (Suboxone) cause opioid withdrawal if injected or used intranasally.

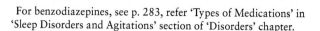

For benzodiazepines, see p. 283, refer 'Types of Medications' in 'Sleep Disorders and Agitations' section of 'Disorders' chapter.

Take-home naloxone
- Pre-filled syringes with naloxone should be provided to patients, carers or hostel staff
- **Prenoxad** is specifically licensed for use in the community
- Provide training for patients and carers: call an ambulance, give rescue breaths if not breathing, place patient in recovery position, administer im naloxone
- Agree on a system for replacing expired naloxone

CHOOSING A MEDICATION
- Exercise caution in prescribing sedative drugs and gabapentinoids in patients who may be using alcohol, opioids or benzodiazepines.
- Drug metabolism is complex in chronic alcohol use, as CYP2E1 and CYP3A4 are induced, but liver failure delays metabolism of many drugs.

Summary of first-line treatments

Drug	Acute intoxication/ overdose	Substitution	Detoxification	Relapse prevention
Alcohol	–	–	Benzodiazepines[BAP]	Acamprosate[BAP] Naltrexone[BAP] Disulfiram[BAP]
Opioids	Naloxone[MPG]	Methadone[BAP] Buprenorphine[BAP]	Methadone[BAP] Buprenorphine[BAP] Lofexidine[BAP]	Naltrexone[BAP]
Benzodiazepines	Flumazenil[MPG]	–	Benzodiazepines (especially diazepam)[BAP]	–

(continued)

Drug	Acute intoxication/ overdose	Substitution	Detoxification	Relapse prevention
Stimulants	(Only if psychotic) Olanzapine[MPG] Haloperidol[MPG]	–	Symptomatic (e.g. hypnotics)[MPG]	–
GHB/ GBL/1,4-BD	–	–	Diazepam +/– baclofen[BAP]	–
Nicotine	–	NRT combination[BAP]	NRT combination[BAP] Bupropion[BAP] Varenicline[BAP]	–

- For drug overdose and withdrawal emergencies, see p. 390, refer 'Alcohol and Drug Withdrawal Syndromes' in 'Emergencies' chapter.

Alcohol

Alcohol dependence

- Generally aim for complete abstinence, although reduced drinking may be a reasonable interim target for those who struggle to attain abstinence.[BAP]
- Use motivational interviewing to help patients recognise problem and to encourage +ve change.[NICE]
- Nalmefene is licensed for ↓alcohol consumption in patients with alcohol dependence who have a high drinking risk level without physical withdrawal symptoms, and who do not require immediate detoxification.[BNF]

Alcohol detoxification

- Should be a planned part of a treatment programme.[BAP]
- Use medications if withdrawal Sx are present.[BAP]
- Do not start medication if patient is currently intoxicated and withdrawal symptoms absent.[MPG]
- Use prophylaxis in those at risk of Wernicke's encephalopathy (see later section).[BAP]

- Benzodiazepines (chlordiazepoxide or diazepam) are the usual choice and are effective for seizure prevention[BAP]:
  - Consider lorazepam or oxazepam if ↓liver function.[MPG]
- Either fixed reducing-dose or symptom-triggered regimen may be used, but adequate monitoring is required if symptom-triggered regimen is used.[BAP]
- Chlordiazepoxide fixed-dose regimen[MPG]:
  - Consider total number of units of alcohol taken in a day and severity of dependence.
  - See examples that follow:

Example fixed-dose chlordiazepoxide regimens[NICE]

Daily EtOH consumption Day	15–25 units		30–49 units		50–60 units
1	15 mg qds	25 mg qds	30 mg qds	40 mg qds	50 mg qds
2	10 mg qds	20 mg qds	25 mg qds	35 mg qds	45 mg qds
3	10 mg tds	15 mg qds	20 mg qds	30 mg qds	40 mg qds
4	5 mg tds	10 mg qds	15 mg qds	25 mg qds	35 mg qds
5	5 mg bd	10 mg tds	10 mg qds	20 mg qds	30 mg qds
6	5 mg nocte	5 mg tds	10 mg tds	15 mg qds	25 mg qds
7		5 mg bd	5 mg tds	10 mg qds	20 mg qds
8		5 mg nocte	5 mg bd	10 mg tds	10 mg qds
9			5 mg nocte	5 mg tds	10 mg qds
10				5 mg bd	10 mg tds
11				5 mg nocte	5 mg tds
12					5 mg bd
13					5 mg nocte

- Chlordiazepoxide symptom-triggered regimen[MPG]:
  - Administer the CIWA (Clinical Institute Withdrawal of Alcohol) Scale regularly

   — Prescribe chlordiazepoxide 20–30 mg up to hourly according to the CIWA score
- For delirium tremens, see p. 390, refer 'Alcohol Withdrawal' in 'Emergencies' chapter.

Alcohol relapse prevention

- All pharmacological Rx should be accompanied by psychosocial support.[BAP]
- Offer pharmacological treatment for moderate-severe alcohol dependence and for those with harmful alcohol use/mild dependence who have not responded to psychosocial interventions alone.[NICE]
- First line: naltrexone or acamprosate.[NICE]
  - Disulfiram may also be used, but certain precautions required (see below).[NICE, BAP]
  - Consider baclofen if aiming for abstinence, high anxiety and initial options ineffective or contraindicated.[BAP]
- Disulfiram inhibits aldehyde dehydrogenase, such that alcohol consumption causes a toxic buildup of acetaldehyde, causing nausea, flushing and palpitations.
  - An option for those aiming at abstinence without any CIs (decompensated HF, CAD, previous CVA, HTN, severe personality disorder, suicidal risk, psychosis).[BAP, SPC]
  - Supervised consumption improves outcome, e.g. friend or relative.[BAP]

Wernicke's encephalopathy (WE)

- Prevention of WE is important during alcohol detoxification but can occur whenever there is a metabolic load on the brain, e.g. infection[BAP]:
  - If at risk (e.g. malnourished or unwell) or other suggestive signs (e.g. peripheral neuropathy), give **Pabrinex** 1 pair im/iv od for 3–5 days
  - If healthy and uncomplicated, give thiamine po 100 mg tds
- Rx of WE (is medical emergency, refer to general hospital):
  - Pabrinex 2 pairs im/iv tds for 3–5 days, then 1 pair od for 3–5 days depending on response[BAP]

Opioids

Opioid dependence

- Treatment options[NICE]:
  - Signposting to self-help groups (e.g. Narcotics Anonymous).
  - Brief opportunistic interventions using motivational interviewing.
  - Psychosocial interventions.
  - Opioid substitution therapy (OST).
  - Opioid detoxification.
- OST can use methadone or buprenorphine, but consider patient choice and safety[BAP, NICE]:
  - Offer alongside a psychosocial intervention.[BAP]
  - Consider buprenorphine/naloxone (Suboxone) if significant concerns Re. injecting.[BAP]
  - Should generally be supervised for ≥ 3 months and only relaxed when compliance is assured.[NICE]
  - Methadone and buprenorphine are controlled drugs, so there are certain additional requirements for prescriptions (see p. 355, refer 'Controlled Drugs' section in 'Miscellaneous' chapter).

Considering OST	
Advantages	**Disadvantages**
• ↑Retention in treatment	• OST diversion
• ↓Drug-related behaviours that risk BBV transmission	• Risk of overdose
• ↓Heroin use	• Injection or snorting of OST
	• Accidental ingestion by children
	• Occupational difficulties
	• Most evidence relies on supervised consumption
	• Can use heroin in addition

Methadone versus buprenorphine	
Methadone	**Buprenorphine**
• Higher retention in treatment • Dose-related QTc prolongation • Cheaper	• Safer in overdose • Lower mortality around initiation • Less prone to CYP interactions • Less sedating

Opioid detoxification

- Can last up to 4 wk as an inpatient or up to 12 wk in the community[NICE]
- Approaches:
  - Taper OST (methadone or buprenorphine)[BAP]
  - Lofexidine may be preferable if short detoxification desired or dependence is mild/uncertain[BAP]
- Accompany pharmacological withdrawal with psychosocial interventions[BAP]

Opioid relapse prevention

- Consider naltrexone po for previously opioid-dependent patients who are highly motivated to remain abstinent[BAP]

Nicotine

- ↓Smoking has uncertain benefit, so aim for cessation.[BAP]
- Medication may be effective alone, but outcomes are superior if combined with behavioural support.[BAP]
- Three main options for pharmacological Rx[BAP,NICE]:
  - NRT.
  - Varenicline.
  - Bupropion.
- Forms of NRT vary by their speed of action:

Slow	Transdermal patch
Medium	Gum, inhalator, lozenge, mouth spray, SL tablet
Rapid	Nasal spray, e-cigarette

- Prescribe a combination of NRT: a transdermal patch + a medium- or rapid-acting form of NRT.[BAP]
- NRT preparations (adapted from [MPG]):

Formulation		Dose	
		<20 cigarettes/day	>20 cigarettes/day or smoking within 30 min of waking
Transdermal patch	16-h formulation	10 mg or 15 mg	25 mg
	24-h formulation	7 mg or 14 mg	21 mg
Nasal spray (0.5 mg/T)		T-TT to each nostril PRN; max 2 sprays/h and 64 sprays/day	
Oral spray (1 mg/T)		T-TT PRN; max 4 sprays/h and 64 sprays/day	
Lozenge (1 mg, 2 mg, 4 mg)		1 mg hourly	2–4 mg hourly; max 60 mg or 15 lozenges/day
Gum (2 mg, 4 mg, 6 mg)		2 mg hourly	4–6 mg hourly; max 60 mg/day
Inhalator (15 mg)		Max 6 cartridges of 15 mg/day	
Sublingual tablet (2 mg)		T-TT hourly	TT hourly; max 40 tablets/day
Mouth strips (2.5 mg)		One strip hourly; max 15 strips/day	

- There is no difference in efficacy between the 16-h and 24-h formulations of transdermal patches, but the 16-h formulations should be removed at bedtime.
- Bupropion has evidence for smoking cessation independent of its antidepressant action.[BAP]
- Varenicline appears to be more effective than single NRT or bupropion, but it is uncertain how it compares to combination NRT.[BAP]

Benzodiazepines

- Benzodiazepine misuse and withdrawal are covered in depth on p. 288, refer 'Stopping' in 'Sleep Disorders and Agitation' section of this chapter]. For benzodiazepine overdose, see p. 382, refer 'Benzodiazepine Overdose' heading in 'Emergencies' chapter.
- Maintenance prescribing is not generally recommended, but consider prescribing as part of a detox.[BAP]
- Manage any co-morbid opioid dependence first.[BAP]

GHB/GBL/1,4-BD

- GHB (and its precursor drugs GBL and 1,4BD) are GABA-B agonists.
- Groups at higher risk of GHB/GBL use: body builders, models, ravers and men who have sex with men (Gonzalez & Nutt, *Psychopharm* 2005; **19**(2): 195–204; Hunter et al., *Postgrad Med J* 2014; **90**(1061): 133–138).
- Intoxication causes relaxation, disinhibition, ataxia and hallucinations:
  - Acute toxicity and overdose can be life-threatening (e.g. coma, respiratory depression, seizures), particularly in combination with other sedatives, e.g. alcohol.
- Withdrawal causes pyrexia, severe anxiety, insomnia, tremors, paranoia and hallucinations, and can progress quickly to severe delirium, seizures and rhabdomyolysis, so consider inpatient admission.[BAP, NEPTUNE]
- Rx of GHB/GBL withdrawal[TOXBASE]:
  1 Ensure clear airway; monitor vital signs, ECG, bloods.
  2 Hydration po/iv.
  3 Diazepam 10–20 mg 2–4 hourly (max 100 mg/24 h) according to Sx.
  4 Baclofen 10–20 mg qds.
  5 Monitor for seizures and delirium.

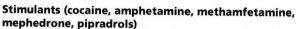

Stimulants (cocaine, amphetamine, methamphetamine, mephedrone, pipradrols)

- No specific medications recommended – symptomatic relief only. Use psychosocial interventions.[BAP]
- For cocaine- or amphetamine-induced psychosis, promote abstinence and give antipsychotics until resolution of Sx. If >1 episode of cocaine-induced psychosis, consider regular low-dose antipsychotic.[NEPTUNE]
- Mephedrone intoxication may be treated with benzodiazepines. Antipsychotics should be used with caution due to risk of seizures.[NEPTUNE]
- Pipradrols have long half-lives, so reassure users that effects do tend to resolve eventually.[NEPTUNE]

Cannabis and synthetic cannabinoid receptor agonists (SCRAs)

- THC in cannabis and SCRAs are agonists at the cannabinoid CB1 receptor, but SCRAs bind with higher affinity. Some SCRAs also have pro-serotonergic activity.
- Cannabis may be detected by routine UDS, but SCRAs cannot: clinical judgment is required.[NEPTUNE]
- Psychosocial interventions should consist of brief advice and interventions in milder cases with consideration of formal psychological therapy and residential treatment for more severe cases.[NEPTUNE]
- In the context of chronic SCRA use:
  - Manage psychosis with antipsychotics (SGAs preferred). If there has been acute SCRA intoxication, perform an ECG due to risk of vomiting-induced hypokalaemia.[NEPTUNE]
  - Manage depression with antidepressants.[NEPTUNE]

'Club drugs' and other novel psychoactive substances (NPSs)

- Psychosocial interventions should consist of brief advice and interventions in milder cases with consideration of formal psychological therapy and residential treatment for more severe cases.[NEPTUNE]

- **Ketamine:** Withdrawal may be assisted with low-dose benzodiazepines, but evidence is very limited.[NEPTUNE]
- **Nitrous oxide:** Stop exposure, check vitamin B12 levels and supplement with vitamin B12. Withdrawal Sx are not significant.[NEPTUNE]
- **MDMA (ecstasy):** In acute anxiety, provide reassurance using benzodiazepines if necessary. Monitor for hyperpyrexia and arrhythmias. Risk of interactions with serotonergic drugs.[NEPTUNE]
- **Hallucinogens (e.g. LSD, psilocybin):** In acute anxiety provide reassurance; benzodiazepines may be used with antipsychotics as second line. There is mixed evidence regarding the existence and treatment of persistent hallucinations following hallucinogen use.[NEPTUNE]

Abuse of prescription medications

- Relevant medications covered in other sections: opioids (p. 299, refer 'Opioids' heading in 'Choosing a medication' in 'Substance Misuse' section), benzodiazepines (p. 288, refer 'Stopping' in 'Sleep disorders and agitation' section), Z-drugs (p. 288, refer 'Stopping' in 'Sleep disorders and agitation' section), stimulants (p. 275, refer 'Starting' in 'ADHD' section), gabapentinoids (p. 248, refer 'Choosing a medication' in 'Anxiety Disorders' section)
- May start with legal prescriptions, but medications may also be purchased online
- General Mx: patient education, collaborative planning (lack of patient involvement may just result in illicit purchase drugs), gradual detoxification, establishing a single prescriber and psychosocial support

Non-pharmacological measures

- Psychosocial intervention is main treatment for patients with harmful substance use but without dependence. In dependence it is an important adjunct to medication.[BAP]

- Change can be conceived as five stages: precontemplation → contemplation → preparation → action → maintenance:
  - Psychosocial interventions can be seen to move patients from one stage to the next.
- **Motivational interviewing** (MI) aims to enhance a patient's motivation to change and can be easily integrated into routine care. It has several core skills:
  - Express empathy.
  - Develop discrepancy with the patient's values and their current behaviour.
  - Reflect back the patient's thoughts, amplifying those that support change.
  - Avoid confrontation.
  - Support confidence that change is possible.

Starting

Acamprosate	Immediately after alcohol detoxification (but may provide neuroprotection during detoxification as well)[BAP]
Naltrexone	Immediately after alcohol detoxification[BAP]
Nalmefene	While drinking, having failed to reduce intake, and not requiring immediate detoxification
Disulfiram	After ≥24 h of abstinence[BAP]
NRT, bupropion, varenicline	Set quit date and start medication 1–2 wk prior to planned quit date[BAP/SPC]
Lofexidine	Treat opioid withdrawal Sx, titrating up according to Sx control and tolerability[MPG]
Methadone, buprenorphine	See algorithm that follows

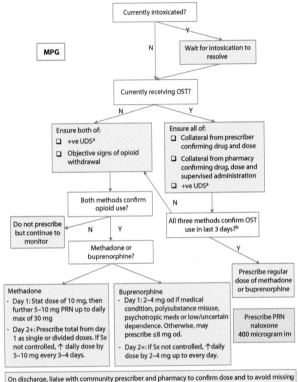

On discharge, liaise with community prescriber and pharmacy to confirm dose and to avoid missing or duplicating a dose. See box on take-home naloxone p. 295, refer 'Take-home naloxone' box.

a Methadone is detected by standard UDS, but buprenorphine requires special kit or laboratory test.

b If OST use has not been supervised within last 72 h, tolerance cannot be guaranteed, so OST must be re-titrated.

Side effects

- **NRT** is pure nicotine without the other components of tobacco smoke. There is no risk of cancer, and it is safe in stable coronary heart disease.[BAP]
- The **NRT nasal spray** can cause nose and throat irritation as well as watering eyes, so it should not be used while driving.[BAP]
- **Varenicline** has sometimes been linked to agitation, depression and suicidal thoughts, but this has not been established.[BAP] Advise patients that if they develop these Sx, they should stop varenicline and seek prompt medical advice.[BNF]
- **Disulfiram**: Must warn patient of potentially severe reaction (flushing, sweating, tachycardia, hypotension, heart failure, arrhythmia, respiratory depression) if they drink alcohol, which can occur ≤7 days after stopping disulfiram.[BAP] Alcohol present in food, perfumes and aerosols can cause a reaction. Disulfiram can also rarely cause hepatotoxicity, so patients should stop taking it if there is a sudden onset of jaundice.[MPG]
- **Naltrexone** has been associated with a reversible ↑in ALT/AST.

Monitoring

Acamprosate, naltrexone, nalmefene	Assess U&Es and LFTs at baseline and follow-up any abnormalities as appropriate[NICE]
Disulfiram	Baseline U&Es & LFTs (including GGT)[NICE]
	Clinical r/v every 2 wk for first 2 months, then every month for the next 4 months, then every 6 months thereafter[BNF]
Bupropion	Monitor BP before and during treatment[BNF]
Varenicline	Closely monitor patients with a Hx of psychiatric disorder[BNF]
Lofexidine	Monitor BP and pulse for ≥72 h or until stable dose achieved, and on discontinuation[BNF]
Methadone	ECG at baseline & annually if dose >100 mg/day or patient at ↑risk of QTc prolongation, e.g. cardiac disease, electrolyte abnormality, other medications[MPG]; monitor baseline LFTs then regularly at 6–9 month intervals[NICE]
Buprenorphine	Monitor baseline LFTs then regularly at 6–9 month intervals[NICE]

Stopping

Acamprosate, naltrexone	Consider stopping after 6 months or if drinking persists beyond 4–6 wk[NICE]
Nalmefene	Stop if no change in drinking behaviour after 4–6 wk
Disulfiram	Consider stopping if no improvement[NICE]
NRT	Continue for ≤8 wk and as long as necessary; no difference in outcome between tapering down versus abrupt discontinuation[BAP]
Bupropion	Discontinuation reaction not expected, but tapering may be considered[SPC]
Varenicline	Risk of relapse, irritability, depression and insomnia; consider tapering dose after 12 wk course[BNF]
Lofexidine	Withdrawal can cause rebound HTN, so withdraw gradually and monitor BP[BNF]
Methadone[1]	Withdraw gradually[BNF]
Buprenorphine[1]	Withdraw gradually[BNF]

[1] If opioids (prescribed or recreational) are stopped or reduced, warn patients that they will lose their tolerance, so it would be extremely dangerous for them to return to taking the same doses they were using before.

Swapping

Between methadone and buprenorphine (see MPG):

- Usually straightforward.
- Swapping from methadone to buprenorphine is important, as it can precipitate opioid withdrawal:

Methadone daily dose	Action[MPG]
<40 mg	Stop methadone abruptly and commence buprenorphine after ≥24 h.
40–60 mg	↓Methadone dose as much as possible without patient becoming unstable, then stop abruptly. Delay buprenorphine until patient in opioid withdrawal (usually 48–96 h).
>60 mg	Aim to ↓methadone dose to ≤30 mg, but if not possible, admit to specialist inpatient unit.

Prescribing in special groups

Children

- Limited evidence, but generally follow adult treatment guidance, adjusting doses accordingly.[BAP]
- Lower threshold for inpatient admission should be used.[BAP]
- **NRT** does not have evidence for effectiveness in adolescents, but it can be considered on an individual basis.[BAP] NRT is recommended in children aged >12 years[NICE] and NRT product licenses permit this.

Elderly

- Limited evidence, but generally follow adult treatment guidance, adjusting doses accordingly.[BAP]
- Offer full physical health screening.[BAP]
- Lower threshold for inpatient admission should be used.[BAP]

Pregnancy

- The UK Chief Medical Officers recommend not drinking alcohol at all during pregnancy.
- Alcohol detoxification should use chlordiazepoxide or diazepam, preferably as an inpatient.[BAP]
- Avoid medications for preventing alcohol relapse.[BAP]
- **NRT** may pose a risk to the foetus, but likely less harmful than smoking. First line: psychosocial interventions. Second line: NRT after risk-benefit analysis. Avoid varenicline and bupropion.[BAP]
- For opioid dependence, offer methadone or buprenorphine substitution (but not buprenorphine/naloxone)[BAP]:
  - Buprenorphine may result in milder neonatal abstinence syndrome compared to methadone.[BAP]
  - Detoxification should be avoided in the first trimester and is cautioned in the third trimester: best time is second trimester.[BAP]

Breastfeeding

- Women on methadone or buprenorphine should still breastfeed, but breastfeeding should not be abruptly withdrawn, as this can precipitate a withdrawal syndrome in infant.[MPG]

- Seek specialist advice for women using crack cocaine or high-dose benzodiazepines.
- Varenicline and bupropion should not be prescribed.[BAP]

Renal impairment
- For maintaining alcohol abstinence, avoid **acamprosate**,[BAP,BNF] but **naltrexone** may be used unless there is severe renal impairment.[BNF]
- For OST, **buprenorphine** is preferred,[BAP] though lower doses should be used.[BNF]
- For smoking, **NRT** should be used with caution in severe renal impairment. ↓Dose of bupropion. ↓Dose of **varenicline** if eGFR <30.

Hepatic impairment
- For alcohol withdrawal, use a short-acting benzodiazepine.[MPG] **Oxazepam** is often preferred. Seek specialist advice.
- **Acamprosate** should be avoided in severe hepatic impairment.[BNF]
- **Naltrexone** should be avoided in acute hepatitis, hepatic failure or severe impairment.[BNF]
- **Methadone** and **buprenorphine** should be avoided or used at a ↓dose.[BNF]

Physical health problems
- **HIV**: Substance misuse can be associated with ↓compliance with antiretrovirals. Some interactions with antiretrovirals can be serious and even fatal.[NEPTUNE]
- NRT and varenicline are safe in Pts with stable cardiac disease.[BAP]

Co-morbid mental health problems
- **Bipolar affective disorder**: Substance misuse or withdrawal may contribute to (hypo)mania. Lithium + valproate may ↓substance misuse. Naltrexone should be first line to ↓alcohol consumption.[BAP] Bupropion is contraindicated dt risk of precipitating mania.
- **Schizophrenia**: Preliminary data suggest clozapine may ↓substance misuse.[BAP]

- **Depression**: Antidepressants with dual serotonergic and noradrenergic profiles may be more effective for depression with substance misuse than SSRIs, but avoid TCAs, as interactions with substances of abuse can cause fatal arrhythmias.[BAP]
- **Anxiety**: Alcohol detoxification should usually be performed before treatment of anxiety disorder, but if this is not possible, follow treatment algorithms for anxiety.[BAP]

Further information

Abdulrahim D & Bowden-Jones O, on behalf of the NEPTUNE Expert Group. *Guidance on the Management of Acute and Chronic Harms of Club Drugs and Novel Psychoactive Substances.* Novel Psychoactive Treatment UK Network (NEPTUNE). London, 2015.

Clinical Guidelines on Drug Misuse and Dependence Update 2017 Independent Expert Working Group. Drug misuse and dependence: UK guidelines on clinical management. London: Department of Health, 2017.

Lingford-Hughes et al., 'BAP updated guidelines: evidence-based guidelines for the pharmacological management of substance abuse, harmful use, addiction and comorbidity. Recommendations from BAP', *J Psychopharmacol* 2012; **26**(7): 899–952.

McAllister-Williams et al., 'British Association for Psychopharmacology consensus guidance on the use of psychotropic medication preconception, in pregnancy and postpartum 2017', *J Psychopharmacol* 2017; **31**(5): 519–52.

NICE, 'Clinical Knowledge Summaries: Opioid Dependence', 2017.

NICE, 'Alcohol-use disorders: diagnosis, assessment and management of harmful drinking and alcohol dependence', 2011.

Non-pharmacological treatments

Non-pharmacological treatments may be alternatives to medications or may complement them. They range from basic communication skills to advanced treatments requiring specialist training.

PSYCHOEDUCATION

Psychoeducation should be part of any treatment plan as it can ↓Sx, ↓relapse rates and ↑compliance. Aim it at the patient and (ideally) carers. It often takes place in routine consultations, but may be formalised in group sessions, courses, patient information leaflets and online resources. Try to **individualise** psychoeducation to the patient in terms of their personal experiences, communication needs and level of education.

Cover:

- Diagnosis
- Symptoms
- Functional impact
- Prognosis
- Treatment
- Self-management
- Medication adherence
- Crisis planning
- Further sources of reliable information

Provide opportunities for questions. Good patient information can be found at https://www.rcpsych.ac.uk/healthadvice.aspx, https://patient.info, https://www.rethink.org/diagnosis-treatment and https://www.mind.org.uk/information-support.

CRISIS PLANNING

Anticipate medication non-adherence, social stressors and symptom breakthrough. Devise a **collaborative** written plan. Templates, such as the following example, can help.

Crisis plan for Joe Bloggs

- My diagnosis is Emotionally Unstable Personality Disorder
- My care coordinator is Sally Perkins (☎ 07999 999999, sally.perkins@mhtrust.uk)
- My carer is Jenny Bloggs (my wife) ☎ 07999 999990
- My warning signs that a crisis is developing:
  Not sleeping well. Relationship difficulties. Thinking too much about my past.
- I can remember that I want to live because:
  I have to be there for my daughter. People think I am a fun person to be with.
- My coping strategies are:
  Using a relaxation exercise. Going out for a walk. Calling a friend.
- If I need help, I can contact:
  My care coordinator (Monday-Friday 09:00-17:00)
  My GP: Dr Jones, Grove Surgery
  Samaritans on 116 123
  NHS helpline on 111
- In an emergency, I can attend my nearest A&E department

LIFESTYLE INTERVENTIONS

DIET

Nutrition is important to mental health in several ways. Specific **deficiencies** of cobalamin (vitamin B12), folate (B9), thiamine (B1), niacin (B3), vitamin D and vitamin C can cause psychiatric symptoms. Obesity is common among psychiatric patient. There is a growing body of research about the role of diet in mental well-being. Antimuscarinic side effects (SEs) of psychotropic meds ⇒ thirst and can contribute to high calorie intake with alcohol and soft drinks.

  Principles for improving diet:

- Balance carbohydrates, fat and protein (see box)
- Eat five portions of fruit/vegetables each day
- Eat ≥2 portions of fish each week

- Eating foods high in omega-3 fatty acids (oily fish, walnuts) may be beneficial in depression and psychosis
- Ensure good calcium intake if ↑PRL in order to ↓risks from osteoporosis
- For serious problems, r/f to dietician

Good options from different food groups	
Carbohydrate	Brown rice, wholemeal bread, fruit, vegetables
Fat	Nuts, vegetable oils, whole grains
Protein	Fish, lean meat, whole grains

Source and for more info: https://www.rcpsych.ac.uk/mental-health/problems-disorders/eating-well-and-mental-health

Occasionally, unwell psychiatric patients may become seriously **malnourished**. For example, this can happen in a patient with severe depression receiving ECT or in a patient with dementia who is self-neglecting. Dieticians generally prefer using 'real' food high in calories, but occasionally supplements may be necessary. Good options are **Complan Shake** (powder to be mixed with full-fat milk) or **Fortisip Compact**. For Complan Shake, prescribe 1–2 sachets/day. For Fortisip Compact, prescribe 1 bottle bd or tds. Give between meals, rather than as a replacement for meals. Prescribe a flavour that patient prefers.

In anorexia nervosa, involve patient, family and multidisciplinary team (MDT) to engage in collaborative approach to diet. NGT feeding sometimes necessary.

EXERCISE

Exercise may be helpful in prevention and treatment of depression and anxiety. It can ↑ sleep, ↑ self-esteem, ↑ concentration and ↓ drug cravings.

Each week, adults should do:

- 150 min of moderate aerobic exercise (e.g. walking, cycling) or 75 min of vigorous exercise (e.g. running, football) +
- Strength exercises on ≥2 days (e.g. lifting weights, press-ups)

For improving mental health, exercise that makes you out of breath is best, but anything is helpful.

Principles for ↑ physical activity:

- Find a form of exercise you enjoy
- Do it in a way you find fun (e.g. with music, with a friend, in an interesting place)
- Build it into your daily routine (e.g. journey to work, sports club)
- Start gently and ↑ gradually
- Avoid exercise close to bedtime, as it can make it harder to wind down

Source and more info: https://www.rcpsych.ac.uk/ mental-health/parents-and-young-people/young-people/ exercise-and-mental-health-for-young-people

SLEEP HYGIENE

See p. 286, refer 'Sleep hygiene techniques' in 'Non-pharmacological Measures' in 'Sleep Disorders and Agitation' part of 'Disorders' chapter.

SOCIAL INTERVENTIONS

CASE MANAGEMENT

Case management or care coordination involves assigning a single member of staff (usually a psychiatric nurse, occupational therapist [OT] or social worker) to care for a patient in the community. Caseloads are typically 10–20 patients. The case manager assesses needs, develops a treatment plan and stays in contact with the patient. The relationship between patient and case manager is very important. Case managers often liaise with other members of the team, primary care, social services, voluntary organisations and employers. There is evidence that case management can ↓ hospital admissions in the most unwell patients.

ACCOMMODATION

A change in accommodation can give stability, protect vulnerable individuals, provide support with activities of daily living (ADLs) or remove a person from a difficult situation (e.g. drugs, abusive relationship, violence). However, accommodation also needs to foster independence.

- Many people even with severe mental illnesses live in **private accommodation**, supported by family and friends. **Local authority housing** and charitable **housing associations** may make more allowances for those with mental health problems.
- **Supported living accommodation** usually provides individuals with their own room and some communal facilities. Support with finances and employment are provided, often with a view to preparing someone for independent living. Staffing is usually 24 h.
- **Hostels** are often a short-term solution for those who are homeless. They often have people with mental health or substance misuse problems. Staffing may vary from working hours only to full 24-h coverage.
- **Therapeutic communities** are typically for patients with personality disorders, psychosis or substance misuse. They may be residential or day units. A range of professionals are involved, but the emphasis is on empowering residents to make collective decisions about how they run the community and to take responsibility for this.
- **Care homes** are commonly designed for those ≥65 yr, but there are specialist care homes that work with younger adults, such as those with learning disabilities, brain injuries or severe mental illnesses. Care homes have 24-h staffing and can provide assistance with washing, toileting, activities and taking most medications. Any nursing interventions must be provided by district nurses.
- **Nursing homes** are care homes that also have 24-h registered nurses. They are suitable for patients who require regular nursing interventions, e.g. wound dressings or administering

injections. Specialist nursing homes exist for those with dementia, Huntington's and Parkinson's. Some have RMNs.

Source (among others) and further info: 'Psychiatric Services' in *Shorter Oxford Textbook of Psychiatry 7E*, 2017.

VOCATIONAL REHABILITATION

Most patients wish to work, but in severe mental illness, unemployment rates are very high. Support may include:

- Training in employable skills
- Voluntary work
- Part-time work
- Special adjustments in the workplace (e.g. time out if experiencing anxiety, a quiet place to rest)

OT is helpful. Sometimes a letter from a health professional can be very persuasive with employers, e.g. in a patient with dissociative seizures, a letter from a psychiatrist stating that the patient needs reassurance and not calling an ambulance might allow the patient to remain in work.

PATIENT SUPPORT GROUPS

Usually helpful in providing peer support. Some are for people with any mental health problem (e.g. Mind, Rethink), others are for a specific disorder (e.g. Bipolar UK) and a few are highly specific (e.g. Maternal OCD). Sometimes groups can be against medication or compulsory treatment. Patients sometimes need a prompt to engage.

CARER SUPPORT

Where possible, involve carers in decision-making and care planning. Provide them with information. They are often keen to know what they can do to help. The Carers Trust provides support for carers. In the United Kingdom, local authorities are obliged to offer a carer's assessment. Financial support is sometimes available.

PSYCHOLOGICAL THERAPIES

COMMON FEATURES

All psychological therapies tend to be based on a confidential therapeutic relationship with active listening and empathy. There is a theoretical rationale for understanding the problem that guides the therapeutic techniques. The therapist's stance can vary from passive (e.g. psychoanalysis) to active (e.g. CBT) depending on the therapy.

Factors to be considered when referring: patient's goals (insight versus problem resolution), ability to form a therapeutic alliance, psychological mindedness, readiness to change and good cognitive function.

COGNITIVE BEHAVIOURAL THERAPY (CBT)

CBT is probably the mostly widely used type of formal psychotherapy and spans 5–20 sessions. Its theoretical model emphasises how a person's interpretations of events shape their emotional and behavioural reactions. Patients learn to recognise and evaluate unhelpful thoughts and identify biases in their perceptions of themselves or the world around them. The behavioural aspect encourages a patient to test their thoughts through behavioural experiments or alter their actions, e.g. with relaxation training, graded exposure or behavioural activation.

COUNSELLING

Counselling tends to be **non-directive** and places an emphasis on **active listening** with **reflecting** back a person's thoughts in order to help a patient better understand their feelings. There may be an element of problem-solving. It is particularly used with relationship problems and bereavement. Counselling typically spans four to six sessions. It is offered by many charities and sometimes in primary care, but its effectiveness is modest. Debriefing after a traumatic event is not recommended,[NICE] as it can actually prolong Sx.

NICE indications for psychological therapies

	CBT	IPT	BA	Couple therapy	Brief psychodynamic	Other
Depression[a]	1st	1st	1st	1st	2nd	2nd Counselling; 2nd MBCT as relapse prevention for recurrent depression
GAD[a]	1st					1st Applied relaxation
Social anxiety disorder	1st				2nd	
Panic disorder ± agoraphobia	1st					
PTSD	1st					1st EMDR
OCD	1st (with ERP)					
BDD	1st (with ERP)					
IBS	1st					1st Hypnotherapy
ME/CFS	1st					1st Graded exercise therapy; 1st Activity management
Schizophrenia	1st					1st Family intervention
Bipolar depression	1st	1st				
Alcohol misuse	1st			1st		1st Behavioural therapies; 1st Social network and environment-based therapies

(continued)

	CBT	IPT	BA	Couple therapy	Brief psychodynamic	Other
ADHD						1st Parental training (children)
Autism						1st Individual or group social learning programme
Dementia						1st Group cognitive stimulation therapy
Borderline PD						Involve Pt in choosing the best intervention for them
Antisocial PD						1st Group cognitive and behavioural interventions
Self-harm						1st Psychological intervention for self-harm (DBT usually used)
Anorexia	1st					1st MANTRA; 1st Specialist supportive clinical management
Bulimia[a]	1st					

Note: 1st, 1st-line intervention; 2nd, 2nd-line intervention; ADHD, attention deficit hyperactivity disorder; BA, behavioural activation; BDD, body dysmorphic disorder; CBT, cognitive behavioural therapy; DBT, dialectic behavioural therapy; EMDR, eye movement desensitisation and reprocessing; ERP, exposure response prevention; GAD, generalised anxiety disorder; IBS, irritable bowel syndrome; IPT, interpersonal therapy; MANTRA, Maudsley Model of Anorexia Nervosa Treatment for Adults; MBCT, mindfulness-based cognitive therapy; ME/CFS, myalgic encephalomyelitis/chronic fatigue syndrome; OCD, obsessive-compulsive disorder; PD, personality disorder; PTSD, post-traumatic stress disorder.

a These disorders may benefit from guided self-help for mild Sx.

SUPPORTIVE PSYCHOTHERAPY

Supportive psychotherapy also emphasises listening skills and is often employed by health professionals in the course of their everyday work. It is supplemented by giving advice and providing hope. It is helpful for patients with enduring illnesses.

PSYCHODYNAMIC THERAPIES

Psychodynamic therapies aim to increase a patient's awareness of the role of unconscious processes on their mind and actions. In practice, this occurs through a close but professional relationship with a therapist in which the patient is encouraged to make **free associations** (say whatever comes into their mind). The therapist offers **interpretations** by linking the patient's current experiences and reactions to the therapist (**transference**) to childhood experiences. There are several forms of psychodynamic therapies:

	Frequency	Position
Psychoanalysis	5× weekly	Patient on a couch; not facing therapist
Psychoanalytic psychotherapy	3× weekly	Patient in chair; facing therapist
Psychodynamic psychotherapy	1× weekly	

Brief psychodynamic psychotherapy can be used where there is a focal problem to be addressed.

INTERPERSONAL PSYCHOTHERAPY

Problems are formulated as grief, role transitions, interpersonal deficits or interpersonal disputes. Specific strategies are then used to address each of these areas, including acknowledging differing expectations, learning to express emotion in alternative ways and examining patterns in relationships.

COGNITIVE ANALYTIC THERAPY (CAT)

CAT takes principles from psychodynamic therapy and CBT. Maladaptive behaviours (or problem procedures) are considered as

traps (a false assumption generates an act that confirms the assumption), **snags** (abandoning appropriate goals because of assumptions about them) or **dilemmas** (false dichotomies in which the only options seen are unhelpful extremes). Treatment involves a written and diagrammatic reformulation of problems, recognising how procedures play out inside and outside the session and homework involving attempting a different behavioural strategy. Treatment spans 16–24 sessions.

DIALECTIC BEHAVIOURAL THERAPY (DBT)

DBT uses principles from CBT and mindfulness and is specifically directed at recurrent self-harm, often in the context of emotionally unstable personality disorder. As well as individual therapy, there are often group sessions with the option for telephone contact in crises. Patients are taught how to manage emotions and use alternative ways out of distressing situations.

GROUP PSYCHOTHERAPY

Group therapy often uses some of the models employed for individual therapy, but there is an emphasis on group members helping each other. There is a psychotherapist and up to eight members of the group. Group therapy may be particularly helpful for those who have difficulties relating to others. Members must be able to commit to attending and participating fully in the group.

THERAPIES FOR PERSONALITY DISORDERS

A number of evidence-based therapies are now available specifically for personality disorders. These include Schema Therapy (developed from CBT), Transference-Focused Psychotherapy and Mentalisation-Based Therapy (derived from psychodynamic therapy).

NEUROSTIMULATION

ELECTROCONVULSIVE THERAPY (ECT)

ECT entails administering a transcranial electric current to induce a generalised tonic-clonic seizure. Various mechanisms have been proposed. It can be an extremely effective acute treatment, but other therapy must be commenced, as Pts often relapse in the weeks following ECT.

In modern practice, a muscle relaxant (e.g. succinylcholine) is administered to ↓ risk of fractures. General anaesthetic is then necessary so that the patient does not consciously experience the paralysis. Propofol is often used, but has the disadvantage of ↑ seizure threshold. ECT is classically given bilaterally; unilateral ECT can be given to the non-dominant hemisphere with the aim of ↓ memory loss, but unilateral ECT requires a higher dose. Typically, 8–12 sessions are required, but this should be carefully titrated to Rx response and SEs.

- Indications: Life-threatening or treatment-resistant cases of catatonia, mania or depression[NICE]
- No absolute contraindications (CIs). Relative CIs: ↑ICP, recent myocardial infarction/cerebrovascular accident, unstable fracture, severe osteoporosis, cerebral aneurysm
- SEs: Headache (Rx: paracetamol, NSAIDs), ↓ memory (especially autobiographical), death from anaesthetic (~1 in 100,000), asystole (ECT ⇒ ↑vagal tone), prolonged seizure (Rx: give more propofol or administer benzodiazepine)
- Workup:
  - Hx, including prior response to ECT, dental problems, personal/family anaesthetic reactions
  - Full physical examination, including inspecting for loose teeth
  - Mini-Mental State Examination (MMSE)
  - Bloods: Full blood count, urea and electrolytes
  - Electrocardiogram

OTHER FORMS OF NEUROSTIMULATION

(Marangell et al., *Acta Psychiatri Scand* 2007; **116**(3): 174–81)

Neurostimulation has mainly been developed in depression, although its use is now expanding to other disorders. None have the robust evidence base of ECT, but they are starting to enter clinical practice in a few centres.

Vagal nerve stimulation (VNS) involves implanting a subcutaneous battery-powered device in the chest wall and connecting it such that it stimulates the vagus nerve in the neck. It has an established role in treatment-resistant epilepsy and has some evidence in depression, presumably by altering the vagal afferent signalling to the brain.

Repetitive transcranial magnetic stimulation (rTMS) uses an electromagnet applied externally to the cranium to induce an electric current in the underlying brain, increasing regional perfusion. It is safer than ECT and very well tolerated, but is less effective.

Deep brain stimulation (DBS) is an invasive form of neurostimulation that was developed for Parkinson's. Like VNS, there is a battery-powered device implanted in the chest wall, but the leads are tunnelled beneath the skull to stimulate the brain. There is emerging evidence of efficacy for Rx-resistant OCD & Tourette's.

Transcranial direct current stimulation (tDCS) simply consists of two electrodes applied externally to the cranium with a current passed between them. Its advantages are its low cost and portability, but it remains investigational.

PSYCHOSURGERY

Psychosurgery gained a bad reputation with historical widespread use of frontal lobotomy for psychiatric disorders. Today, psychosurgery is rare, with only a few centres offering it with specific criteria for very severe and treatment-resistant cases. A few procedures have a limited evidence base:

Procedure	Indications
Anterior capsulotomy	OCD
Anterior cingulotomy	Depression, BPAD, OCD
Subcaudate tractotomy	Depression, BPAD, anxiety, OCD
Limbic leucotomy	Depression, BPAD, OCD

Source: Patel et al., *World Neurosurgery* 2013; 80(3–4): S31.e9–S31.e16
Note: BPAD, bipolar affective disorder; OCD, obsessive-compulsive disorder.

Basic psychopharmacology

Pharmacokinetics is what the body does to a drug.
Pharmacodynamics is what a drug does to the body.

PHARMACOKINETICS

Pharmacokinetics has four stages: (**ADME**) absorption →
distribution → metabolism → excretion.

ABSORPTION

- Absorption is the process of drug entry into the circulation from
  the site of administration.
- Drugs given intravenously are directly administered into the
  circulation.
- Oral drugs are absorbed through the gut mucosa, mostly in
  the small intestine, but some acidic drugs are absorbed in the
  stomach.
- If basic drugs (e.g. diazepam, imipramine, methadone) are taken
  after a meal, absorption is reduced, whereas absorption of acidic
  drugs (e.g. aspirin, ibuprofen) is accelerated.
- Some very lipophilic drugs require bile to emulsify them.
- Formulations can be engineered so that the release of active
  compounds is prolonged, which can make a drug with a short
  $t_{1/2}$ into one that can be given od. These are known as **modified
  release (MR), extended release (ER)** or **sustained release (SR)**.
- Intramuscular drugs are absorbed almost completely, and speed
  depends on the chemical properties of the injection.
- Long-acting injections (LAIs) or 'depots' use oil-based vectors
  which take longer periods to reach circulation where the active
  drug is cleaved from the long-chain fatty acid. Shorter fatty acid
  chains (e.g. in zuclopenthixol acetate [Clopixol Acuphase])
  serve to deliver the drug more quickly.

DISTRIBUTION

- Distribution is the process of drug partitioning into body tissues from circulation.
- In the bloodstream, drugs are often partially bound to proteins:
  - Acidic and neutral drugs bind to **albumin**. Basic drugs bind to α_1-**acid glycoprotein**.
  - Only the unbound drug is active.
  - If a drug binds to the same place on a protein as another drug, it can displace it → ↑unbound (active) drug.
- Distribution to organs depends on (1) the blood supply to that organ and (2) how lipophilic the drug is.
  - **Hydrophilic** molecules tend to stay in the blood. **Lipophilic** drugs tend to distribute in adipose tissue.
- To diffuse across the blood-brain barrier, drugs must be (1) small molecules and (2) lipophilic. Some drugs are transported across the blood-brain barrier by transporter proteins, e.g. amisulpride and gabapentin.
- In the elderly, relative to body mass, there are higher levels of fat but lower water and albumin. Therefore, there is an ↑ volume of distribution for lipophilic drugs (→ ↑$t_{1/2}$), a ↓ volume of distribution for hydrophilic drugs (→ ↑initial levels) and ↑ free levels of drugs that are highly bound to albumin.

METABOLISM

- Metabolism is the conversion of drugs to (usually) inactive, hydrophilic compounds which can then be excreted by the kidneys. Metabolism occurs in the liver.
- Hydrophilic drugs (e.g. lithium) can be eliminated unchanged by the kidneys. Others must undergo **hepatic metabolism**.
- Two phases of drug metabolism:
  - Phase 1: **Modification**: alteration by oxidation, reduction, etc. This may result in a compound that is pharmacologically active.

- Phase 2: **Conjugation**: addition of polar group to make drug hydrophilic, e.g. glucuronide or sulphate. Products are pharmacologically inactive.
- The **cytochrome P450 (CYP)** enzyme system is the most important in drug metabolism, the most significant being CYP1A2, CYP2C9, CYP2C19, CYP2D6, CYP2E1 and CYP3A4. Some drugs have significant metabolism via other routes though.
  - CYP2D6 is the most genetically variable cytochrome enzyme: 7% of Caucasians are poor metabolisers and up to 29% of Black people are very fast metabolisers (Davies & Nutt, *Psychiatry* 2007; **6**(7): 268–72).
  - Up to 25% of East Asians are CYP2C19 poor metabolisers (Davies & Nutt, *Psychiatry* 2007; **6**(7): 268–72).
  - See p. 341, refer 'Enzyme Interactions' heading in this chapter for specific cytochrome interactions.
- Drugs are carried from the gastrointestinal (GI) tract to the liver via the hepatic portal vein before reaching systemic circulation. During this stage, they undergo **first pass metabolism**. Extensive first pass metabolism can make the oral route unsuitable.
- In **liver disease**, both first pass metabolism and elimination metabolism are often impaired, leading to higher plasma concentrations of some drugs.
- Metabolites are sometimes pharmacologically active. In a few cases, the administered medication is a **pro-drug** for the active metabolite. Lofepramine is an example of a pro-drug that is metabolised to desipramine.
- In children, side effects may be more marked and less predictable, so it is advisable to start at lower doses relative to weight than in adults. However, due to children's faster metabolism, their final dose may be higher in terms of mg drug/ kg body weight.

EXCRETION

- Excretion is the loss of a drug or its metabolites from the body.
- Drugs and their metabolites may be excreted by the kidneys into urine, via the faeces (e.g. clozapine) or by the liver into bile, which can lead to some drugs being re-absorbed from the GI tract (e.g. oral contraceptives).
- Most psychotropic drugs undergo some hepatic metabolism prior to excretion, but **lithium, amisulpride, sulpiride** and **paliperidone** are prominent examples of psychotropic drugs that are renally excreted unchanged.
- Renal impairment → accumulation of renally excreted drugs.
- There are two patterns for drug elimination kinetics.
  - **Zero-order kinetics**: A fixed *amount* of drug is eliminated per unit of time, e.g. 10 mg in the first hour, then 10 mg in the second hour, etc., until it is fully eliminated. A few psychotropic drugs follow zero-order kinetics, notably **ethanol, fluoxetine, paroxetine** and **phenytoin**. Small increases in doses can lead to unpredictably large increases in plasma levels.
  - **First-order kinetics**: A fixed *proportion* of drug is eliminated per unit of time; e.g. for a starting concentration of 20 mg, 10 mg may be eliminated in the first hour, then 5 mg in the second hour, then 2.5 mg in the third hour, etc. The vast majority of drugs follow first-order kinetics.
  - However, enzymes that usually metabolise drugs with first-order kinetics can be **saturated** at high doses, resulting in zero-order kinetics.
- In first-order kinetics, **half-life** ($t_{1/2}$) is the time it takes for a drug to reach half its plasma concentration. The $t_{1/2}$ is constant, such that after $2 \times t_{1/2}$, a quarter of the original concentration will remain, etc.
- Drugs reach a steady state in plasma after $4–5 \times t_{1/2}$.
- In the elderly, renal function tends to be reduced, resulting in slower excretion of many drugs.

PHARMACODYNAMICS

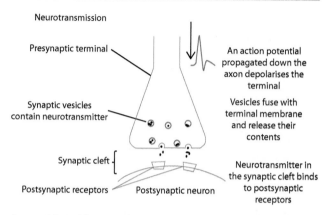

Source: Adapted from *Fundamentals of Clinical Psychopharmacology*, Anderson & McAllister-Williams 2015.

THE SYNAPSE

Neurotransmission starts with an electrical impulse in an axon. This causes calcium influx in the presynaptic terminal, resulting in exocytosis of vesicles containing neurotransmitters. These neurotransmitters may cross the synapse and bind to postsynaptic or presynaptic receptors. The receptor may open an ion channel or activate a G-protein, resulting in an intracellular enzyme cascade. Neurotransmitter is removed from the synapse, either by breakdown by an enzyme or by re-uptake into the presynaptic terminal. Breakdown may also occur in the presynaptic neuron. Neurotransmitters in the presynaptic terminal can then be packaged into vesicles ready for exocytosis.

DRUG TARGETS

- Psychotropic drugs have four main mechanisms:
  1 Influencing receptor activation
  2 Enzyme inhibition
  3 Transporter interference
  4 Ion channel stabilisation

Receptor binding

The target for a drug is a neurotransmitter receptor. Postsynaptic receptors mediate a response in the postsynaptic neuron. Presynaptic receptors are usually **autoreceptors** that exert a negative feedback effect on release of the neurotransmitter. There are several possible actions on a receptor:

- An **agonist** binds the receptor in the same location, and stimulates the receptor to the same degree, as the neurotransmitter; e.g. methadone is an agonist at the μ opioid receptor.
- An **antagonist** binds the receptor in the same location as the neurotransmitter, but it does not stimulate it, blocking the neurotransmitter from acting; e.g. most antipsychotics are antagonists at the dopamine D_2 receptor.
- A **partial agonist** binds the receptor in the same location as the neurotransmitter, but it stimulates it to a lower degree than the neurotransmitter. If levels of the neurotransmitter are low, a partial agonist will increase the postsynaptic response by providing some receptor stimulation. If levels of the neurotransmitter are high, a partial agonist will reduce the postsynaptic response by blocking the neurotransmitter from binding the receptor. For example, aripiprazole is a partial agonist at the dopamine D_2 receptor, and buspirone is a partial agonist at the serotonin 5-HT_{1A} receptor.
- A **positive allosteric modulator** binds to a different site on the receptor from the one that the neurotransmitter binds to; it increases the response of the receptor to the neurotransmitter. For example, benzodiazepines bind to the $GABA_A$ receptor at a site different from the GABA binding site and facilitate the opening of the chloride channel by GABA.

- A **negative allosteric modulator** binds to a different site on the receptor from the one that the neurotransmitter binds to; it reduces the response of the receptor to the neurotransmitter. For example, ketamine binds to the ion channel of the glutamatergic NMDA receptor, reducing its activity.

Although drugs are often labelled as having activity at one particular receptor, in reality they often bind to multiple receptors. This can account for SEs of a medication. For example, olanzapine is principally used as a dopamine D_2 antagonist and causes extrapyramidal symptoms (EPSEs) and ↑prolactin due to D_2 antagonism; however, it also has antihistaminergic and antimuscarinic SEs.

Once a receptor is stimulated, it activates a downstream signalling cascade by one of these mechanisms:

- **Ligand-gated ion channels**: Some receptors are coupled to an **ion channel**. When the receptor is activated, the ion ion channel opens, allowing influx or efflux of an ion. For example GABA acts on the $GABA_A$ receptor to open a Cl^- channel, resulting in Cl^- influx and consequent hyperpolarisation of the cell membrane.
- **G protein-coupled receptors**: Receptors are coupled to a 'G protein'. When the receptor is activated, it causes a conformational change in the G protein, which then changes the activity of an enzyme or an ion channel. The effect depends on which G protein is coupled to the receptor.
  - G_s stimulates adenylyl cyclase → ↑cAMP synthesis → ↑transcription of specific genes
  - G_i inhibits adenylyl cyclase → ↓cAMP synthesis → ↓transcription of specific genes
  - G_q stimulates phospholipase C → IP_3 and DAG signalling → opening of Ca^{2+} channels
  - G proteins may also couple to ion channels, e.g. the $5\text{-}HT_{1A}$ receptor couples to potassium and calcium channels (as well as to G_i)

Enzyme inhibition

- Drugs may inhibit enzymes that **degrade** neurotransmitters. For example, monoamine oxidase inhibitors reduce the activity of the enzyme monoamine oxidase, which is responsible for the breakdown of 5-HT, DA and NA.

Transporter interference

- Drugs may block the **reuptake transporters** that remove neurotransmitters from the synapse, e.g. selective serotonin reuptake inhibitors (SSRIs) block the serotonin reuptake transporter, SERT/5-HTT.

Ion channel modulation

- Some ion channels in the cell membrane open in response to a **depolarisation**, allowing an influx of ions.
- Drugs can block these ion channels. For example lamotrigine and carbamazepine bind voltage-gated sodium channels and stabilise them in the inactive state; gabapentin and pregabalin bind to the presynaptic voltage-gated potassium channel, reducing release of neurotransmitters.

NEUROTRANSMITTER SYSTEMS

Many neurotransmitters involved in psychopharmacology are known as **monoamines** because they contain a single amine group. They include the **catecholamines** (dopamine [DA], noradrenaline [NA] and adrenaline), **tryptamines** (serotonin [5-HT] and melatonin) and histamine. Glutamate, GABA and opioid systems are also important.

DOPAMINE (DA)

Synthesis and inactivation

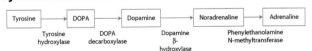

As well as being a neurotransmitter, DA is also a precursor to adrenaline and noradrenaline. DA is either inactivated in the extracellular space by catechol-O-methyl-transferase (**COMT**) or taken up into the presynaptic terminal by the dopamine transporter (**DAT**). In the presynaptic terminal, it may be repackaged into vesicles or broken down by monoamine oxidase (**MAO**) A or B.

Pathways

Name	From	To	Function	Effect of blockade
Mesolimbic	Ventral tegmental area	Nucleus accumbens	Motivation, reward	Antipsychotic
Mesocortical	Ventral tegmental area	Prefrontal cortex	Cognition, emotion	Cognitive impairment, blunted affect
Nigrostriatal	Substantia nigra	Striatum	Movement initiation	EPSEs
Tuberoinfundibular	Hypothalamus	Anterior pituitary	Inhibits prolactin release	↑prolactin

Receptors

The five dopamine receptors (D_1, D_2, D_3, D_4 and D_5) are categorised as the D_1 type (D_1 and D_5) and the D_2 type (D_2, D_3 and D_4).

Receptor	Group	Target	Synaptic location	Brain location
D_1	D_1 type	G_s	Postsynaptic	Limbic system
D_2	D_2 type	G_i	Pre- and postsynaptic	Limbic system, basal ganglia, pituitary
D_3	D_2 type	G_i	Pre- and postsynaptic	Limbic system, basal ganglia
D_4	D_2 type	G_i	Pre- and postsynaptic	Limbic system
D_5	D_1 type	G_s	Postsynaptic	Basal ganglia, hypothalamus

Example drugs

Most antipsychotics act by antagonism at the D_2 receptor, although aripiprazole is a D_2 receptor partial agonist. Some also bind to the D_3 receptor, such as amisulpride, a D_2/D_3 antagonist and cariprazine, a D_2/D_3 partial agonist. The antiemetics metoclopramide and domperidone are also D_2 receptor antagonists.

SEROTONIN (5-HT)

Synthesis and inactivation

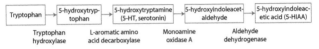

Tryptophan	5-hydroxytryptophan	5-hydroxytryptamine (5-HT, serotonin)	5-hydroxyindoleacetaldehyde	5-hydroxyindoleacetic acid (5-HIAA)
	Tryptophan hydroxylase	L-aromatic amino acid decarboxylase	Monoamine oxidase A	Aldehyde dehydrogenase

Serotonin action in the synapse is terminated by its reuptake into the presynaptic terminal via the serotonin transporter (**SERT/5-HTT**). Here it can be packaged into vesicles or degraded by **MAO-A**.

Receptors

Receptor	Location	Target	Function
5-HT$_1$ (5-HT$_{1A}$, 5-HT$_{1B}$, 5-HT$_{1D}$)	Raphe nuclei, hippocampus, smooth muscle	G_i	Autoreceptors on 5-HT neurons, vasoconstriction
5-HT$_2$	Central nervous system (CNS), platelets, smooth muscle	G_q	GI motility, platelet aggregation, CNS excitation/inhibition
5-HT$_3$	Area postrema, PNS	Na$^+$/K$^+$/Ca^{2+} ion channel	Vomiting, nociception
5-HT$_4$	GI tract, CNS	G_s	Cognition
5-HT$_5$	Olfactory bulb	G_s	Unknown
5-HT$_6$	Hippocampus	G_s	↑ ACh release
5-HT$_7$	CNS, GI tract, blood vessels	G_s	Circadian rhythms

Example drugs

SSRIs and some tricyclic antidepressants (TCAs) block SERT, causing ↑ levels of synaptic 5-HT. Monoamine oxidase inhibitors

(MAOIs) cause ↓5-HT breakdown. Atypical antipsychotics usually have some antagonism at 5-HT_2 receptors. The anxiolytic drug buspirone is a partial agonist at the 5-HT_{1A} receptor. The antiemetic ondansetron is a 5-HT_3 receptor antagonist. For migraine, the 5-HT_2 antagonist pizotifen is used in prophylaxis, while the $5\text{-HT}_{1B/D}$ agonists are effective in acute treatment.

HISTAMINE

Synthesis and inactivation

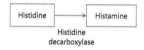

There is no presynaptic transporter for histamine, so its breakdown is dependent on one of two enzymes: histamine methyltransferase (**HMT**) and diamine oxidase (**DAO**).

Receptors

Receptor	Location	Target	Function
H_1	Mast cells, CNS	G_q	Inflammatory response (vasodilatation, ↑ vascular permeability); wakefulness
H_2	Stomach, neutrophils	G_q	↑ Gastric acid
H_3	Presynaptic terminals in CNS and PNS	G_i	↓ Release of other neurotransmitters
H_4	Mast cells, eosinophils, monocytes	G_i	Modulates allergic response

Example drugs

The first-generation 'antihistamines' (e.g. chlorphenamine, promethazine) are antagonists at the H_1 receptor, so can treat various allergic conditions; however, they cross the blood-brain barrier, so they also cause drowsiness. Second-generation H_1

antagonists (e.g. cetirizine, loratadine) are less prone to crossing the blood-brain barrier, so they cause less drowsiness. H_2 antagonists (e.g. cimetidine, ranitidine) are a second-line Rx for GORD.

MELATONIN

Synthesis

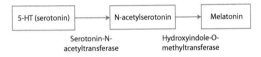

| 5-HT (serotonin) | → | N-acetylserotonin | → | Melatonin |

Serotonin-N-acetyltransferase   Hydroxyindole-O-methyltransferase

Synthesis only occurs in the pineal gland.

Receptors

Receptor	Function	Location	Target
MT$_1$	↓ SCN activity, promotes sleep	SCN, retina, cardiovascular system	G$_i$
MT$_2$	Shifts circadian rhythms		

Example drugs
Synthetic melatonin is an MT$_1$ and MT$_2$ agonist; it is used as a hypnotic. Agomelatine is an antidepressant that also has MT$_1$ and MT$_2$ agonism, so it tends to promote sleep.

GLUTAMATE
Glutamate is the brain's main excitatory neurotransmitter.

Synthesis and inactivation

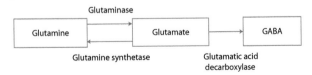

Glutaminase

| Glutamine | → | Glutamate | → | GABA |

Glutamine synthetase   Glutamatic acid decarboxylase

Receptors

Receptor	Location		Target	Function
AMPA	CNS	Postsynaptic	Cation channel	Fast excitatory neurotransmission
Kainate		Postsynaptic		
NMDA		Postsynaptic		Slow excitatory neurotransmission, long-term potentiation
Metabotropic (**mGlu$_{1-8}$**)	Pre- and postsynaptic		G_q/G_i	Modify glutamate release and the response to other glutamate receptors

Example drugs

Memantine is a voltage-dependent NMDA antagonist used in
Alzheimer's disease to block putative neuronal excitotoxicity.
The recreational drugs ketamine and PCP are non-voltage-
dependent NMDA antagonists that can cause euphoria and
psychosis. Esketamine, the *S*-enantiomer of ketamine, is a novel
antidepressant.

GAMMA-AMINO-BUTYRIC ACID

GABA is the brain's major inhibitory neurotransmitter.

Synthesis and inactivation

GABA is synthesised from glutamate (see above). The **GABA
transporter** (**GAT**) can remove it from the synapse, and **GABA
transaminase** may then degrade it.

Receptors

Receptor	Location	Target	Function
GABA$_A$	CNS	Cl$^-$ channel	Hyperpolarises cell membrane → sedative, myorelaxant and anxiolytic effects
GABA$_B$	CNS	G_i	Slow hyperpolarisation

Example drugs

Benzodiazepines and Z-drugs are positive allosteric modulators at the GABA$_A$ receptor, enhancing the action of endogenous GABA. The anticonvulsant and mood stabiliser sodium valproate inhibits GABA transaminase, reducing GABA breakdown.

OPIOID
Synthesis

Endogenous opioids (**endorphins**) are synthesised in the anterior pituitary gland from a precursor molecule **POMC**. They preferentially act on the μ-opioid receptors.

Receptors

Receptor	Location	Target	Function
μ	Brain, spinal cord, GI tract	G$_i$	Analgesia, respiratory depression, euphoria, ↓ GI motility, sedation
δ	Brain, GI tract	G$_i$	Analgesia, respiratory depression, ↓ GI motility
κ	Brain, spinal cord, GI tract	G$_i$	Dysphoria, sedation, analgesia

Example drugs

Classic opioids (such as morphine, diamorphine and methadone) are agonists at the μ-opioid receptor. Naloxone and naltrexone are antagonists at all three opioid receptors, with highest affinity for the μ-receptor. Buprenorphine is a μ partial agonist and a δ/κ antagonist. Nalmefene is a μ/δ antagonist and a κ partial agonist.

ACETYLCHOLINE (ACh)

Synthesis and inactivation

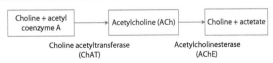

Choline + acetyl coenzyme A → Acetylcholine (ACh) → Choline + actetate

Choline acetyltransferase (ChAT)   Acetylcholinesterase (AChE)

Receptors

Receptor	Location	Target	Function
Nicotinic (nAChR)	CNS and neuromuscular junction	$Na^+/K^+/Ca^{2+}$ ion channel	(*in CNS*) Cognition, memory, reward; (*at neuromuscular junction*) muscle contraction
Muscarinic (mAChR)	Smooth muscle, myocardium, CNS	G_q/G_i	Exocrine secretion, GI motility, urination, bradycardia, cognition

Example drugs

Nicotine in tobacco products is an agonist at the nAChR, while varenicline is a partial agonist. Many drugs for Alzheimer's disease (donepezil, rivastigmine and galantamine) inhibit acetylcholinesterase. Many psychotropic medications (e.g. TCAs, SGAs) have antimuscarinic SEs, causing dry mouth, urinary retention and constipation.

DRUG INTERACTIONS

ENZYME INTERACTIONS

- Drug interactions can be due to changes in the activity of an enzyme that metabolises one or both drugs. The CYP system is most commonly implicated.
- Drugs may be **substrates** of an enzyme (they are metabolised by it), **inhibitors** of an enzyme (they ↓ its activity) or **inducers** of an enzyme (they ↑ its activity).
- Enzyme inhibition tends to happen immediately and resolves promptly after stopping the inhibiting drug. The effects of induction can take days to weeks to appear, as induction involves production of new enzymes. When the drug is withdrawn, the enzymes need to be broken down for the effect to be reversed, which also takes days to weeks.
- CYP interactions can have serious consequences. They should be considered when **starting** and **stopping** a drug. For example:
  - The OCP is metabolised by CYP3A4. Carbamazepine and St John's wort induce CYP3A4, so they can cause failure of the OCP.

- Tobacco smoking (not NRT) induces CYP1A2, which metabolises clozapine. Stopping smoking (e.g. on admission to hospital) can cause clozapine toxicity.
- Fluvoxamine inhibits several CYP enzymes that metabolise Warfarin, so it can result in a raised INR.
- Carbamazepine induces its own metabolism: after a few weeks from an initial dose, the serum level can be much lower. It therefore requires dose adjustments after initial dosing.

Below are some of the most important interactions of psychotropic medications, along with a few important interactions of non-psychotropic medications. This table is **not** exhaustive.

Class	Drug	CYP1A2	CYP2C9	CYP2C19	CYP2D6	CYP2E1	CYP3A4
Antidepressants and anxiolytics	Agomelatine	M					
	Amitriptyline		M	M	↓M		M
	Bupropion				↓		
	Buspirone						M
	Citalopram			M	M		M
	Clomipramine				M↓		
	Duloxetine	M			M↓		
	Escitalopram			M	↓		
	Fluoxetine				M↓		↓
	Fluvoxamine	M↓	↓	↓	M		↓
	Imipramine				M		M
	Mirtazapine						M
	Nortriptyline				M		
	Paroxetine				↓		↓
	Reboxetine						M
	St John's wort		↑	↑			↑
	Trazodone						M
	Venlafaxine				M		M
	Vortioxetine				M		
Antipsychotics	Aripiprazole				M		M
	Clozapine	M			↓		

(continued)

Class	Drug	CYP1A2	CYP2C9	CYP2C19	CYP2D6	CYP2E1	CYP3A4
	Haloperidol				M↓		M
	Lurasidone						M
	Olanzapine	M			M		
	Quetiapine						M
	Risperidone				M		
	Zuclopenthixol				M		
Anticonvulsants	Carbamazepine	↑	↑	↑			M↑
	Lamotrigine		M				
	Phenytoin	↑	M	M			M↑
	Valproate		M				
Sedatives	Alprazolam						M
	Clonazepam						M
	Diazepam			M			M
	Melatonin	M					
	Midazolam						M
	Nitrazepam						M
	Z-drugs						M
Substance misuse	Alcohol (acute)[1]					M↓	M↓
	Alcohol (chronic)[1]					M↑	↑
	Buprenorphine						M
	Caffeine	M					
	Codeine[2]				M		
	Disulfiram					↓	
	Methadone						M
	Tobacco (**not** NRT)	↑					
Cognitive enhancers / stimulants	Amphetamines				M		
	Atomoxetine				M		
	Donepezil						M
	Galantamine				M		M
	Modafinil		↓	↓			M
Cardiovascular	Amiodarone	↓	↓		↓		↓
	ARBs		M				
	Diltiazem/verapamil						M
	PDE inhibitors						M
	Statins						M
	Warfarin	M	M	M			M

(continued)

Class	Drug	CYP1A2	CYP2C9	CYP2C19	CYP2D6	CYP2E1	CYP3A4
GI	Cimetidine	↓		↓	↓		↓
	Omeprazole			M↓			
Antibiotics	Azole antifungals		↓	↓			↓
	Ciprofloxacin	↓					↓
	Clarithromycin/ erythromycin						M↓
	Cobicistat				M↓		M↓
	Efavirenz	↓	↓	↑			↑
	Metronidazole		↓				
	Protease inhibitors (not ritonavir)						M↓
	Rifampicin	↑	↑	↑			↑
	Ritonavir			↑	↓		M↓
Other	Calcineurin inhibitors						M
	Cyclophosphamide			**M**			
	Grapefruit juice	↓					↓
	NSAIDs		M				
	OCP						M
	Tamoxifen[2]				M		M
	Theophylline	M					

Source: **MPG**, Flockhart DA. 2007. *Drug Interactions: Cytochrome P450 Drug Interaction Table*. Indiana University School of Medicine. Available from https://drug-interactions.medicine.iu.edu. Accessed 15/10/2018.

Note: M, substrate of the enzyme (see 'metab by **P450**' in common drugs section entries); ↓, inhibitor of the enzyme; ↑, inducer of the enzyme. Interactions in **bold** are considered important by the sources that follow, but note that the potency of many interactions is not known.

[1] In occasional drinkers, the main enzyme responsible for metabolising *alcohol* is alcohol dehydrogenase, but in heavy drinkers, CYP2E1 is induced and has the greatest effect on alcohol metabolism.

[2] *Codeine* and *tamoxifen* are pro-drugs that *require* metabolism by CYP2D6 to become active. Pharmacological inhibition of CYP2D6 has been shown to ↓ the effectiveness of tamoxifen and ↑ risk of Ca recurrence.

Interactions with non-medicinal products

These are commonly used and easily forgotten about when taking a drug history or explaining how to take a medication.

- St John's wort (*Hypericum perforatum*) induces CYP2C9, CYP2C19 and CYP3A4. This can cause the OCP to fail.

- Drinking **alcohol** as a one-off inhibits CYP2E1 and CYP3A4, but chronical alcohol use induces these enzymes. Patients who return from a one-off binge should have their medications reviewed before being administered (a) to avoid compounding respiratory depression and (b) to ensure there is no important pharmacokinetic interaction. In chronic alcoholism, dosing is complex because some cytochrome enzymes are induced, but active drug concentrations may be higher because of lower blood proteins.
- **Tobacco** induces CYP1A2, but NRT does not have this effect. Therefore, active smoking reduces clozapine levels, but smoking cessation causes an increase in clozapine levels.
- **Grapefruit juice** inhibits CYP1A2 and CYP3A4, so should generally be avoided by patients taking medications that are metabolised by these pathways.

OTHER IMPORTANT INTERACTIONS

- Many pharmacodynamic interactions are additive from multiple drugs with similar effects. Such interactions are often responsible for QTc prolongation, sedation and respiratory depression.
- **MAOIs** can cause a hypertensive crisis if taken in combination with foods high in tyramine or some nasal decongestants (see p. 236, refer 'MAOI tyramine effect' in 'Depression' part of 'Disorders' chapter).
- Serotonin syndrome usually occurs in patients taking >1 medication with pro-**serotonergic activity** (see p. 389, refer 'Serotonin Syndrome' heading in 'Emergencies' chapter).
- **Lithium** is renally excreted. **Diuretics, NSAIDs** and **ACEIs** can directly or indirectly impair lithium excretion, raising serum levels. Acetazolamide can increase lithium excretion.
- **Carbamazepine** has an active metabolite, carbamazepine-10,11-epoxide, which mediates many of the adverse effects of the drug. **Valproate** inhibits the enzyme that degrades it, increasing levels of carbamazepine-10,11-epoxide and worsening SEs.
- **Lamotrigine** is metabolised by UGT2B7, which is inhibited by valproate. If valproate is co-prescribed with lamotrigine, the dose of lamotrigine should be halved.

SIDE EFFECT PROFILES

Knowledge of these, together with a drug's mechanism(s), will simplify learning and allow anticipation of drug SEs.

Cholinoceptors

ACh stimulates nicotinic and muscarinic receptors. Anticholinesterases $\Rightarrow \uparrow$ ACh and $\therefore$ stimulate both receptor types and have 'cholinergic fx'. Drugs that $\downarrow$ cholinoceptor action do so mostly via muscarinic receptors (antinicotinics used only in anaesthesia) and are $\therefore$ more accurately called 'antimuscarinics' rather than 'anticholinergics'.

Cholinergic fx	Antimuscarinic fx
Generally $\uparrow$ secretions	*Generally $\downarrow$ secretions*
Diarrhoea	**C**onstipation
Urination	**U**rinary retention
Miosis (constriction)	**M**ydriasis $\downarrow$ accommodation[2]
Bronchospasm/bradycardia[1]	**B**ronchodilation/tachycardia
Excitation of CNS (and muscle)	**D**rowsiness, **D**ry eyes, **D**ry skin
Lacrimation $\uparrow$	
Saliva/sweat $\uparrow$	
Commonly caused by	
Anticholinesterases:	Atropine, ipratropium (Atrovent)
MG Rx, e.g. pyridostigmine	Antihistamines (including cyclizine)
Dementia Rx, e.g. rivastigmine, donepezil	Antidepressants (especially TCAs)
	Antipsychotics (especially 'typicals')
	Hyoscine, Ia antiarrhythmics

[1] Together with vasodilation $\Rightarrow \downarrow$ BP.

[2] $\uparrow$ blurred vision and $\uparrow$ IOP.

Adrenoceptors

α generally excites sympathetic system (except*):

- $\alpha_1 \Rightarrow$ GI smooth-muscle relaxation*, otherwise contracts smooth muscle: vasoconstriction, GI/bladder sphincter constriction (uterus, seminal tract, iris [radial muscle]). Also $\uparrow$ salivary secretion, $\downarrow$ glycogenolysis (in liver).

- $\alpha_2 \Rightarrow$ inhibition of neurotransmitters (especially NA and ACh for feedback control), Pt aggregation, contraction of vascular smooth muscle, inhibition of insulin release. Also prominent adrenoceptor of CNS (inhibits sympathetic outflow).

β generally inhibits sympathetic system (except*):

- $\beta_1 \Rightarrow \uparrow$ HR*, $\uparrow$ contractility* (and $\uparrow$ salivary amylase secretion).
- $\beta_2 \Rightarrow$ vasodilation, bronchodilation, muscle tremor, glycogenolysis (in hepatic and skeletal muscle). Also $\uparrow$ renin secretion, relaxes ciliary muscle and visceral smooth muscles (GI sphincter, bladder detrusor, uterus if not pregnant).
- $\beta_3 \Rightarrow$ lipolysis, thermogenesis (of little pharmacological relevance).

Serotonin (5-HT)

Relative excess: 'Serotonin syndrome'; seen with antidepressants at $\uparrow$ doses or if swapped without adequate 'tapering' or 'washout period'. Initially causes restlessness, sweating and tremor, progressing to shivering, myoclonus and confusion, and, if severe enough, convulsions/death.

Relative deficit: 'Antidepressant withdrawal/discontinuation syndrome' occurs when antidepressants stopped too quickly; likelihood depends on $t_{\frac{1}{2}}$ of drug. Causes 'flu-like' symptoms (chills/sweating, myalgia, headache and nausea), shock-like sensations, dizziness, anxiety, irritability, insomnia, vivid dreams. Rarely $\Rightarrow$ movement disorders and $\downarrow$ memory/concentration.

Dopamine (DA)

Relative excess: Causes behaviour changes, confusion and psychosis (especially if predisposed, e.g. schizophrenia). Seen with L-dopa and DA agonists used in Parkinson's (and some endocrine disorders, e.g. bromocriptine).

Relative deficit: Causes extrapyramidal fx (see later text), $\uparrow$prolactin (sexual dysfunction, female infertility, gynaecomastia), neuroleptic malignant syndrome. Seen with DA antagonists, especially antipsychotics and certain antiemetics such as metoclopramide, prochlorperazine and levomepromazine.

Extrapyramidal effects

Abnormalities of movement control arising from dysfunction of basal ganglia.

- *Parkinsonism:* Rigidity and bradykinesia ± tremor.
- *Dyskinesias* (= abnormal involuntary movements); commonly:
  - *Dystonia* (= abnormal posture): dynamic (e.g. oculogyric crisis) or static (e.g. torticollis).
  - *Tardive (delayed onset) dyskinesia:* Especially orofacial movements.
  - *Others:* Tremor, chorea, athetosis, hemiballismus, myoclonus, tics.
- *Akathisia* (= restlessness): Especially after large antipsychotic doses.

All are commonly caused by antipsychotics (especially older 'typical' drugs) and are a rare complication of antiemetics (e.g. metoclopramide, prochlorperazine – especially in young women). Dyskinesias and dystonias are common with antiparkinsonian drugs (especially peaks of L-dopa doses).

Most respond to stopping (or ↓dose of) the drug – if not possible, does not work or immediate Rx needed add antimuscarinic drug (e.g. procyclidine) but does not work for akathisia (try β-blocker) and can worsen tardive dyskinesia: seek neurology ± psychiatry opinion if in doubt. See p. 194, refer Extrapyramidal Side Effects' section in 'Psychosis' part of 'Disorders' chapter.

Cerebellar effects

Especially antiepileptics (e.g. phenytoin, valproate) and alcohol.

- **Dysdiadochokinesis, dysmetria** (= past-pointing) and rebound
- **Ataxia of gait** (wide-based, irregular step length) ± trunk
- **Nystagmus:** Towards side of lesion; mostly coarse and horizontal
- **Intention tremor** (also titubation = nodding-head tremor)
- **Speech:** Scanning dysarthria – slow, slurred or jerky
- **Hypotonia** (less commonly hyporeflexia or pendular reflexes)

FURTHER READING

Anderson & McAllister-Williams, *Fundamentals of Clinical Psychopharmacology*, 2016: endorsed by the BAP, this book contains everything that the psychiatrist should know about basic psychopharmacology.

See also:

Ritter et al., *Rang & Dale's Pharmacology*, 8e, 2015.

Stahl, *Stahl's Essential Psychopharmacology: Neuroscientific Basis and Practical Applications*, 2013.

Davies & Nutt, *Psychiatry* 2004; **3**(7): 268–72.

Miscellaneous

PRESCRIBING IN THE PERINATAL PERIOD

Here we cover general principles: disorder-specific guidance is given in the relevant chapters.

- With a few exceptions, most prescribing decisions are a balance of risks and benefits in the context of an individual patient, rather than simple instructions.[BAP]
- Data on safety of psychotropic drugs in pregnancy should be considered with caution as the evidence is generally based on observational studies rather than randomised controlled trials (RCTs). There are significant risks of confounding variables (e.g. smoking and alcohol use). Efficacy is usually generalised from studies in the non-perinatal populations.[BAP]
- Discuss treatment and prevention options with woman including potential benefits of treatment, consequences of no treatment, harms associated with treatment and what might happen if treatment is changed/stopped.[NICE]
- Poor mental health in pregnancy predicts mental illness post-partum, but it is possible that effective treatment might ↓ this risk.[BAP]
- Untreated mental illness can have a negative impact on pregnancy outcome, specifically due to higher rates of substance misuse, poor self-care and suboptimal use of antenatal care.[BAP]
  - Untreated antenatal depression may be associated with low birth wt, preterm delivery and emotional problems in the child.[BAP]
  - Antenatal stress and anxiety may be associated with behavioural and mental health problems in the child.[BAP]
  - Eating disorders ↓ fertility. Anorexia nervosa is associated with ↓ birth wt. Bulimia nervosa is associated with ↑ birth wt.[BAP]
- General factors to consider in management: Accuracy of diagnosis, illness factors (course, severity, risk), comorbidities, relapse frequency/triggers, (F)Hx of perinatal relapses, treatment Hx, social function.[BAP]
- Minimise number and dose of medications but avoid subtherapeutic doses.[BAP]

- Using a drug with known efficacy in this patient may be preferable to one of unknown efficacy with a possible lower pregnancy risk.[BAP]
- Explore and address substance misuse, including smoking.[BAP]

PRECONCEPTION

- Discuss family planning issues and the risks/benefits related to conception and contraception options with all women of childbearing potential taking psychotropic medications.[BAP]
- Particular concerns centre on valproate and carbamazepine, which can cause adverse effects before pregnancy is confirmed.[BAP] See p. 223, refer 'Pregnancy' heading in 'Bipolar Affective Disorder' section of 'Disorders' chapter.

DURING PREGNANCY

- Pregnancy does not protect against mental illness.[BAP]
- Women with severe mental illness should be managed as high-risk pregnancies. If taking medications associated with high risk of malformation, they should be offered additional USS.[BAP]
- Discuss risks/benefits of psychotropic medications as soon as possible on confirmation of pregnancy.[BAP]
- Generally avoid suddenly stopping medications on confirmation of pregnancy, as this can precipitate relapse.[BAP]
- Generally avoid switching medications in pregnancy, unless benefits outweigh risks.[BAP]
- Monitor more closely for gestational diabetes mellitus in women on second-generation antipsychotics (SGAs).[BAP]
- If folate-lowering drugs are used, Px folic acid 5 mg od.[BAP]
- In late pregnancy, consider risks of neonatal adaption syndromes (multiple drugs) and persistent pulmonary hypertension of the newborn (SSRIs).[BAP]
- Ensure multidisciplinary input, involving midwives, obstetricians, mental health team and social services, as appropriate.

- The website http://www.uktis.org has useful information on medicines in pregnancy for professionals. http://www.medicinesinpregnancy.org has similar information designed for patients.

INTRAPARTUM

- In women with severe mental illnesses, it is recommended that delivery is in hospital.[BAP]
- Ensure midwives are aware of any changes in medication around delivery.[BAP]

BREASTFEEDING

- In general, the World Health Organization (WHO) recommends exclusive breastfeeding for first 6 months.
- Sedative medications are cautioned due to impaired care for baby and feeding.[BAP]
- Relative infant dose (box) is used to give an indication of the extent to which a drug enters the breast milk.

Relative Infant Dose (RID)

$$RID = \frac{Infant\ dose/kg/day}{Maternal\ dose/kg/day}$$

<10% of maternal dose is generally considered acceptable

- If no clear evidence on difference in safety between drugs, usually best not to switch.[BAP]
- Do not recommend specific timing of feeding or discarding breastmilk.[BAP]
- Monitor infant for adverse effects, e.g. sedation, poor feeding.[BAP]
- Exercise additional caution for premature/sick infants or in polypharmacy.[BAP]

PRESCRIBING IN AUTISM

No medications have sufficient evidence to justify their routine use
for the core Sx of autism, but there are some possible treatments
directed at comorbidities.

Disorder	Adult Rx[BAP]	Child Rx[BAP]
Core Sx of autism	–	–
Depression	Standard guidelines[a]	SSRIs
Anxiety disorders	Standard guidelines[a]	
Sleep problems	Standard guidelines[a] with early consideration of melatonin	Melatonin
Irritability	Consider trial of risperidone, aripiprazole or an SSRI, but behavioural/educational interventions should be tried first and continued	Consider trial of risperidone or aripiprazole, but behavioural/educational interventions should be tried first and continued
ADHD	Standard guidelines[a]	1. Methylphenidate 2. Atomoxetine 3. Clonidine/lofexidine
Tic disorders	Consider clonidine or guanfacine on a case-by-case basis	

[a] For these patients, cautiously follow the relevant guidelines for these conditions in the general
population, starting with low-dose treatment wherever possible.

PRESCRIBING IN PERSONALITY DISORDERS

The *International Classification of Diseases 11th Revision*
(ICD-11) no longer codes specific personality disorders, opting
instead for 'prominent personality traits or patterns'. However,
the following are used in current National Institute for Health and
Care Excellence (NICE) guidelines.

BORDERLINE PERSONALITY DISORDER

- Medications should not generally be used for the disorder or its
  symptoms, although medications may be used for comorbidities,

which are common. Antipsychotics should not be used in the medium or long term.[NICE]

- For crises, consider cautious use of sedative medications (e.g. promethazine) up to 1 wk. Avoid polypharmacy. Consider the potential for overdose and the possibility of concurrent substance misuse.[NICE]
- For insomnia, first-line treatment is sleep hygiene. If this is unsuccessful, general sleep guidance may be followed, but consider the potential for hypnotic abuse; promethazine is a better option.[NICE]
- When prescribing, consider the often increased risk of overdose when deciding on drug, dose and quantity in each script.

ANTISOCIAL PERSONALITY DISORDER

- Do not routinely prescribe medications for the disorder or any associated aggression, but medications may be used for comorbidities.[NICE]

CONTROLLED DRUGS (CDs)

In the United Kingdom, special 'prescription requirements' apply to 'schedule 2 or 3 drugs. *NB: Special Home Office license is needed to prescribe Schedule 1 CDs.* The Department of Health recommends that quantity prescribed should not exceed 30 days.

Selected CDs

- Ketamine
- Midazolam
- Some opioids (morphine, diamorphine, fentanyl, methadone, buprenorphine, oxycodone)
- Stimulants (methylphenidate, lisdexamfetamine)
- Gabapentin and pregabalin (as of April 2019)

There must be a handwritten signature (if electronic prescribing used may accept advanced electronic signature). The following must be written 'so as to be indelible, e.g. written by hand, typed or computer generated':

- Date signed (CD prescriptions valid for 28 days from the date signed).
- Patient's full name and address and, where appropriate, age.
- Drug name + form* + strength (when >1 strength available). If multiple strengths, then prescribe each one separately.
- Dosing regimen. 'As directed' is not acceptable, but '10 mg up to one hourly as required' is acceptable.
- Total amount of drug to be dispensed *in words and figures.***
- Prescriber's address must be specified (should already be on the prescription form, e.g. hospital address) and should be within the United Kingdom.

*Omitting the form (e.g. tablet/liquid/patch) is a common reason for an invalid prescription. It is often assumed to be obvious from the prescription (e.g. fentanyl as a patch or Oramorph as a liquid), but it still has to be written even if only one form exists.

** For tabs and other discrete formulations, state total number (in words and figures) of dose units to be supplied, e.g. '8 (eight) tablets of 10 mg'. For liquids, state total volume (in words and figures), e.g. '80 (eighty) mL'.

If prescribing PRN, must be very specific, e.g. take ONE or TWO tablets PRN.

These requirements *do not* apply to schedule 4 drugs (e.g. most benzodiazepines) and schedule 5 drugs (e.g. codeine, dihydro-codeine). For full details on controlled drug guidance in the United Kingdom, see https://www.gov.uk/government/publications/information-about-controlled-drugs-regulations.

OFF-LICENSE PRESCRIBING

(Royal College of Psychiatrists & British Association for
Psychopharmacology, 'Use of licensed medicines for unlicensed
applications in psychiatric practice, 2e', 2017)

All medications have a market authorisation that specifies
indications and doses that a medication may be used for, as
described in a summary of product characteristics (SPC) (at https://
www.medicines.org.uk/emc). The BNF takes account of the market
authorisation as well as expert guidance. In the United Kingdom,
the Medicines Act 1968 permits doctors to prescribe off-license,
and guidelines sometimes recommend this (e.g. sertraline for
anxiety). There are five reasons that prescribing may fall outside a
product license: Demographic (e.g. age range, pregnancy), Disorder,
Dosage, Duration, Domain (different country).
 Recommendations:

- Check that any licensed alternatives be excluded either on
  clinical grounds or due to a therapeutic trial.
- Be familiar with the evidence base for the off-license medication,
  including effectiveness, acceptability, side effects (SEs) and
  interactions.
- Obtain advice from another prescriber with expertise in this area
  (± specialist pharmacist) if you lack the expertise yourself, there is
  not an extensive evidence base or you have particular concerns.
- Consider and document potential risks and benefits, including
  considering children, elderly, childbearing potential, medical
  comorbidity, impaired capacity.
- Discuss with patient and carers. Explain risks and benefits. If
  use is supported by authoritative guidance, explain in general
  terms why medicine is unlicensed. Otherwise, give a more
  detailed explanation. Obtain consent or consider lack of
  capacity. Document discussion.
- Start at a low dose and monitor carefully, involving other health
  professionals.
- If lack of benefit or risks outweigh benefits, withdraw the
  medication.

PSYCHIATRIC SIDE EFFECTS OF MEDICATIONS

(Sidhu & Balon, *Current Psychiatry* 2008; 7(4): 61–74)

Many non-psychotropic drugs can have neurobehavioural SEs. We highlight some of the most important here.

Drug/Class	Psychotropic SEs
ACEIs	↑ Arousal, psychomotor agitation
Anabolic steroids	Paranoia, aggression, mania, delirium
β-blockers	Sleep disorders, delirium, hallucinations, sedation
Corticosteroids	Depression, mania, psychosis, dependence
Efavirenz	Depression, mania, suicidal ideation
H₂ receptor antagonists	Depression, irritable withdrawal syndrome
Interferon	Depression
Isotretinoin	Depression, suicidal behaviour
Isoniazid	Mania, psychosis, serotonin syndrome
Levetiracetam	Depression, psychosis
Oestrogens and prostagens	Variable effects on mood
Valproate	Confusion, agitation

MEDICATION ADHERENCE

Medication non-adherence is a major risk factor for relapse. To optimise adherence, consider the following[BAP]:

- Devise a collaborative treatment plan
- Offer choices of medications, where possible
- Keep regimen simple: ↓frequency of dosing and ↓number of tablets
- Proactively monitor for and treat SEs
- Regularly check adherence by asking patient
- If there is a Hx of non-adherence, consider checking adherence with pill counting or drug plasma levels
- Consider long-acting injections, where available

Dossette boxes may also help if forgetting medications is a problem, but they do not help if lack of insight or motivation is the problem. Some medications (e.g. valproate, orodispersible formulations) are unsuitable for dossette boxes.

RISK ASSESSMENT

(Adapted from Harrison et al., *Shorter Oxford Textbook of Psychiatry*, 7E, 2018)

All psychiatric assessments should include an evaluation of risk. Risk to self includes suicide, deliberate self-harm, deterioration in physical health, deterioration in mental health, absconding, substance misuse and self-neglect. Risk to others includes violence, neglect of children or vulnerable adults and driving. Risk from others includes violence and neglect (particularly for children and vulnerable adults). We give some general principles and cover the topics of suicide/self-harm and violence in more depth.

General principles:

- Obtain a collateral history
- Include patient and carers in plan
- Include views of more than one professional
- Look for patterns of behaviour

SUICIDE AND SELF-HARM
(Adapted from Bouch & Marshall, *Adv Psychiatr Treat* 2005; **11**(2): 84–91)

Stable risk factors
- FHx of suicide
- Older age
- Male
- Single
- Childhood adversity
- Previous self-harm
- Seriousness of prior suicidality
- Previous hospitalisation

- Known mental disorder
- Known substance misuse disorder
- Personality disorder/traits

Dynamic risk factors
- Mental state
  - Active psychological Sx
  - Hopelessness
  - Suicidal ideation, communication and intent
  - Problem-solving deficits
- Substance use
- Poor treatment adherence
- Time around psychiatric admission and discharge
- Psychosocial stress

Future risk factors
- Access to preferred method (e.g. tablets, weapon, railway)
- Future stress
- Poor engagement
- Poor treatment response

VIOLENCE
(Adapted from the Douglas et al., *HCR-20V3: Assessing Risk for Violence – User Guide*, 2013. Burnaby, Canada: Mental Health, Law, and Policy Institute, Simon Fraser University.)

Historical risk factors
- Violence
- Other antisocial behaviour
- Unemployment
- Substance use
- Major mental disorder (e.g. psychotic, mood)
- Personality disorder (e.g. antisocial, psychopathic)
- Traumatic experiences
- Poor response to treatment

Dynamic risk factors
- Poor insight
- Violent ideation or intent

- Symptoms of major mental disorder
- Instability
- Poor response to treatment

Future risk factors
- Poor engagement and compliance
- Lack of support in living situation
- Stress or difficulty coping

PSYCHIATRIC CLASSIFICATION

In the broadest terms, psychiatric disorders may be classified as:

- Psychotic (e.g. schizophrenia, schizoaffective disorder, delusional disorder)
- Neurotic (e.g. depression, anxiety, obsessive-compulsive disorder)
- Cognitive (e.g. Alzheimer's disease, frontotemporal dementia, learning disability)

The most commonly used classification systems worldwide are the *ICD-11* and the *Diagnostic and Statistical Manual of Mental Disorders* (DSM-5).

ICD-11
Produced by the WHO, the latest version of *ICD* was released in 2018. *ICD* covers conditions across every branch of medicine and gives broad clinical descriptions for each. Chapter 6 *Mental, behavioural or neurodevelopmental disorders* includes most of the conditions diagnosed in psychiatry.

Within each category, there are more descriptive specifiers, e.g. 06 Mental, behavioural or neurodevelopmental disorders

> 6A2 Schizophrenia or other primary psychotic disorders
>> 6A20 Schizophrenia
>>> 6A20.0 Schizophrenia, 1st episode
>>>> 6A20.00 Schizophrenia, 1st episode, currently symptomatic.

Y codes designate other *specified* subclasses (e.g. 6A2Y Other specified schizophrenia or other primary psychotic disorders), while Z codes designate *unspecified* subclasses (e.g. 6A2Z Schizophrenia or other primary psychotic disorders, unspecified).

The diagnostic groups within Chapter 6 are as follows.

Code	Diagnostic group	Important examples
GA0	Neurodevelopmental disorders	6A02 Autism spectrum disorder, 6A05 Attention deficit hyperactivity disorder
6A2	Schizophrenia or other primary psychotic disorders	6A20 Schizophrenia, 6A23 Acute and transient psychotic disorder
6A4	Catatonia	6A40 Catatonia associated with another mental disorder; 6A41 Catatonia induced by psychoactive substances, including medications
6A6	Bipolar or related disorders	6A60 Bipolar type I disorder, 6A61 Bipolar type II disorder
6A7	Depressive disorders	6A70 Single episode depressive disorder, 6A71 Recurrent depressive disorder
6B0	Anxiety or fear-related disorders	6B00 Generalised anxiety disorder, GB03 Specific phobia
6B2	Obsessive-compulsive or related disorders	6B20 Obsessive-compulsive disorder, 6B23 Hypochondriasis
6B4	Disorders specifically associated with stress	6B40 Post traumatic stress disorder, 6B43 Adjustment disorder
6B6	Dissociative disorders	6B60 Dissociative neurological symptom disorder, 6B64 Dissociative identity disorder
6B8	Feeding or eating disorders	6B80 Anorexia nervosa, 6B81 Bulimia nervosa
6C0	Elimination disorders	6C00 Enuresis, 6C01 Encopresis
6C2	Disorders of bodily distress or bodily experience	6C20 Bodily distress disorder
6C4	Disorders due to substance use	6C40 Disorders due to use of alcohol, 6C43 Disorders due to use of opioids

(*continued*)

Code	Diagnostic group	Important examples
6C5	Disorders due to addictive behaviours	6C50 Gambling disorder, 6C51 Gaming disorder
6C7	Impulse control disorders	6C70 Pyromania
6C9	Disruptive behaviour or dissocial disorders	6C90 Oppositional defiant disorder
6D1	Personality disorder and related traits	6D10.2 Severe personality disorder
6D3	Paraphilic disorders	6D32 Pedophilic disorder
6D5	Factitious disorders	6D50 Factitious disorder imposed on self, 6D51 Factitious disorder imposed on another
6D7	Neurocognitive disorders	6D70 Delirium
6D8	Dementia	6D80 Dementia due to Alzheimer's disease, 6D81 Vascular dementia
6E2	Mental or behavioural disorders associated with pregnancy, childbirth and the puerperium	6E21 Mental or behavioural disorders associated with pregnancy, childbirth or the puerperium, with psychotic symptoms
6E4	Psychological or behavioural factors affecting disorders or diseases classified elsewhere	6E40.3 Maladaptive health behaviours affecting disorders or diseases classified elsewhere
6E6	Secondary mental or behavioural syndromes associated with disorders or diseases classified elsewhere	6E61 Secondary psychotic syndrome, 6E62 Secondary mood syndrome

It is easily browsed online: https://icd.who.int/browse11.

DSM-5

DSM is produced by the *American Psychiatric Association* and, as well as being used by mental health professionals in the United States, it is also commonly used for research worldwide. It takes the form of a manual with three sections: I – development of *DSM-5* and its organisation; II – diagnostic classes and their criteria; III – cultural considerations, conditions for further study and an alternative dimensional model for personality disorders.

There are 19 diagnostic classes, as follows. Unlike *ICD-11*, the definitions in *DSM-5* are highly specific and operationalised.

- Neurodevelopmental Disorders
- Schizophrenia Spectrum and Other Psychotic Disorders
- Bipolar and Related Disorders
- Depressive Disorders
- Anxiety Disorders
- Obsessive-Compulsive and Related Disorders
- Trauma- and Stressor-Related Disorders
- Dissociative Disorders
- Somatic Symptom Disorders
- Feeding and Eating Disorders
- Elimination Disorders
- Sleep-Wake Disorders
- Sexual Dysfunctions
- Gender Dysphoria
- Disruptive, Impulse Control and Conduct Disorders
- Substance Use and Addictive Disorders
- Neurocognitive Disorders
- Personality Disorders
- Paraphilic Disorders
- Other Mental Disorders and Additional Codes
- Medication-Induced Movement Disorders and Other Adverse Effects of Medication
- Other Conditions That May Be a Focus of Clinical Attention

MENTAL HEALTH ACT (MHA) IN ENGLAND AND WALES

The MHA in England and Wales was passed in 1983 and is regularly revised. The MHA allows (1) detention of people suffering from mental disorder and then (2) their treatment, potentially against their will. For brevity, we do not include mental health legislation in Scotland and Northern Ireland.

COMMONLY USED SECTIONS

See Table 5.1.

Sections 2 (s2) and 3 (s3)

Patient must have mental disorder of a 'nature' (type of disorder) and/or 'degree' (severity) that makes it necessary for the patient

Table 5.1 Summary of most frequently used MHA sections

Section	Aim	Maximum duration[a]	Authorised by	May apply to
2	Assessment and/or treatment	28 days	AMHP + 2 doctors (one must be s12 approved; in practice often both are s12 approved)	Inpatients or outpatients
3	Treatment	6 months[b]		
4	Emergency assessment	72 h	AMHP + doctor	
5(2)	Doctor's holding power	72 h	Doctor	Inpatients
5(4)	Nurse's holding power	6 h	Nurse	
17	Leave		RC	Patients detained under MHA
17A	CTO	6 months[b]	RC	Patients detained under s3
135	Conveyance to a place of safety by police	24 h	Magistrate	Patients in a place authorised by a magistrate (which may include private residences)
136		24 h	Police	Patients anywhere other than in a private residence

Note: AMHP, Approved Mental Health Practitioner, usually a social worker; CTO, Community Treatment Order, which allows the RC to place certain conditions on a patient's discharge from an s3 or 37; the patient may be recalled to hospital if they breach these conditions and there is significant risk or relapse; RC, Responsible Clinician, the professional with overall responsibility for the patient's care, usually a consultant psychiatrist.

[a] Sections should always be used for the miminum necessary time.

[b] s3 and a CTO last for 6 months in the first instance, but the RC may renew the Section with the agreement of another member of the team (s3) or an AMHP (CTO).

to be detained in hospital for their health, their safety or the protection of others for the purposes of:

- s2: assessment or assessment followed by treatment
- s3: treatment, and appropriate medical treatment is available

Pts detained under s3 may be considered for a CTO, and the patient may be recalled to hospital if they do not abide by the terms of the CTO and there is significant risk or relapse.

Section 5(2)

This is the most relevant section for junior doctors to allow emergency detention long enough for assessment for s2/3 if appropriate. The 72 h limit is to cover bank holiday weekends, but s2/3 assessments should be organised as soon as is practicable and the section reviewed regularly by the ward team.

Important points re s5(2):

- Patients must already be admitted: it only applies to inpatients (*not* emergency department or outpatient departments, although 'clinical decisions units' may count as inpatient setting).
- For use in emergencies only; when not possible or safe to wait for completion of an assessment for s2 or 3.
- Appropriate least restrictive measures must have been considered and tried/failed.
- Give full address (including postcode) for hospital in which patient is to be detained. Incorrect/incomplete info can invalidate form.
- Appropriate sentence must be deleted regarding whether: (1) the clinician in charge of the treatment of the patient is filling in the form, or (2) a 'nominee' (a junior member of the team or the on-call clinician covering this team) is filling in the form.
- Give full reasons why informal treatment is no longer appropriate; include mental state abnormalities and potential risks to the patient and/or others.
- Form must be filed in the patient's notes and hospital MHA office informed. Generally, the MHA office holds the originals of detention papers. (Figure 5.1 presents example of completed form.)
- Reasons for using s5(2) should be documented clearly in patient's notes.

FORM H1 *Regulation 4(1)(g)*
Section 5(2) – report on hospital in-patient
Mental Health Act 1983

PART 1
(To be completed by a medical practitioner or an approved clinician qualified to do so under section 5(2) of the Act)

To the managers of *(name and address of hospital)*

> St Elsewhere Hospital, London, S18 9GE

I am *(PRINT full name)*

> Dr Anthony Mally

and I am *(Delete (a) or (b) as appropriate)*

(a) ~~the registered medical practitioner/the approved clinician (who is not a registered medical practitioner~~ *(delete the phrase which does not apply)*

(b) a registered medical practitioner/~~an approved clinician (who is not a registered medical practitioner)~~* who is the nominee of the registered medical practitioner ~~or approved clinician (who is not a registered medical practitioner)~~ *(*delete the phrase which does not apply)*

in charge of the treatment of *(PRINT full name of patient)*

> John Smith

who is an in-patient in this hospital and not at present liable to be detained under the Mental Health Act 1983.

It appears to me that an application ought to be made under Part 2 of the Act for this patient's admission to hospital for the following reasons-
(The full reasons why informal treatment is no longer appropriate must be given)

> This patient with a history of paranoid schizophrenia and with current active psychosis (auditory hallucinations and persecutory delusions) is trying to leave hospital despite having severe physical health problems (femoral and pelvic fractures, pneumonia). He lacks insight into his mental and physical health problems and is suspicious/unstrusting of staff advice and intentions.

(If you need to continue on a separate sheet please indicate here ( ) and attach that sheet to this form)

continue overleaf

Figure 5.1 Example of completed s5(2) form. (Reproduced from *BMJ*, Humphreys et al., 348, 2043, 2014, with permission from BMJ Publishing Group Ltd.)

Section 5(4)

Like s5(2), s5(4) applies only to patients admitted to hospital. A nurse who is suitably qualified, experienced and competent may detain a patient if a doctor cannot attend immediately and the patient is suffering from a mental disorder to such a degree that it is necessary for the patient to be detained. An s5(4) can detain a patient for up to 6 h or until a doctor can attend.

CONSENT TO TREATMENT

For patients who are not detained under the MHA, the Mental Capacity Act (see following section) applies regarding consent to treatment. This also applies to patients detained under s5(2) or s5(4).

Treatment of informal patients is like that for a physical health problem – authority to treat flows either from the patient's capacitous consent or using the procedures set out in the MCA (see following section). Authority to treat mental disorder for *detained patients* may be given under Part 4 of the MHA (Part 4A for CTO patients), but Part 4 does **not** apply to s5(2), s135(1) and s136 patients. *Treatment* includes nursing, psychological intervention, specialist mental health habilitation, rehabilitation and care; its purpose must be to alleviate, or prevent a worsening of, the disorders or its symptoms or manifestations.

If electroconvulsive therapy (ECT) is administered at any point or medication is given beyond the first **3 months** of detention, special certification requirements apply.

After 3 months, s58 of the MHA stipulates that treatment can only be given if there is either:

a. A completed **Form T2** certifying that the patient has **consented** to the treatment and is capable of understanding its nature, purpose and likely effects; or
b. A completed **Form T3** certifying that a **second opinion appointed doctor (SOAD)** agrees that the treatment is appropriate, and either the patient lacks capacity (according to MCA criteria) to consent to the treatment or the patient has capacity to consent to the treatment and is refusing it. The SOAD agrees a treatment plan and may amend the treatment plan of the Responsible Clinician (or Approved Clinician in charge of treatment); the SOAD then issues the T3.

Regardless of the time period, s58A of the MHA stipulates that adult patients may only be given ECT if there is either:

a. A completed **Form T4** certifying that the patient has **consented** to the treatment and is capable of understanding its nature, purpose and likely effects; or
b. A completed **Form T6** certifying that a **SOAD** agrees that (i) the treatment is appropriate, (ii) the patient has capacity to consent to the treatment and (iii) there is no prohibition on ECT by any advance decision or lasting power of attorney.

ECT at any point or other treatment beyond 3 months of detention may be given in **emergency** situations under **s62** MHA if the treatment is:

a. Immediately necessary to save the patient's life, or
b. Reversible and immediately necessary to prevent a serious deterioration, or
c. Reversible, not hazardous and immediately necessary to alleviate the patient's serious suffering, or
d. Reversible, not hazardous, immediately necessary and represents the minimum interference necessary to prevent the patient being a danger to himself or others.

s62 criteria: a) or b) must be met for urgent ECT – a), b), c) or d) must be met for medication.

MENTAL CAPACITY ACT (MCA) IN ENGLAND AND WALES

For the sake of concision, we do not include mental capacity legislation in Scotland and Northern Ireland. Also, consider that this legislation is in the process of being updated. The up-to-date act can be found at https://www.legislation.gov.uk/ukpga/2005/9/contents, and the official Code of Practice is at https://www.gov.uk/government/publications/mental-capacity-act-code-of-practice. The MCA in England and Wales was passed in 2005. It provides a legal framework and a code of practice for assessing capacity and making decisions on behalf of those who lack capacity. Importantly it only applies to patients aged 16 and over.

Principles of the MCA:

- *Assumption of capacity*: A person must be assumed to have capacity unless it is established to be lacking.
- *Optimise decision-making*: A person is not to be treated as unable to make a decision unless all practicable steps to help him or her to do so have been taken without success.
- *Unwise decisions*: An unwise decision does not mean a lack of capacity.
- *Best interests*: Acts done, or decisions made, for incapacitous individuals must be in their best interests.
- *Use least restrictive options*: The least restrictive action or decision should always be employed.

Lack of capacity requires demonstrating both:

1 Impairment of, or disturbance in, functioning of the mind or brain
2 Because of (1), the person is unable to make a decision for himself or herself because he or she is unable to:
   - Understand the information relevant to the decision
   - Retain that information
   - Use or weigh that information as part of the process of making the decision
   - Communicate his or her decision (whether by talking, using sign language or any other means)

If a patient lacks capacity, a decision should be made to treat them in their best interests. This should take account of the patient's preferences, views of those close to the patient and the possibility of the patient regaining capacity. See the decision-making algorithm in Figure 5.2.

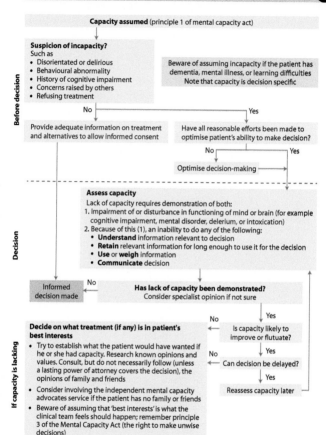

Figure 5.2 Assessment of Capacity. (Adapted by permission from Nicholson et al., *BMJ* 2008; **336**: 322–5.)

Emergencies

Most psychiatric emergencies require transfer to a general hospital for definitive treatment, though some mild cases may occasionally be managed in a psychiatric setting. Emergency management may also be required prior to transfer. In all cases, include the following specific management as part of an **ABCDE** assessment.

RAPID TRANQUILISATION (RT)

RT is parenteral pharmacological intervention with the goal to achieve a state of calmness without sedation, sleep or unconsciousness, but sedation may be considered an appropriate interim strategy.[BAP] There are several phases of the management of acute disturbance[BAP]:

- Pre-RT – de-escalation
- Pre-RT – by mouth (po)/inhaled (inh)/buccal treatment
- RT – intramuscular (im) treatment
- RT – im combinations
- RT – intravenous (iv) treatment

Some degree of physical restraint will often be required to administer RT safely.[BAP]

DE-ESCALATION

Should precede and accompany RT[NICE]

De-escalation techniques[BAP]:

- Continual risk assessment
- Self-control techniques (ensure own emotional regulation)
- Avoidance of provocation (be aware of known triggers)
- Respect patient space (↓ perceived threat)
- Management of environment (move other patients away or move patient to a more appropriate space)
- Passive intervention and watchful waiting (minimise cognitive load)
- Empathy (verbal and non-verbal)
- Reassurance
- Respect and avoidance of shame
- Appropriate use of humour

- Identification of patient needs (seeking to resolve them)
- Distraction
- Negotiation
- Reframing events (provide alternative interpretations)
- Non-confrontational limit setting (prevent a choice within certain boundaries)

MEDICATIONS

Adverse effects are frequently dose related, with higher doses and combinations having higher risks. Parenteral dosing is more likely to cause side effects compared with oral dosing. The following gives a list of drugs covered in this section; not all are recommended for RT.

Medication[BAP]	Route	Bioavailability	T_{max}	Side effects (SEs)
Promethazine	po	25%	2–3 h	Antimuscarinic fx, sedation, drowsiness, agitation, confusion, central nervous system (CNS) depression, hypotension, ↓seizure threshold, rarely extrapyramidal symptoms (EPS) and rarely neuroleptic malignant syndrome (NMS)
	im	100%	2–3 h	
Lorazepam	po	100%	2 h	↓ GCS, over-sedation, drowsiness, hypotension with risk of falls, **respiratory depression**, ataxia, cardiovascular collapse, amnesia, disinhibition (rare), dependence, tolerance (may ↓ efficacy)
	im	100%	1–1.5 h	
	iv	100%	sec–min	
Midazolam	Buccal	75%	30 min	
	im	>90%	30 min	
	iv	100%	sec–min	
Clonazepam	po	90%	1–4 h	
	im	93%	3 h	
Diazepam	po	76%	30–90 min	
	iv	100%	≤15 min	

(continued)

Medication[BAP]	Route	Bioavailability	T_{max}	Side effects (SEs)
Loxapine	inh	91%	2 min	Antimuscarinic fx,
Aripiprazole	po	87%	3–5 h	hypotension (particularly
	im	100%	1 h	olanzapine and
Haloperidol	po	60–70%	2–6 h	benzodiazepines
	im	100%	20–40 min	combination), dystonia,
	iv	100%	sec–min	akathisia, oculogyric crisis,
Olanzapine	po	Unknown	5–8 h	Parkinsonism, QTc
	im	Unknown	15–45 min	prolongation (particularly
	iv	100%	sec–min	haloperidol), NMS (see
Quetiapine	po	Unknown	1.5 h	p. 386, refer 'Neuroleptic
Risperidone	po	67%	1–2 h	Malignant Syndrome'
Droperidol	po	75%	1–2 h	section in this chapter)
	im	100%	≤30 min	Loxapine can ⇒
	iv	100%	sec–min	bronchospasm (consider
Zuclopenthixol acetate (Clopixol Acuphase)[SPC]	im	100%	36 h	prescribing prn salbutamol)

Source: Schwinghammer et al., *Biopharm Drug Dispos* 1984; **5**(2): 185–94; Beradis et al., *Int J Mol Sci* 2017; **18**(2): 349.

T_{max} is the time taken to reach maximum plasma concentration of a drug, although some effect (usually level of sedation) is usually observed earlier than this point.

Do not normally exceed BNF max doses (**including regular medication**) and only do so under direction of a senior doctor.[NICE]

Avoid prescribing multiple antipsychotics (including regular) where possible.

> **Akathisia** is a feeling of restlessness and an inability to stay still. It is a SE of antipsychotics and can resemble agitation. Avoid giving further RT as additional antipsychotics may worsen it.[BAP]

PO/INH/BUCCAL TREATMENT

- No difference in efficacy between typical and atypical antipsychotics.[BAP]
- Do not use oral **clonazepam** or **diazepam** acutely: no evidence for efficacy and they can accumulate.[BAP]
- Buccal midazolam may have a more rapid onset of action and be associated with greater sedation and respiratory depression than other benzodiazepines, but is shorter acting.
- Orodispersible formulations act no more quickly than normal tablets, but it is easier to ensure compliance.[BAP]
- Electrocardiogram (ECG) advisable before giving haloperidol.[SPC]
- Inhaled **loxapine**[BAP]:
  - Requires some patient cooperation.
  - Due to the risk of bronchospasm, it is contraindicated in respiratory distress or active airways disease (e.g. asthma, chronic obstructive pulmonary disease [COPD]).
  - Assess respiratory function before administering: exclude active respiratory pathology, e.g. wheeze, active COPD/asthma.
  - Have a salbutamol inhaler to hand in case of bronchospasm (often within 1 h).

IM TREATMENT

- **Haloperidol** can cause acute dystonia, so should not be used as monotherapy, but the addition of promethazine $\Rightarrow \downarrow$ EPSEs, so the combination is an option. Haloperidol + lorazepam is also an option.[BAP]
- Leave 1 h between im **olanzapine** and im **benzodiazepine** due to risk of hypotension and respiratory depression.[BAP]
- High doses of antipsychotics do not cause more rapid or effective sedation, but they $\uparrow$ SEs.[BAP]
- **Lorazepam** may cause respiratory depression: flumazenil must be immediately available.
- **Haloperidol** or **droperidol** in any formulation should only be used with a pre-treatment ECG.[BAP]
- **Droperidol** is structurally similar to haloperidol, but is more sedative. It was withdrawn from use in the United Kingdom in

2001 due to QTc prolongation, although there is some recent evidence supporting its use.[BAP]

- **Promethazine** is useful in benzodiazepine-tolerant patients.[BAP]

IV TREATMENT

- Only use iv treatment in settings where resuscitation equipment and clinicians trained for medical emergencies are available.[BAP]
- If giving iv **diazepam**:
  - Flumazenil must be confirmed as immediately available.
  - Use emulsified formulation (Diazemuls), not the aqueous solution.[BAP]
  - It can accumulate.[BAP]
  - Give 1 mL/min (not bolus).[BAP]
  - Keep patient supine for ≥ 1 h after administration.[BAP]
- Only give iv **haloperidol** or droperidol with continuous cardiac monitoring to detect QTc prolongation and arrhythmias.[BAP]
- iv **olanzapine** is effective, but should be used with caution due to risk of respiratory depression and lack of reversal agent.[BAP]

ZUCLOPENTHIXOL ACETATE
(CLOPIXOL ACUPHASE)

- im injection form of the typical antipsychotic, often known by its brand name **Clopixol Acuphase**. It must be distinguished from the long-acting depot zuclopenthixol *decanoate*.
- Not a form of RT as the sedative effect can take several hours to develop and has a prolonged duration, but it is sometimes an option once RT options have been exhausted.[BAP]
- Main advantage is $\downarrow$ number of injections.[BAP]
- However, marked risks, including coma and fatal arrhythmia. Do not give if patient accepting po treatment, antipsychotic naïve, sensitive to EPSEs, unconscious, pregnant or with hepatic/renal/cardiac disease. Do not give at the same time as other parenteral antipsychotics or benzodiazepines (wait at least 1 h for im, 15 min for iv before giving Acuphase).
- Perform an ECG before use.[BAP]

BAP/NAPICU ALGORITHM

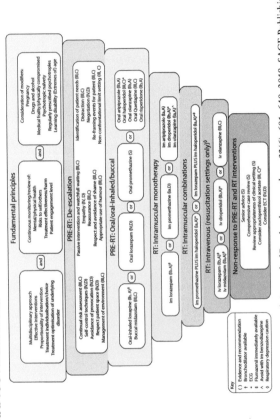

(Reprinted from Patel & Sethi et al. *Journal of Psychopharmacology*, 32(6), 601–640, 2018, SAGE Publishing, https://doi.org/10.1177/0269881118776738.)

- When deciding between options, consider patient preference, health problems/pregnancy, intoxication, previous response, SEs, interactions and total dose prescribed.[NICE]
- For im RT, use lorazepam rather than an antipsychotic if no info about previous response, no ECG, pre-existing cardiac disease or antipsychotic-naïve.[NICE]

PREGNANCY

- Complex area, so seek senior advice.
- Try to avoid medications, but weigh against risks of untreated illness and/or physical restraint.[BAP]
- Medications with short half-lives are recommended.
- No contraindications for promethazine, lorazepam or haloperidol.[BAP]
- Giving meds immediately before birth should be avoided. When given in late pregnancy, benzos ⇒ floppy baby syndrome, while antipsychotics ⇒ neonatal EPSEs.[BAP]
- If RT is required during labour, an iv benzodiazepine with an anaesthetist and paediatrician present should be considered.

MINIMUM MONITORING POST-INTERVENTIONS

Intervention		Physical monitoring[BAP]	Psychiatric observations[BAP]
Pre-RT		News hourly for ≥1 h	Hourly
im RT[a]	Most patients	News every 15 min for ≥1 h	Every 15 min
	Patient over-sedated, asleep or physically unwell	News every 15 min for ≥1 h + continuous pulse oximetry until ambulatory	Continuous (within eyesight)
iv RT		Continuous monitoring with availability of resuscitation facilities	Continuous (within arm's length)

[a] Buccal midazolam and loxapine may require monitoring according to im schedule due to risk of respiratory dysfunction.

DRUG TOXICITY SYNDROMES

Unless you are familiar with the up-to-date management of the specific overdose (OD) in question, the following sources should always be consulted:

- *Toxbase website (https://www.toxbase.org):* Authoritative and updated regularly. Should be used in the first instance to check clinical features and Mx of the poison(s) in question. If you use the website, you will need to sign in under your departmental account; if your department is not registered, contact your accident and emergency (A&E) department to obtain a username and password. An app now exists and requires an nhs. net email address to register.
- *National Poisons Information Service (NPIS):* If in the United Kingdom, phone 0344 892 0111 (if in Republic of Ireland 01 809 2566) for advice if unsure of Toxbase instructions and for rarer/mixed ODs.

Check paracetamol and aspirin levels in all patients who are unable to give an accurate history or if any suspicion.

OPIOID OVERDOSE

(Thanacoody, *BMJ Best Practice* 2018, https://bestpractice.bmj. com/topics/en-gb/339)

Signs: Respiratory depression (e.g. RR <12 when awake) and failure, miosis, ↓ consciousness.

Measure arterial blood gas (ABG): If ABG not immediately available, give naloxone.

NB: Hypercapnia is commonly present; clinically significant hypoxia is a terminal event.

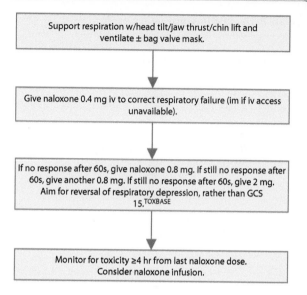

Support respiration w/head tilt/jaw thrust/chin lift and
ventilate ± bag valve mask.

↓

Give naloxone 0.4 mg iv to correct respiratory failure (im if iv access
unavailable).

↓

If no response after 60s, give naloxone 0.8 mg. If still no response after
60s, give another 0.8 mg. If still no response after 60s, give 2 mg.
Aim for reversal of respiratory depression, rather than GCS
15.[TOXBASE]

↓

Monitor for toxicity ≥4 hr from last naloxone dose.
Consider naloxone infusion.

- In the case of cardiac arrest, administer naloxone while giving
  CPR.
- Examine the patient for opioid patches, which may be causing
  the toxicity.
- Be aware naloxone may not be fully effective in reversing
  buprenorphine and tramadol overdosage due to their complex
  pharmacology.
- Naloxone is generally safe and has no contraindications.
  However, it only lasts for 30–90 min – much less than the
  duration of many opioids, so it is common for toxicity to return
  once naloxone has worn off.
- Naloxone will precipitate withdrawal in dependent individuals,
  but opioid withdrawal is not fatal per se. Very rarely, cardiac
  arrest has occurred following naloxone administration.

BENZODIAZEPINE OVERDOSE^{TOXBASE}

Signs: ↓Consciousness, mild respiratory depression, ataxia

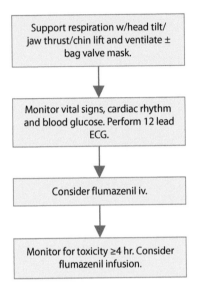

- Unlike naloxone, **flumazenil** can only be given iv and should not be given in those with epilepsy, benzodiazepine dependence or who have co-ingested proconvulsant drugs (e.g. tricyclic antidepressants, clozapine) due to risk of causing seizures.
- Flumazenil will induce withdrawal in benzodiazepine-dependent individuals.
- Flumazenil should be given iv (not im) over 15 sec. Aim for airway protection and ventilation, not GCS 15. First dose: 0.5 mg. If inadequate response after 30 sec, give 0.5 mg again. If inadequate response after 30 sec, give 1 mg.
- Flumazenil lasts for ~1 h, so toxicity often recurs.

PARACETAMOL OVERDOSE

Significant OD is >75 mg/kg in any 24 h period (toxicity may occur if >150 mg/kg, toxicity uncommon if 75–150 mg/kg).

If paracetamol OD is suspected, urgent assessment is required, as treatment must be commenced within 8 h.

Initial management

This depends on time since ingestion. 0–8 h post-ingestion:

- *Activated charcoal:* If within 1 h of significant OD.
- *Acetylcysteine:* Wait until 4 h post-ingestion before taking urgent sample for paracetamol concentration (results are meaningless until this time). If patient presents at 4–8 h post-ingestion, take sample ASAP.

If levels above the treatment line (see Figure 6.1), give the following acetylcysteine: first bag over 1 h, second bag over 4 h, third bag over 16 h.

> Do not delay acetylcysteine beyond 8 h post-ingestion if waiting for paracetamol concentration and if OD is >150 mg/kg (beyond 8 h, efficacy ↓s substantially) – ivi can be stopped if levels come back as below treatment line and international normalised ratio (INR), alanine (-amino) transferase (ALT) and creatinine normal.

8–24 h post-ingestion:

- *Acetylcysteine:* Give regimen as previously stated ASAP if >150 mg/kg OD taken. Do not wait for urgent paracetamol concentration.

>24 h post-ingestion:

- Acetylcysteine is controversial when presenting this late. Check creatinine, liver function tests (LFTs), INR, glucose and paracetamol concentration, and consult Toxbase or NPIS for individual cases.

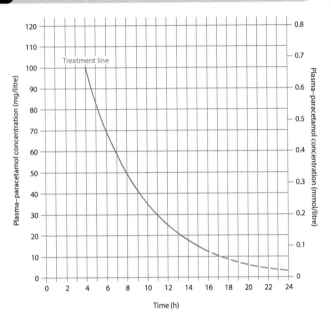

Figure 6.1 Treatment lines for acetylcysteine treatment of paracetamol overdose. (Reproduced with permission of the MHRA under the terms of the Open Government Licence (OGL) v3.0.)

Medical clearance

Patients may be *medically* fit for discharge once acetylcysteine ivi is completed, and INR, ALT, creatinine and HCO_3^- ($\pm$ pH) are normal (or recovering in two successive checks if additional acetylcysteine has been administered). In patients with laboratory abnormalities despite acetylcysteine, consult Toxbase $\pm$ NPIS for advice on further acetylcysteine and specialist referral.

ANTIPSYCHOTIC OVERDOSE^{TOXBASE}

Features: CNS depression, acute dystonia, blurred vision, fluctuating mental state. Less commonly, ↓/↑blood pressure (BP), ↓/↑heart rate (HR), seizures, renal failure, coma. NMS (see next section) can occur at any point in Rx, but it is **not** especially common in overdose.

Clozapine toxicity is increased in clozapine-naïve patients. Features can persist for several days.

Serotonin syndrome (p. 389, refer 'Serotonin Syndrome' heading in this chapter) may occasionally occur in overdose of atypical antipsychotics.

Patients require a medical assessment (in addition to a psychiatric assessment) if dose > toxic dose (see table below), ≥2 drugs taken, symptomatic or phenothiazine taken by a patient who does not usually take phenothiazines.

Drug	Suggested toxic po dose
Haloperidol	0.5 mg/kg
Chlorpromazine	6 mg/kg
Sulpiride	25 mg/kg
Trifluoperazine	0.4 mg/kg
Flupentixol	0.13 mg/kg
Fluphenazine	0.2 mg/kg
Zuclopenthixol	0.6 mg/kg
Olanzapine	1.5 mg/kg
Risperidone	1 mg/kg
Paliperidone	0.4 mg/kg
Quetiapine	15 mg/kg

(continued)

Drug	Suggested toxic po dose
Amisulpride	25 mg/kg
Clozapine	10 mg/kg
Lurasidone	10 mg/kg
Aripiprazole	1 mg/kg

Mx includes: Consideration of activated charcoal (if presenting within 1 h), provided airway can be protected. 12-lead ECG, checking for QT prolongation. Magnesium sulphate for torsade de pointes, VF or VT preceded by prolonged QT. For seizures, a single brief seizure does not need treatment; otherwise use benzodiazepines. Procyclidine or diazepam for acute dystonia. Fluids for hypotension.

Observe for ≥6 h post-ingestion (≥12 h for clozapine). Following clozapine overdose, full blood count (FBC) must be monitored weekly for ≥3 wk to check for agranulocytosis.

Acute dystonia may rarely occur some days after overdose in naïve patients. Patients should be warned of this possibility and advised to seek treatment if this occurs.

NEUROLEPTIC MALIGNANT SYNDROME (NMS)

(TOXBASE Gurrera, *BMJ Best Practice* 2017, https://bestpractice.bmj.com/topics/en-gb/990)

- *Risk factors:* Parkinson's, alcohol-related brain damage, learning disability, agitation, dehydration, high-potency first-generation antipsychotics, rapid antipsychotic dose ↑, multiple antipsychotics, abrupt withdrawal of anticholinergics
- *Clinical features:* Muscle rigidity, fever, altered consciousness and autonomic instability, usually with an insidious onset
- *Blood markers:* ↑creatine kinase (CK), ↑white cell count (WCC), ↓iron and ↑LFTs

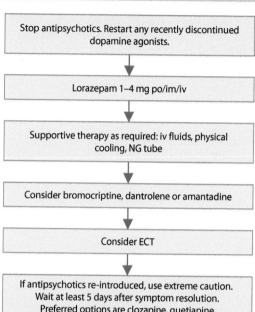

Stop antipsychotics. Restart any recently discontinued dopamine agonists.

↓

Lorazepam 1–4 mg po/im/iv

↓

Supportive therapy as required: iv fluids, physical cooling, NG tube

↓

Consider bromocriptine, dantrolene or amantadine

↓

Consider ECT

↓

If antipsychotics re-introduced, use extreme caution. Wait at least 5 days after symptom resolution. Preferred options are clozapine, quetiapine and aripiprazole. Avoid high potency or structurally similar antipsychotics.

ANTIDEPRESSANT OVERDOSE^{TOXBASE}

Features: Tremor, agitation, tachycardia, QTc prolongation (more with citalopram), torsade de pointes, ↑/↓ BP, rhabdomyolysis, serotonin syndrome (see next section).

In addition, tricyclic antidepressants (TCAs) can cause antimuscarinic fx (sinus tachycardia, confusion, drowsiness, dry mouth and dilated pupils), convulsions, coma, ↑tone and hyperreflexia. Arrhythmias can occur shortly after ingestion.

Patients require a medical assessment (in addition to psychiatric assessment) if dose>toxic dose (see table below), ≥2 drugs taken or symptomatic.

Fatalities are rare when selective serotonin reuptake inhibitors (SSRIs) or mirtazapine are taken alone. TCAs and monoamine oxidase inhibitors (MAOIs) can be very dangerous.

Mx includes: Consideration of activated charcoal (if presenting within 1 h), provided airway can be protected. Magnesium sulphate for torsade de pointes, VF or VT preceded by prolonged QT. Monitoring of ABGs, urea and electrolytes (U&Es), blood glucose and SpO_2. Treat seizures and agitation with benzodiazepines. For TCAs, consider iv sodium bicarbonate.

Observe for ≥6 h post-ingestion.

Drug	Suggested toxic dose	Drug	Suggested toxic dose
Citalopram	2 mg/kg	Doxepin	4 mg/kg
Escitalopram	1 mg/kg	Trimipramine	5 mg/kg
Sertraline	7 mg/kg	Mirtazapine	5 mg/kg
Fluoxetine	6 mg/kg	Mianserin	4 mg/kg
Fluvoxamine	15 mg/kg	Trazodone	15 mg/kg
Paroxetine	3 mg/kg	Phenelzine	2.5 mg/kg
Duloxetine	5 mg/kg	Tranylcypromine	0.4 mg/kg
Venlafaxine	7 mg/kg	Isocarboxazid	0.6 mg/kg
Clomipramine	4 mg/kg	Moclobemide	30 mg/kg
Amitriptyline	3 mg/kg	Vortioxetine	1 mg/kg
Dosulepin	3 mg/kg	Reboxetine	0.5 mg/kg
Imipramine	4 mg/kg	Bupropion	6 mg/kg
Nortriptyline	2.5 mg/kg	Agomelatine	3 mg/kg
Lofepramine	4.5 mg/kg		

SEROTONIN SYNDROME

(Boyer & Shannon, *NEJM* 2005; **352**(11): 1112–20; Ellahi, *BJPsych Adv* 2015; **21**(5): 324–32)

- Occurs in up to 1% of patients on SSRI monotherapy but 15% of those with antidepressant overdose.
- Drugs responsible (often in combination or with CYP inhibition): serotonergic antidepressants, lithium, St John's wort, some opioids (tramadol, pethidine, fentanyl, buprenorphine, dextromethorphan), certain Abx (linezolid, isoniazid), selegiline, some recreational drugs (cocaine, amphetamine, MDMA), carbamazepine, methylphenidate, certain antipsychotics (risperidone, olanzapine), triptans.
- *Features:* Agitation, (myo)clonus, autonomic instability, pyrexia, hyperreflexia, tremor, diaphoresis, diarrhoea, rigors and rigidity, usually with a rapid onset. Death can occur within 24 h.

Management:

- Stop serotonergic drugs. Look for and remove opioid patches.
- Avoid physical restraint, as can worsen lactic acidosis.
- Diazepam for agitation.
- Cyproheptadine (5-HT$_{2A}$ antagonist) po 12 mg stat, then 2 mg every 2 h for ongoing Sx.
- Physical cooling.

LITHIUM TOXICITY

([TOXBASE] Haussmann et al., *Int J Bipolar Disord* 2015; **3**(1): 23)

If a patient on lithium has accidentally taken twice their daily dose, advise them to omit their next dose and then continue as normal. In all other cases of lithium overdose, a patient should have medical assessment, including an urgent lithium concentration measurement.

- *Risk factors:* Dehydration, hyponatraemia, renal impairment, certain drugs (non-steroidal anti-inflammatory drugs [NSAIDs], ACE-i, thiazide diuretics)

- *Features:* Coarse tremor, nausea, drowsiness, confusion,
  diarrhoea, seizures, ECG changes (heart block, bradycardia,
  ST elevation)

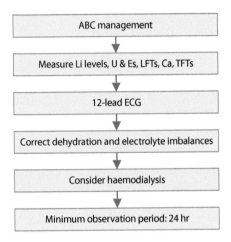

Activated charcoal is not helpful in lithium toxicity.

Symptoms may be delayed and repeat lithium levels are necessary
(see TOXBASE). Lithium toxicity is often more profound in those
already established on lithium, as lithium has saturated their tissues.

ALCOHOL AND DRUG WITHDRAWAL SYNDROMES

ALCOHOL WITHDRAWAL
(Shuckit, *NEJM* 2014; **371**(22): 2109–113)

This covers more severe alcohol withdrawal and delirium tremens.
For milder Sx, see p. 296, refer 'Alcohol detoxification' heading in
'Substance Misuse' part of 'Disorders' chapter.

The diagnostic criteria for alcohol withdrawal are met when two or more of the following are present:

- Autonomic hyperactivity (e.g. sweating or pulse rate greater than 100 beats per minute)
- Increased hand tremor
- Insomnia
- Nausea or vomiting
- Transient visual, tactile or auditory hallucinations or illusions
- Psychomotor agitation
- Anxiety
- Grand mal seizures

Withdrawal begins 10–72 h after last drink.

The revised Clinical Institute Withdrawal Assessment for Alcohol (CIWA-Ar) scale should be used to determine both the severity of withdrawal and the need for treatment. If drug treatment is required, patients should ideally be treated with regimens that are patient-specific and flexible to respond to changes in severity of withdrawal (symptom triggered). Fixed treatment schedules, where the patient is given a standard regimen irrespective of their symptoms, are inappropriate.

The American Society of Addiction Medicine produced an evidence-based Practice Guideline recommending that treatment should be initiated using a symptom-triggered regimen when the CIWA-Ar score is >8; this will benefit the patient symptomatically. When the CIWA-Ar score is ≥15, the use of a symptom-triggered regimen reduces the risk of major complications developing.

- Consider transfer to intensive care unit.
- Bloods: U&E, FBC, LFTs.
- Monitor CIWA-Ar score and vital signs at least every 30 min.
- Pabrinex iv, one pair of ampoules daily for 3–5 days. Consider regular thiamine and vitamin B compound strong after.
- Rehydration po/iv.
- Benzodiazepines (preferably iv), e.g. diazepam 10–20 mg iv, repeated as required to control features. Initially, doses may be needed every few minutes if diagnosis has been delayed.

- If antipsychotic effect required, use haloperidol 0.5–5 mg po/im. Many other antipsychotics should be avoided due to proconvulsant effect.
- Provide reorientation (see Delirium p. 300, refer 'Opioid detoxification' heading in 'Disorders' chapter).

OPIOID WITHDRAWAL

Features: Yawning, sweating, salivation, lacrimation, urination, defaecation, abdominal pain, muscle cramps
  Opioid withdrawal can be extremely unpleasant, but it is not life-threatening. See p. 300, refer 'Opioid detoxification' heading in 'Disorders' chapter for Mx.

BENZODIAZEPINE WITHDRAWAL

(Puening et al., *J Emerg Med* 2017)

- *Features:* Anxiety, panic, tremor, hallucinations, hyperventilation, generalised tonic-clonic seizures. Timing dependent on $t_{\frac{1}{2}}$ of the benzodiazepine.
- Normally managed in the community (see p. 288, refer 'Stopping' heading in 'Sleep disorders and agitation' section of 'Disorders' chapter), but if there is abrupt discontinuation, delirium, seizures or psychosis can develop, requiring hospitalisation.
- Treat symptomatically with po diazepam (iv if patient unable to swallow). Re-evaluate regularly.
- May use haloperidol (as in delirium tremens) if psychosis does not respond to benzodiazepines.

GHB/GBL WITHDRAWAL[TOXBASE]

- *Features:* Agitation, insomnia, confusion, hallucinations, seizures, rigidity. $t_{\frac{1}{2}}$ <1 h, so withdrawal can be rapid and severe. Withdrawal resembles alcohol withdrawal with more prominent neuropsychiatric features, and may be more prolonged (up to 2 wk).

- *Management:*
  - Ensure clear airway, monitor vital signs, ECG and bloods
  - Hydration po/iv
  - Diazepam 10–20 mg 2–4 hourly (max 100 mg/24 h) according to Sx
  - Baclofen 10–20 mg qds
  - Monitor for seizures

CATATONIA

(Fink & Taylor, *Catatonia: A Clinician's Guide to Diagnosis and Treatment*, 2003; Clinebell et al., *J Clin Psychiatry* 2014; 75(6): 644–51)

Catatonia is a severe psychomotor disorder that can be caused by depression, psychosis, mania and a large range of other psychiatric and medical disorders.

International Classification of Diseases, 11th Revision (ICD-11) criteria: 'several' of stupor, catalepsy, waxy flexibility, mutism, negativism, posturing, mannerisms, stereotypies, psychomotor agitation, grimacing, echolalia and echopraxia. It can appear in another mental disorder, be induced by psychoactive medications or be due to another medical condition.

- *Management:* Management should be simultaneously directed at the underlying disorder (e.g. depression, infection), the catatonic syndrome and the complications of catatonia.
  - Delirium and NMS should be excluded.
  - If diagnosis of catatonia is unclear, try the **lorazepam challenge test**: assess baseline mental state (ideally with a catatonia rating scale), give lorazepam 1 mg iv/im/po, wait

5/15/30 min (depending on route of administration) and re-assess mental state.

— Often the underlying psychopathology is not readily apparent. Treatment with benzodiazepines may clarify this.

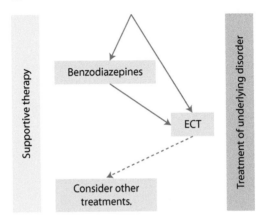

Benzodiazepines and ECT are similarly effective. ECT may be indicated first-line in life-threatening cases. **Lorazepam** is the preferred benzodiazepine, but note that patients with catatonia may both tolerate and require high doses of benzodiazepines for effective treatment. Start at 2 mg lorazepam po/im/iv and carefully titrate up to 20–30 mg, monitoring for efficacy, sedation and respiratory depression. Amantadine and memantine are gaining an evidence base in treatment-resistant catatonia in case reports.

- The role of antipsychotics is complex and controversial. On the one hand, catatonic patients are at ↑risk of NMS. On the other, underlying psychosis may require treatment. If antipsychotics are used, avoid high-potency drugs and monitor carefully.

Complications	Prevention/management
Dehydration	Fluid monitoring, iv fluids
Poor food intake	Lorazepam 30–60 min before meals
Pressure sores	Pressure mattress, repositioning
Contractures	Mobilisation, physiotherapy
Venous thromboembolism (deep vein thrombosis, pulmonary embolism)	TED stocking, low molecular weight heparin
NMS (catatonia is a strong risk factor)	Caution with antipsychotics

DELIRIUM

Diagnosis: Confusion Assessment Method (CAM) or 4AT

Confusion Assessment Method (CAM)
(Inouye et al., *Ann Intern Med* 1990; 15; **113**(12): 941–8)

1 Acute onset and fluctuating course
2 Inattention
3 Disorganised thinking
4 Altered level of consciousness

Diagnosis requires 1 and 2 and either 3 or 4.

4AT (Maclullich et al., 2011)
1 Alertness
    − Fully alert but not agitated −0
    − Mild sleepiness for <10 sec after waking −0
    − Clearly abnormal −4
2 AMT4 (age, DoB, location, year)
    − No mistakes −0
    − 1 mistake −1
    − 2+ mistakes −2
3 Attention (months of the year backwards)
    − 7+ months correctly −0
    − Starts but scores <7 months or refuses to start −1
    − Untestable (as too unwell, drowsy or inattentive) −2
4 Acute change or fluctuating course in alertness, cognition or other mental function

- No –0
- Yes –4
- 4+ Possible delirium ± cognitive impairment
- 1–3 Possible cognitive impairment
- 0 Delirium or severe cognitive impairment unlikely

Causes of delirium: **DDELIRIUMM** – Drugs (especially opioids, benzodiazepines, anticholinergics), Discomfort (i.e. pain), Electrolytes (especially ↓Na^+, ↑/↓Ca^{2+}, ↑urea), Lungs (↓O_2, ↑CO_2), Infection, Respiratory failure (hypoxia, hypercapnia), Impaction (of stools), Urinary retention, Metabolic (↓/↑glucose, ↓/↑thyroid), Myocardial infarction

Management[NICE]:

- If doubt about role of dementia, Rx delirium first.[NICE]
- Identify underlying cause(s) and Rx.[NICE]
- Reorientation (e.g. frequent explanations, clocks, photos).[NICE]
- Involve family and friends.[NICE]
- Consistency of staff.[NICE]
- Minimise moving room or ward.[NICE]
- Pharmacological treatments:
  - If delirium is the context of alcohol withdrawal or benzodiazepine withdrawal, give a benzodiazepine (see p. 390, refer 'Alcohol Withdrawal' heading in this chapter).
  - For other forms of delirium, there are no licensed drugs. If agitated, try non-pharmacological de-escalation first. If unsuccessful, may give haloperidol 0.5–2 mg or olanzapine 2.5–5 mg. Minimise length of treatment. Avoid antipsychotics in Parkinson's or Lewy body dementia.[NICE] Some new evidence suggests antipsychotics may not ↓duration of delirium (Girard et al., *NEJM* 2018; **379**(26): 2506–16). Benzodiazepines should generally be avoided as they may worsen confusion, so only use as last resort or if antipsychotics contraindicated.
  - De-prescribing (e.g. of anticholinergics, opioids, anticonvulsants) is often more important than prescribing.

SEIZURES (EPILEPTIC AND DISSOCIATIVE)

(Adapted from Mellers J, *Postgrad Med J* 2005; **81**(958): 498–504)

	Dissociative seizure	Epileptic seizure
Distinguishing features		
Timing		
• Gradual onset	Common	Rare
• Waxing and waning	Common	Very rare
• Duration >5 min	Common	Rare (but serious)
Motor		
• Side-to-side head movement	Common	Rare
• Asynchronous thrashing movements	Common	Very rare
• Pelvic thrusting	Occasional	Rare
Eyes		
• Eyes closed	Common	Rare
• Unreactive pupils	Rare	Common
• Henry and Woodruff sign (eyes switch side to look downwards when patient repositioned)	Occasional	Very rare
Post-ictal		
• Recall for unresponsive period	Common	Very rare
Acute management[a]	• Avoid benzodiazepines (worsen dissociation) and other anticonvulsants	(SIGN 143) *Initial management:* • Secure airway • High-flow O_2 • Vital signs • Obtain iv access • Time seizure

(*continued*)

	Dissociative seizure	Epileptic seizure
	• Hold a mirror up to patient and wait for gaze convergence – may terminate seizure • Grounding exercises to challenge the dissociation: encourage patient to think of five things they can hear/see/feel or perform some repetitive mental arithmetic (e.g. serial 7s)	*If seizure persists >5 min give one of:* • Midazolam 10 mg buccal/intranasal (preferred option) • Lorazepam 4 mg iv (if midazolam not available) • Diazepam 10 mg pr/iv (if other options not available) *If no response within 10 min, may repeat dose of benzodiazepine and transfer to A&E for iv anticonvulsant (e.g. phenytoin, levetiracetam, valproate).* Exclude or treat reversible metabolic causes, especially ↓O$_2$, ↓glucose (give thiamine as well as glucose in alcoholic or malnourished patient)

[a] If type of seizure is uncertain, treat as an epileptic seizure and seek a specialist opinion.

NB:

• Patients can, and often do, have both epileptic and dissociative seizures, so identifying one type does not exclude other types occurring, too. Ensure history taken from patient ± collateral of multiple seizure types.
• Many psychotropics (serotonergics, antipsychotics) can lower seizure threshold and should be reviewed if epileptic seizures occur or are suspected.
• Clozapine is particularly prone to inducing seizures during titration and after dose increases.

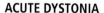

ACUTE DYSTONIA

More common with typical antipsychotics (can occur with atypicals and antidepressants) and takes several forms: **laryngeal dystonia** (stridor, dyspnoea and respiratory distress), **torticollis** (twisted neck), **opisthotonus** (back arching), **trismus** (limited jaw opening), **blepharospasm** (eyelids forced shut) and **oculogyric crisis** (eyes fixed in upward gaze). Onset can be delayed by hours or a few days. May be more common in younger patients, and those antipsychotic-naïve.

Management:

- Secure airway (rarely needed)
- Consider procyclidine 5–10 mg im/iv stat
- Review antipsychotic prescription

CLOZAPINE-INDUCED AGRANULOCYTOSIS

(Young et al., *Schizophr Bull* 1998; **24**(3): 381–90)

- The threshold for stopping clozapine is substantially higher than the clinical definition of significant neutropenia/agranulocytosis:
  - Neutrophils: Stop if <1.5 × 10⁹/L ("red result").
  - WCC: Stop if <3 × 10⁹/L ("red result").
- Twice weekly monitoring is required if neutrophils <2 × 10⁹/L or WCC <3.5 × 10⁹/L ("amber result") until recovery.
- Haematological effects are most likely in first year (especially in first 4 months of therapy), and they are not dose dependent.
- Patient with benign ethnic neutropenia may have different thresholds.
- *Warning signs:* Sore throat, fever, any other Sx of infection ⇒ check WCC for agranulocytosis.

Management of agranulocytosis:

- Immediate discontinuation of clozapine. Daily FBC until patient has a 'green' result.

- Consult haematologist for consideration of reverse isolation, prophylactic Abx and GCSF.
- Note on patient record to contraindicate future clozapine.

HIV POST-EXPOSURE PROPHYLAXIS (PEP)

(Cresswell et al., 'UK guideline for the use of HIV Post-Exposure Prophylaxis Following Sexual Exposure', *Int J STD AIDS* 2015; **27**(9): 713–38)

Risky sexual practices are common in mania and acute psychosis. Needle sharing may occur in IVDUs.

When to give PEP:

	Source HIV status		
	HIV+		High-risk group with unknown HIV status
	Viral load >200/mL or unknown	On ART with sustained viral load <200/mL	
Receptive anal sex	✓	✗	✓
Insertive anal sex	✓	✗	C
Receptive vaginal sex	✓	✗	C
Insertive vaginal sex	C	✗	C
Needle sharing	✓	✗	C

Note: ✓, give PEP; C, consider PEP; ✗, do not give PEP.

High-risk groups in the United Kingdom are men who have sex with men, intravenous drug users (IVDUs) from high-risk countries (e.g. Eastern Europe and Central Asia) and immigrants from countries where HIV prevalence >1% (e.g. Sub-Saharan Africa).

PEP is not generally recommended following oral sex or human bites. Ideally, start PEP within 24 h of exposure, but it can be considered up to 72 h. Prescribe **Truvada (tenofovir disoproxil fumarate 245 mg and emtricitabine 200 mg) 1 tab OD + raltegravir 400 mg every 12 h for 28 days**. These drugs have multiple interactions (including with

psychotropic drugs), so check at https://www.hiv-druginteractions.
org/checker.

Baseline bloods should include HIV/hep B/hep C/syphilis serology,
hep B sAg, U&E, LFT. Also perform baseline sexually transmitted
infections (STIs) screen, urinalysis and pregnancy test (for women).
Pregnancy does not contraindicate PEP, but testing allows an
informed discussion.

PEP may be initiated out-of-hours by a non-specialist, but
there should be prompt discussion with an HIV specialist with
arrangement for follow-up.

Attempt to gain history from source if confirmed HIV+: current
treatment and resistance may, rarely, warrant deviation from
standard PEP.

HANGING

1. **Call for help,** particularly if you are on your own, but minimise
   delays to step 2.
2. **Remove any ligature** from around neck. If patient still
   suspended, support the body while doing this. Support the
   C-spine as best you can.

> C-spine injuries are only common if patient has dropped
> from more than their body height. In practice, most
> attempted hangings have not generated forces likely
> to injure the bony spine. Though C-spine injury should
> always be considered, airway compromise and asphyxia,
> and reduced cerebral perfusion are the most likely causes
> of injury and death. Restoring the airway and circulation
> is therefore the highest priority of First Aid in attempted
> hanging, over C-spine control.

3. Standard **ABC assessment** and management, considering the
   following:
   a. *Airway:* Lie patient on floor and assess. Support airway
      if necessary, preferentially with a **jaw thrust,** to avoid
      destabilising the C-spine.

With the patient supine, this is achieved by approaching the patient from behind (cranially, with their body directed away from you). The heels of the hands grasp the sides of the patient's head as a solid base of support, and the index fingers are placed behind the mandible, to displace it anteriorly. Specifically try to avoid the 'Head tilt, chin lift' technique of opening a compromised airway – this technique tends to extend the neck, which may be unsafe in the setting of cervical spinal injury. However, if a jaw thrust is unsuccessful, other airway-opening techniques should be employed, to prevent death from asphyxiation. More is to be lost by inadequately managing an airway than the unlikely event of destabilising an injury of the cervical spine.

b. *Breathing and circulation:* If not breathing, or pulseless, initiate Basic Life Support (BLS). The patient may be apnoeic but have a pulse, in which case rescue breaths are indicated. Continue to administer BLS until help arrives. If breathing and circulation are intact, place the patient in the recovery position. This is best achieved by two people, with one attempting to maintain the C-spine in an anatomically neutral position, neither flexed, nor extended. This position may be supported manually, until help arrives. Ensure that breathing and circulation are maintained.

Petechiae in the face and conjunctivae are common.

SELF-LACERATION

Often superficial with only simple dressing required. Occasionally, there is risk of significant haemorrhage. The principles of haemorrhage control in first aid are *pressure* and *elevation*. Most commonly, bleeding of the limbs can be controlled by these measures alone. Penetrating injuries to the torso, thighs (particularly groin), head or neck, require urgent specialist assessment.

● Ensure your own safety – do not proceed if there is a risk of injury to yourself.

- Apply gloves.
- Remove any clothing necessary to expose the wound.
- If there is an object in the wound, do not remove it, but apply pressure to either side of it. Apply direct pressure to wound, with gauze and a bandage. If not available, use any material to hand, particularly if bleeding is brisk.
- Raise the affected limb with the injury higher than the heart to reduce blood flow. Lie the patient flat.
- If bleeding is not controlled, ensure that pressure is being properly applied over the wound. Sometimes, in the urgency to control haemorrhage, pressure is ineffectively applied, and then masked by a bandage. A cool head, and recommencing an assessment from scratch, is often the most effective strategy. Thereafter, try to disturb the wound as little as possible.

Lacerations to specific areas

- *Limb:* If bleeding remains uncontrolled despite firm local pressure and elevation, a tourniquet may be applied, proximal to (above) the bleeding point. This is uncommonly required but may be lifesaving in acute, severe haemorrhage. A tourniquet may be a belt or any ligature, tied tightly enough that the bleeding is controlled, in combination with local pressure and elevation. Facilitate urgent transfer to A&E by ambulance. Ensure that all parties are aware that a tourniquet has been applied.
- *Torso/abdomen:* Apply pressure to control external haemorrhage. It will not be possible to control internal haemorrhage. Lie the patient flat and facilitate urgent transfer to A&E by ambulance.
- *Neck:* Sitting the patient up can decrease bleeding, particularly from veins, and often provides effective haemorrhage control, in combination with manually applied, local pressure. Sitting the patient up achieves elevation of the injury – be aware that lying the patient flat may increase bleeding. However, if the patient's level of consciousness drops, suggestive of cerebral hypoperfusion, the patient should be laid flat. Never apply a circumferential bandage to the neck, for obvious reasons.

- Complete ABCDE assessment – Part of E is ensuring that all penetrating injuries are accounted for. You may have perfectly managed their superficial wrist wounds, but is there an occult, penetrating wound to the abdomen?

ACUTE CORONARY SYNDROMES (ACS)

Clues: Angina, N&V, sweating, LVF, arrhythmias, Hx of IHD. Remember atypical pain and silent infarcts in DM, elderly or if ↓GCS.

ACS encompasses the following:

1 **STEMI:** ST elevation myocardial infarction.
2 **NSTEMI:** Non-ST elevation MI; troponin (T or I) +ve.
3 **UA(P):** Unstable angina (pectoris); troponin (T or I) −ve.

FOR ALL ACS

- Do not routinely administer O_2, but monitor O_2 saturation using pulse oximetry as soon as possible, to guide the use of supplemental oxygen to maintain levels >94%.
- *Aspirin:* 300 mg po stat (chew/dispersible form) unless CI. If in A&E, check has not been given already by paramedics or GP.
- *Clopidogrel:* 300 mg po (some give 600 mg, especially if immediate PCI planned). Prasugrel (60 mg po loading dose) and ticagrelor 180 mg po loading dose are alternatives – see local guidelines for which to use.
- *Opiate: in United Kingdom most centres give diamorphine 2.5–5 mg iv + antiemetic (e.g. metoclopramide 10 mg iv),*

Date/Time	Infusion fluid	Vol-ume	Additives if any drug and dose	Rate of admin	Dura-tion	Dr's signature	Time star-ted	Time compl-eted	Set up by sig-nature	Batch No.
25/12	N. saline	50 mL	50 mg GTN	0–10 mL / h*		TN				
	*TITRATE TO PAIN: Stop if systolic BP<100 mmHg									

Figure 6.2 Drug chart showing how to write up GTN ivi.

repeat diamorphine iv according to response. Morphine is an alternative, initially 3–5 mg iv, repeating every few minutes until pain free.

- *GTN:* one to two sprays or sl tablets (300 micrograms–1 mg). If pain continues or LVF develops, set up ivi, titrating to BP and pain.
  NB: can $\Rightarrow$ ↓BP; do not give if systolic ≤100 mm Hg or inferior infarct (i.e. suspected RV involvement).

Consider:

- β-*blocker (cardioselective):* Unless CI (see propranolol, p. 142, refer 'Propranolol' in 'Common Drugs' chapter), especially beware 💀 asthma, acute LVF 💀, ↓BP (systolic <100 mm Hg), ↓HR (<60/min), second-/third-degree HB; get senior help if in doubt.
  - *Can be given iv or po:* It is often recommended to give iv for STEMI and po for NSTEMI and UAP. In acute settings, metoprolol is often drug of choice as short $t_{1/2}$ (if chronic LVF use bisoprolol) means it wears off quickly if acute LVF develops. Consult local protocol or get senior advice if unsure.
  - *Iv:* e.g. metoprolol 1–5 mg iv, giving 1–2 mg aliquots at a time while monitoring BP and HR. Repeat to max 15 mg, stopping when BP ≤100 mm Hg or HR ≤60. Then consider starting metoprolol po.
  - *Po:* For example, metoprolol 25–50 mg bd-tds. If cardiodynamically stable 24 h later, change to long-acting β-blocker e.g. bisoprolol 5–10 mg od.
  - If already on β-blocker, ensure dose adequate to control HR.
  - If β-blocker CI and ↑HR consider Ca^{2+} blocker (e.g. diltiazem SR 60–120 mg bd; beware – also CI in LVF) and get senior ± cardiology advice.
- *Insulin:* For all type I DM and type II DM or people without a history of diabetes with CBG >11 on admission. Give conventional sliding scale or GIK ivi (e.g. DIGAMI) if local protocol exists; contact CCU for advice.

- *iv fluids:* If RV infarct. *Clues:* ↓BP with no pulmonary oedema, inferior or posterior ECG changes (especially ST elevation ≥1 mm in aVF) and ↑JVP. If suspected, do right-sided ECG and look for ↑ST in V4. Avoid vasodilating drugs (especially nitrates and ACE-i). Care with β-blockers (can ⇒ HB).

IF STEMI

- *Reperfusion therapy:* Primary PCI is the preferred option, if unavailable or CI consider thrombolysis. *NB:* Starting one or the other ASAP is paramount ('time = myocardium'!) ∴ if appropriate, initiate/organise during previously mentioned steps.
- *Heparin:* iv heparin is given with *recombinant* thrombolytics for 24–48 h to avoid the rebound hypercoagulable states they can cause but is *not* needed with *streptokinase*. If ongoing chest pain or unresolving ECG changes, get senior advice on further anticoagulation and arrange rescue PCI.
- Consider (consult local protocol/cardiology on-call if unsure):
  - *Glycoprotein IIb/IIIa inhibitor:* Especially if not thrombolysed (CI or presentation too late) or PCI planned and still unstable. Use with caution (especially <48 h post-thrombolysis).
  - *Rescue PCI:* Especially if thrombolysis given and chest pain persists for ≥90 min or non-resolving or worsening (e.g. ≤50% reduction in) ST elevation on ECG.

IF NSTEMI OR UAP

- *Heparin:* LMWH, e.g. enoxaparin 1 mg/kg bd sc or fondaparinux 2.5 mg od sc especially if PCI planned in first 24–36 h after symptom onset.
- Consider (consult local protocol/cardiology on-call if unsure):
  - *Glycoprotein IIb/IIIa inhibitor:* If high risk* (defined by ACC/ESC as: haemodynamic or rhythm instability, persistent pain, acute or dynamic ECG changes, TIMI risk score >3

[see following], ↓left ventricular function, ↑troponin) and/or ongoing chest pain/ECG changes.

TIMI risk score for UA/NSTEMI. (Source: Antman E et al. JAMA 2000; 284:835–842.)

One point for presence of each of the following:

- Age ≥65 yr
- ≥3 of following risk factors for IHD: FHx of IHD, ↑BP, ↑cholesterol, DM, current smoker
- Prior coronary stenosis (≥50% occlusion)
- Aspirin use in past 7 days
- Severe angina (≥2 episodes within 24 h)
- ST segment deviations (↑ or ↓) at presentation
- +ve serum cardiac markers (troponin)

Score >3 indicates ↑risk* of developing cardiac events and death.

SECONDARY PREVENTION

For all ACS unless CI or already started:

- *Next day:* Aspirin 75 mg od, 'statin' (atorvastatin 80 mg od see NICE/BNF for reasons of down arrow dose) and clopidogrel 75 mg od (for 1 yr^NICE). If prasugrel used (instead of clopidogrel) 10 mg od unless >75 yr or <60 kg in which case use 5 mg od. If ticagrelor used, 90 mg bd po for 1 yr
- *When stable cardioselective:* β-blocker (if not already started, e.g. bisoprolol 1.25 mg od once any LVF clears; see previous for CI) and ACE-i (e.g. ramipril 2.5 mg bd po started at least 48 h after MI, then 5 mg bd after 3 days if tolerated). Consider addition of aldosterone antagonist eplerenone in established LVF (EF <40% on echocardiogram) and signs of HF after 3 days (closely monitor U&Es).
- *ASAP:* Diet/lifestyle changes (↓Wt, diet changes, ↑exercise, ↓smoking, etc.).

ACUTE ASTHMA

Clues: SOB, wheeze, peak expiratory flow (PEF) <50% of best**, RR ≥25/min, heart rate (HR) ≥110/min, cannot complete sentences in one breath, SaO_2 ≥94%.

- Attach pulse oximeter
- 40%–60% O_2 through high-flow mask, e.g. Hudson mask
- Salbutamol 5 mg neb in O_2: repeat up to every 15 min if life-threatening
- Ipratropium 500 micrograms neb in O_2: repeat up to every 4 h if life-threatening or fails to respond to salbutamol
- Prednisolone 40–50 mg po od for at least 5 days. Hydrocortisone 100 mg qds iv can be given if unable to swallow or retain tablets.

Both prednisolone and hydrocortisone can be given if very ill.

> ### Life-threatening features
> - PEF <33% of best**
> - O_2 sats <92%
> - PaO_2 <8 kPa, $PaCO_2$ >4.6 kPa or pH <7.35
> - Silent chest, cyanosis or ↓respiratory effort
> - ↓HR, ↓blood pressure (BP) or dysrhythmia
> - Exhaustion, confusion or coma
>
> **Or predicted best

If life-threatening features (☠ *NB*: patient may not always *appear* distressed ☠), get senior help and consider the following:

- *$MgSO_4$ ivi*: 1.2–2 g over 20 min (8 mmol = 2 g = 4 mL of 50% solution) unlicensed indication.
- *Aminophylline iv*: attach cardiac monitor and give loading dose* of 5 mg/kg iv over 20 min then ivi at 500–700 micrograms/kg/h (300 micrograms/kg/h if elderly). ☠ **If already on maintenance po aminophylline/theophylline, omit loading dose* and check levels ASAP to guide dosing** ☠.

- *Ivi salbutamsol:* 5 micrograms/min initially (then up to 20 micrograms/min according to response): back-to-back or continuous nebs now often preferred. Monitor K^+.
- Call anaesthetist for consideration of intensive therapy unit (ITU) care or intubation. Initiate this during the previously mentioned steps if deteriorating.

CHRONIC OBSTRUCTIVE PULMONARY DISEASE EXACERBATION

Clues: SOB, wheeze, RR >25/min, HR >110.

- *Attach sats monitor* and do baseline arterial blood gases (ABGs) for patients with O_2 saturation <94% on air, or requiring O_2 to achieve this.
- *Use controlled/targeted O_2 to achieve O_2 saturation >94% via a venturi (eucapnic patients) or 88%–92% (hypercapnic patients);* should be *prescribed on drug chart.* ↑Dose cautiously if hypoxia continues, but repeat ABGs to ensure CO_2 not ↑ing and (more importantly) pH not ↓ing.
- *Ipratropium 500 micrograms neb* in O_2: Repeat up to every 4 h if very ill.
- *Salbutamol 5 mg neb* in O_2: Repeat up to every 15 min if very ill (seldom necessary >hourly).
- *Prednisolone 30 mg po* then od for ≤2 wk (often 7–10 days). Some give first dose as hydrocortisone 200 mg iv – rarely used now unless unable to swallow.
- *Antibiotics* if 2 out of 3 of Hx of ↑ing SOB, ↑ing volume or ↑ing purulence of sputum.

If no improvement, consider:

- *Aminophylline ivi:* see Mx of asthma (p. 408, refer 'Acute Asthma' section) for details.
- *Respiratory support:* Continuous positive airway pressure (CPAP) and high-flow nasal cannulae for type 1 respiratory failure if just ↓PaO$_2$ or NIV (BIPAP) if also ↑PaCO$_2$; consider doxapram if NIV not available.
- *Intubation:* Discuss with ITU/anaesthetist.

PULMONARY EMBOLISM

Clues: Usually RR >20 and PaO$_2$ <10.7 kPa (or ↓O$_2$ sats).

- 60%–100% O$_2$ if hypoxic. Care if type 2 respiratory failure (e.g. COPD).
- *Analgesia:* if xs pain or distress, try paracetamol/ibuprofen first; consider opiates if severe or no response (☠ can ⇒ respiratory depression ☠).
- *Anticoagulation:* LMWH, e.g. dalteparin or enoxaparin. Once PE confirmed, load with warfarin or treat with DOAC. Consider iv heparin if surgery being contemplated, or rapid reversal may be required.*

If massive PE, worsening hypoxia or cardiovascular instability (↓BP, RV strain/failure), seek senior help and consider:

- *Fluids ± inotropes:* if systolic BP <90 mm Hg.
- *Thrombolysis (e.g. alteplase):* if ↓BP ± collapse.
- *Embolectomy*:* seek urgent cardiothoracic opinion.

SEPSIS (SEVERE OR SEPTIC SHOCK)

Clues: Evidence of infection + ↓blood pressure (BP) (mean arterial pressure [MAP] <65 mm Hg), serum lactate >4 mmol/L, ↓urine output, ↑creatinine, ↑bilirubin and ↑international normalised ratio (INR); further hemodynamic assessment (including cardiac function) to determine type of shock if clinical examination does not lead to clear diagnosis.

- Start treatment (Rx) and resuscitation immediately.
- *Oxygen:* 100% via non-rebreathe mask aiming for O$_2$ saturation 94%–98%; caution – aim for 88%–92% in chronic obstructive pulmonary disease (COPD)/at risk of up arrow CO$_2$ respiratory failure.
- Take bloods including cultures, full blood count (FBC), urea and electrolytes (U&Es), liver function tests (LFTs), clotting, serum blood glucose (BG), C-reactive protein (CRP), blood gas, lactate.

- *Fluid:* For sepsis-induced hypoperfusion, give 500 mL Hartmann's iv in 15 min (if not contraindicated) and aim for ≥30 mL/kg of iv crystalloid fluid within first 3 h; 1 L of crystalloid over 30 min; if still ↓BP consider further iv fluids (20 mL/kg) to achieve urine output >0.5 mL/kg/h (caution if LVF). Use albumin in addition to crystalloids for initial resuscitation and subsequent intravascular volume replacement when patients require large amounts of crystalloids. Response to fluids can also be monitored by resolution of up arrow HR tachycardia, altered consciousness, oliguria and hyperlactatemia.

- *Vasopressors:* If systolic BP <90 mm Hg after fluid resuscitation, senior clinician may start noradrenaline, delivered via a dedicated lumen on central line at initial dose 0.05–0.15 micrograms/kg/min. Monitor MAP by arterial line, by dedicated central line to maintain MAP >65 mm Hg. Measure mixed venous O_2 saturation and if <65%–70% need further fluid/packed red blood cells (RBCs) to achieve haematocrit >30%.

- Identify source of infection and any need for source control (chest X-ray ± other imaging, e.g. computerised tomography, echo; removal of infected devices/tissue/fluid; surgery/interventional radiology).

- *Antibiotics:* As appropriate, call Microbiology/see local trust guidelines ASAP (within 1 h) ensuring all cultures taken first from infected tissue/fluid (e.g. sputum/stool/urine/pus/cerebrospinal fluid/joint fluid/pleural aspirate) (unless significantly delays antibiotics); include at least two sets of blood cultures (aerobic and anaerobic). Narrow antimicrobial therapy once pathogen identification and sensitivities established and/or adequate clinical improvement. Daily assessment for de-escalation of antimicrobial therapy. Perform and document review of antimicrobial Rx within 48 h of first dose.

- *Blood products:* To maintain normal coagulation and aim for Hb ≥70g/L to maximise tissue perfusion; >100 g/L if other indications, e.g. myocardial ischemia, severe hypoxemia, or acute hemorrhage.

- *Blood glucose:* Aim for <10 mmol/L using validated insulin sliding scale.
- *Venous thromboembolism prophylaxis:* Od low-dose low-molecular-weight heparin (e.g. enoxaparin 40 mg sc od) unless contraindicated.
- *Stress ulcer prophylaxis:* H_2 antagonist or proton pump inhibitor for patients who have bleeding risk factors, patients on corticosteroids and those on nil by mouth.
- Remove iv access devices that are possible source of sepsis as soon as other vascular access established.
- *Steroids:* Senior staff in critical care to consider iv hydrocortisone (50 mg 6 hourly) when ↓BP responds poorly to adequate fluid resuscitation and vasopressors.

Adapted from Surviving Sepsis Campaign: International guidelines for management of severe sepsis and septic shock: 2016. *Intensive Care Medicine* 2017;**43**:304–377.

DIABETIC KETOACIDOSIS (DKA)

Clues: Ketotic breath, Kussmaul's (deep/rapid) breathing, dehydration, confusion/↓Glasgow Coma Scale, gastric stasis/abdominal pain.

The Joint British Diabetes Societies Inpatient Care Group has published UK guidelines for the Mx of DKA in adults (https://www.diabetes.org.uk/resources-s3/2017-09/Management-of-DKA-241013.pdf). These involve using a fixed-rate insulin ivi rather than a sliding scale, using blood ketone measurement to guide treatment, using bedside glucose and ketone meters when available and using venous rather than arterial blood gases. This guidance is increasingly being incorporated into local guidelines, and this section has been updated to reflect it. *NB: Follow local diabetes team protocols where applicable; the following guidance is an example of a guideline for DKA Mx.*

- *Diagnostic criteria:* Serum blood glucose (BG) >11.1 mmol/L, pH <7.3 and/or HCO_3 <15 mmol/L, +ve ketones (serum ≥3 mmol/L or urine dipstick ≥2+).
- *Initial measures:* O_2 if hypoxic, weigh patient (if possible), two wide-bore iv cannulae. Consider nasogastric tube (NGT) (if coma) and central line (especially if ↓↓pH or Hx of HF), but urinary catheter often sufficient.
- *Initial Ix:* Blood ketones, capillary blood glucose (CBG), venous BG, urea and electrolytes (U&Es), venous blood gases (arterial blood gas [ABG] if hypoxic), full blood count (FBC), C-reactive protein (CRP), blood cultures, electrocardiogram (ECG), chest X-ray, urinalysis and culture.
- *Biochemical monitoring:* Hourly CBG and ketones (bedside if available), venous blood gas (for pH, bicarbonate and K^+) at 1, 2, 4, 6, 12, 18 and 24 h.
- *iv fluids:* Initially 0.9% saline according to individual patient needs (guided by pulse, blood pressure [BP], urine output, biochemistry ± central venous pressure).
  The following is a guide:
  - *If systolic BP <90 mm Hg:* 500 mL over 15 min. If BP remains <90 mm Hg, repeat this but call for senior help.
  - *Otherwise* give more slowly, e.g. 1 L over 1 h, 2 L over 4 h, then 2 L over 8 h.
  - Add KCl once K^+ <5.5 mmol/L, as can ↓ rapidly dt insulin (but do not give KCl in first litre unless K^+ <3.5 mmol/L). Roughly 40 mmol needed per litre during rehydration: adjust to individual response with regular checks (quickest done with blood gas machines: most give K^+ levels; can use venous samples as long as put in ABG or other heparinised syringe).
- *Insulin:* As soluble insulin ivi (e.g. **Actrapid**). Use a fixed-rate ivi 0.1 units/kg/h (estimate Wt if necessary). Fx: ↓BG (aim ↓BG by 3 mmol/L/h), ↓ketogenesis (aim ↓blood ketones 0.5 mmol/L/h; if no ketone measurement: aim ↑bicarbonate 3 mmol/L/h), ↓K^+ (keep between 4 and 5 mmol/L). If delay in ivi availability, give 0.1 units/kg im stat (↓dose if BG <20 mmol/L). If patient takes long-acting (basal analogue) insulin sc (e.g. **Tresiba**, **Lantus**

or **Levemir**), continue this at usual dose/time. If blood ketones not ↓ing to target, ↑insulin ivi rate by 1 unit/h. Once BG <14, add 10% glucose 125 mL/h alongside 0.9% saline. If BG <7 do not stop insulin but ↑rate of glucose ivi. Continue insulin ivi until blood ketones <0.6 mmol/L, pH >7.3 and patient eating/drinking; pH normal and eating/drinking; then switch to sc regimen.

- *Heparin:* Give low-molecular-weight heparin (LMWH) until mobile (Px dose unless Rx dose indicated); follow local guidelines.

Consider:

- *Antibiotics:* Search for and treat infection.
- *Diabetes specialist team:* Involve ASAP.
- *Pregnancy test:* For presentation of gestational diabetes.
- *High dependency unit (HDU)/intensive therapy unit (ITU):* For one-to-one nursing ± ventilation if required.
- *Bicarbonate:* If severe acidosis (e.g. pH <7); very rarely needed and potentially dangerous. Get senior help if concerned.

Watch for complications: *electrolyte changes* (especially ↓K^+, ↓Na^+, ↓Mg^{2+}, ↓PO_4), TE (especially DVT/PE), *cerebral oedema* (↓GCS, papilloedema, false-localising, cranial nerve palsies), adult respiratory distress syndrome (ARDS), *infections* (especially aspiration pneumonia).

↓GLUCOSE

Treat if BG <3 mmol/L or symptoms and BG <4 mmol/L: ↑sympathetic drive (↑HR, sweating, aggression/behavioural changes), seizures or confusion/↓GCS.

- *Glucose orally:* 15–20 g quick acting carbohydrates especially sugary drinks, mouth gel (e.g. **hypostop/glucogel/dextrogel**) or dextrose tablets. Miss this step if severe, but useful if delays in iv access.

- *Glucose 150–200 mL* of 10% glucose ivi or 75–100 mL of 20% glucose ivi (over 10–15 min); beware of fluid overload if HF.
- *Glucagon 1 mg* im/iv stat: If very low glucose or no iv access. Give oral carbohydrate within 10–30 min to prevent recurrence.

NB: Think of and correct any causes, especially xs DM Rx, alcohol withdrawal, liver failure, aspirin OD (rarely Addison's disease, $\downarrow T_4$). If dt sulphonylureas, relapse is common; consider admission (See JBDS 2018 guidance).

Reference information

GUIDELINES

British Association for Psychopharmacology (BAP)

The British Association for Psychopharmacology produces Consensus Guidelines for treatment of many psychiatric disorders, updated at regular intervals. They are extensively referenced in this book with [BAP]. They are freely available at https://www.bap.org.uk/guidelines.

Topic	BAP guideline	Publication date
Anxiety disorders	Evidence-based pharmacological treatment of anxiety disorders, post-traumatic stress disorder and obsessive-compulsive disorder: a revision of the 2005 guidelines from the British Association for Psychopharmacology	2014
Attention deficit hyperactivity disorder (ADHD)	Evidence-based guidelines for the pharmacological management of attention deficit hyperactivity disorder: update on recommendations from the British Association for Psychopharmacology	2014
Autism	Autism spectrum disorder: consensus guidelines on assessment, treatment and research from the British Association for Psychopharmacology	2018
Benzodiazepines	Benzodiazepines: risks and benefits. A reconsideration	2013
Bipolar affective disorder	Evidence-based guidelines for treating bipolar disorder: revised third edition recommendations from the British Association for Psychopharmacology	2016
Dementia	Clinical practice with anti-dementia drugs: a revised (third) consensus statement from the British Association for Psychopharmacology	2017

(continued)

Topic	BAP guideline	Publication date
Depression	Evidence-based guidelines for treating depressive disorders with antidepressants: a revision of the 2008 British Association for Psychopharmacology guidelines	2015
Metabolic side effects	BAP guidelines on the management of weight gain, metabolic disturbances and cardiovascular risk associated with psychosis and antipsychotic drug treatment	2016
Off-license prescribing	Use of licensed medicines for unlicensed applications in psychiatric practice, 2nd edition	2017
Off-license prescribing	BAP Position Statement: off-label prescribing of psychotropic medication to children and adolescents	2016
Perinatal psychiatry	British Association for Psychopharmacology consensus guidance on the use of psychotropic medication preconception, in pregnancy and postpartum 2017	2017
Rapid tranquilisation	Joint BAP NAPICU evidence-based consensus guidelines for the clinical management of acute disturbance: de-escalation and rapid tranquillisation	2018
Schizophrenia	Evidence-based guidelines for the pharmacological treatment of schizophrenia: recommendations from the British Association for Psychopharmacology	2011
Sleep disorders	British Association for Psychopharmacology consensus statement on evidence-based treatment of insomnia, parasomnias and circadian rhythm disorders	2010
Substance misuse	BAP guidelines: evidence-based guidelines for the pharmacological management of substance abuse, harmful use, addiction and comorbidity: recommendations from BAP	2012

National Institute for Health and Care Excellence (NICE)
Many NICE guidelines are also relevant to mental health and
may be found at https://www.nice.org.uk/guidance/lifestyle-
and-wellbeing/mental-health-and-wellbeing. In addition, several
'pathways' serving as interactive ways to navigate the guidelines
may be found at this link. These and some NICE evidence articles
are referenced with NICE.

Topic	NICE guideline	Code	Publication date
ADHD	Attention deficit hyperactivity disorder: diagnosis and management	NG87	2018
Alcohol	Alcohol-use disorders: diagnosis, assessment and management of harmful drinking and alcohol dependence	CG115	2011
Anxiety disorders	Generalised anxiety disorder and panic disorder in adults: management	CG113	2011
ASPD	Antisocial personality disorder: prevention and management	CG77	2009
Autism	Autism spectrum disorder in adults: diagnosis and management	CG142	2012
Autism (children)	Autism spectrum disorder in under 19s: recognition, referral and diagnosis	CG128	2011
Borderline PD	Borderline personality disorder: recognition and management	CG78	2009
BPAD	Bipolar disorder: assessment and management	CG185	2014
Care transition	Transition between inpatient mental health settings and community or care home settings	NG53	2016
Common mental health problems	Common mental health problems: identification and pathways to care	CG123	2011

(continued)

Topic	NICE guideline	Code	Publication date
Conduct disorder	Antisocial behaviour and conduct disorders in children and young people: recognition and management	CG158	2013
Delirium	Delirium: prevention, diagnosis and management	CG103	2010
Dementia	Dementia: assessment, management and support for people living with dementia and their carers	NG97	2018
Depression	Depression in adults: recognition and management	CG90	2009
Depression	Depression in adults with a chronic physical health problem: recognition and management	CG91	2009
Depression (children)	Depression in children and young people: identification and management	CG28	2005
Eating disorders	Eating disorders: recognition and treatment	NG69	2017
Forensic mental health	Mental health of adults in contact with the criminal justice system	NG66	2017
Learning disability	Mental health problems in people with learning disabilities: prevention, assessment and management	NG54	2016
Learning disability	Challenging behaviour and learning disabilities: prevention and interventions for people with learning disabilities whose behaviour challenges	NG11	2015
OCD and BDD	Obsessive-compulsive disorder and body dysmorphic disorder: treatment	CG31	2005
Perinatal mental health	Antenatal and postnatal mental health: clinical management and service guidance	CG192	2014

(*continued*)

Topic	NICE guideline	Code	Publication date
Psychosis	Psychosis and schizophrenia in adults: prevention and management	CG178	2014
Psychosis (children)	Psychosis and schizophrenia in children and young people: recognition and management	CG155	2013
Psychosis and substance misuse	Coexisting severe mental illness (psychosis) and substance misuse: assessment and management in healthcare settings	CG120	2011
PTSD	NG116 Post-traumatic stress disorder	CG26	2018
Rapid tranquilisation	Violence and aggression: short-term management in mental health, health and community settings	NG10	2015
Self-harm	Self-harm in over 8s: short-term management and prevention of recurrence	CG16	2004
Social anxiety disorder	Social anxiety disorder: recognition, assessment and treatment	CG159	2013

Other

Topic	Guideline	Publication date	Reference
Club drugs and novel psychoactive substances	Novel Psychoactive Treatment: UK Network (NEPTUNE) (http://neptune-clinical-guidance.co.uk)	2015	**NEPTUNE**
Prescribing in psychiatry	*The Maudsley Prescribing Guidelines in Psychiatry*, 13th edition	2018	**MPG**
Various	Scottish Intercollegiate Guidelines Network (SIGN) (https://www.sign.ac.uk)	Various	**SIGN**

USEFUL CONTACTS

CRISIS CONTACTS

Contact	Description	Website	Telephone number
CALM (Campaign Against Living Miserably)	For men in crisis	https://www.thecalmzone.net	0800 58 58 58 (5 p.m.–midnight)
ChildLine	Emergency counselling service	https://www.childline.org.uk	0800 1111 (24/7)
NHS 111	Helpline for urgent medical problems; can connect patients to onward care	https://111.nhs.uk	111 (24/7)
PAPYRUS	Suicide prevention line; accepts calls from concerned others	https://www.papyrus-uk.org	0800 068 4141 (Monday–Friday, 10 a.m.–10 p.m. and weekends 2 p.m.–10 p.m.)
Samaritans	Crisis line for any issues	https://www.samaritans.org.uk	116 123 (24/7)

PATIENT INFORMATION/SUPPORT

See also Psychoeducation (p. 313), refer 'Psychoeducation' heading in 'Non-pharmacological treatments' chapter

Contact	Description	Website	Telephone number
NHS Patient Information	Reliable information on common mental health problems	https://www.nhs.uk/conditions	–
Mind	Mental health information and support	https://www.mind.org.uk	0300 123 3393 (Monday–Friday, 9 a.m.–6 p.m.)

(continued)

Contact	Description	Website	Telephone number
Alcoholics Anonymous	Peer support network for those wishing to stop drinking	https://www.alcoholics-anonymous.org.uk	0800 9177 650 (24/7)
Narcotics Anonymous	Peer support network for those wishing to stop using drugs	https://ukna.org	0300 999 1212 (daily, 10 a.m. until midnight)
Alzheimer's Society	Support for those with all types of dementia and their carers	https://www.alzheimers.org.uk	0300 222 1122 (Monday–Wednesday, 9 a.m.–8 p.m., Thursday and Friday, 9 a.m.–5 p.m. and weekends, 10 a.m.–4 p.m.)
BEAT Eating Disorders	Support for those with eating disorders	https://www.beateatingdisorders.org.uk	Adults: 0808 801 0677; students: 0808 801 0811; young people: 0808 801 0711 (Monday–Friday, 12 p.m.–8 p.m., weekends, 4 p.m.–8 p.m.)
Mencap	Support for those with a learning disability and their families	https://www.mencap.org.uk	0808 808 1111 (Monday–Friday, 9 a.m.–5 p.m.)

PROFESSIONAL

Contact	Description	Website	Telephone number
National Poisons Information Service (NPIS)	Comprehensive information on management of drug overdoses	https://www.toxbase.org (requires institutional login)	0344 892 0111 (24/7)

(continued)

Contact	Description	Website	Telephone number
UK Teratology Information Service (UKTIS)	Drug monographs with detailed information on use in pregnancy	http://www.uktis.org	0344 892 0909 (Monday–Friday, 9 a.m.–5 p.m.)
UK Drugs in Lactation Advisory Service (UKDILAS)	Advice on prescribing in breastfeeding women	https://www.sps.nhs. uk/articles/ukdilas	0121 424 7298 (Monday–Friday, 9 a.m.–5 p.m.)
LactMed	Comprehensive U.S. resource for prescribing in breastfeeding women	https://toxnet.nlm. nih.gov/newtoxnet/ lactmed.htm	+1 301 496 1131
Specialist Medicines Information Service for Psychiatry at the Maudsley Hospital	Advice from specialist mental health pharmacists for UK health professionals	–	020 3228 2317 (Monday–Friday, 9 a.m.–5 p.m.)
Medscape	Free professional medical information	https://reference. medscape.com	–
Mental Elf	Blog distilling mental health research	https://www. nationalelfservice. net/mental-health	–

REFERENCE VALUES

NB: normal ranges often vary between laboratories. The ranges given here are deliberately narrow to minimise missing abnormal results, but this means that your result may be normal for your laboratory's range, which should always be checked if possible.

Biochemistry

Na$^+$	135–145 mmol/L
K$^+$	3.5–5 mmol/L
Urea	2.5–6.5 mmol/L
Creatinine	70–110 micromole/L
Ca^{2+}	2.15–2.65 mmol/L
PO$_4$	0.8–1.4 mmol/L
Albumin	35–50 g/L
Protein	60–80 g/L
Mg^{2+}	0.75–1.0 mmol/L
Cl$^-$	95–105 mmol/L
Glucose (fasting)	3.5–5.5 mmol/L
LDH	70–250 iu/L
CK	25–195[a] units/L ($\neq$ in blacks)
Trop I	<0.4 ng/mL (= microgram/L)
Trop T	<0.1 ng/mL (= microgram/L)
D-dimers	<0.5[b] mg/L
Bilirubin	3–17 micromole/L
ALP	30–130 iu/L
AST	3–31 iu/L
ALT	3–35 iu/L
GGT	7–50[a] iu/L
Amylase	0–180 units/dL
Cholesterol	3.9–5.2 mmol/L
Triglycerides	0.5–1.9 mmol/L
LDL	<2 mmol/L
HDL	0.9–1.9 mmol/L
Urate	0.2–0.45 mmol/L
CRP	0–10 mg/L

[a] Sex differences exist: females occupy the lower end of the range.

[b] D-dimer normal range can vary with different test protocols: check with your lab.

Haematology

Hb male	13.5–17.5 g/dL
Hb female	11.5–15.5 g/dL
Pt	150–400 × 10^9/L
WCC	4–11 × 10^9/L
NØ	2–7.5 × 10^9/L (40%–75%)
LØ	1.3–3.5 × 10^9/L (20%–45%)
EØ	0.04–0.44 × 10^9/L (1%–6%)
PCV (Hct)	0.37–0.54[a] L/L
MCV	76–96 fl
ESR	<age in years *(+10 in women)/2*
HbA$_{1c}$	<48 mmol/mol

[a] Sex differences exist: females occupy the lower end of the range.

Clotting

APTT	35–45 sec
APTT ratio	0.8–1.2
INR	0.8–1.2

Haematinics

Iron	11–30 micromole/L
Transferrin	2–4 g/L
TIBC	45–72 micromole/L
Serum folate	1.8–11 microgram/L
B$_{12}$	200–760 pg/mL (5 ng/L)

Arterial blood gases

PaO$_2$	>10.6 kPa
PaCO$_2$	4.7–6 kPa
pH	7.35–7.45

Arterial blood gases

HCO_3^-	24–30 mmol/L
Lactate	0.5–2.2 mmol/L
Base xs	±2 mmol/L

Thyroid function

Thyroxine (total T_4)	70–140 nmol/L
Thyroxine (free T_4)	9–22 pmol/L
TSH	0.5–5 mU/L

INDEX